New Strategies for Treatment of Sepsis

New Strategies for Treatment of Sepsis

Editors

Antonio Mirijello
Alberto Tosoni

MDPI • Basel • Beijing • Wuhan • Barcelona • Belgrade • Manchester • Tokyo • Cluj • Tianjin

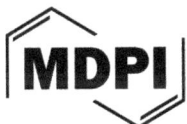

Editors
Antonio Mirijello
Department of Medical Sciences
Internal Medicine Unit
Casa Sollievo della Sofferenza
IRCCS
San Giovanni Rotondo
Italy

Alberto Tosoni
Department of Internal Medicine
and Gastroenterology
Fondazione Policlinico
Universitario "A. Gemelli"
IRCCS
Rome
Italy

Editorial Office
MDPI
St. Alban-Anlage 66
4052 Basel, Switzerland

This is a reprint of articles from the Special Issue published online in the open access journal *Medicina* (ISSN 1648-9144) (available at: www.mdpi.com/journal/medicina/special_issues/treatment_sepsis).

For citation purposes, cite each article independently as indicated on the article page online and as indicated below:

LastName, A.A.; LastName, B.B.; LastName, C.C. Article Title. *Journal Name* **Year**, *Volume Number*, Page Range.

ISBN 978-3-0365-2483-2 (Hbk)
ISBN 978-3-0365-2482-5 (PDF)

© 2021 by the authors. Articles in this book are Open Access and distributed under the Creative Commons Attribution (CC BY) license, which allows users to download, copy and build upon published articles, as long as the author and publisher are properly credited, which ensures maximum dissemination and a wider impact of our publications.

The book as a whole is distributed by MDPI under the terms and conditions of the Creative Commons license CC BY-NC-ND.

Contents

About the Editors vii

Preface to "New Strategies for Treatment of Sepsis" ix

Antonio Mirijello, Alberto Tosoni and on behalf of the Internal Medicine Sepsis Study Group
New Strategies for Treatment of Sepsis
Reprinted from: *Medicina* **2020**, *56*, 527, doi:10.3390/medicina56100527 1

Matteo Rossetti, Gennaro Martucci, Christina Starchl and Karin Amrein
Micronutrients in Sepsis and COVID-19: A Narrative Review on What We Have Learned and What We Want to Know in Future Trials
Reprinted from: *Medicina* **2021**, *57*, 419, doi:10.3390/medicina57050419 5

Alfredo Aisa-Alvarez, María Elena Soto, Verónica Guarner-Lans, Gilberto Camarena-Alejo, Juvenal Franco-Granillo, Enrique A. Martínez-Rodríguez, Ricardo Gamboa Ávila, Linaloe Manzano Pech and Israel Pérez-Torres
Usefulness of Antioxidants as Adjuvant Therapy for Septic Shock: A Randomized Clinical Trial
Reprinted from: *Medicina* **2020**, *56*, 619, doi:10.3390/medicina56110619 19

Salvatore Lucio Cutuli, Simone Carelli, Domenico Luca Grieco and Gennaro De Pascale
Immune Modulation in Critically Ill Septic Patients
Reprinted from: *Medicina* **2021**, *57*, 552, doi:10.3390/medicina57060552 33

Giuseppe Bertozzi, Aniello Maiese, Giovanna Passaro, Alberto Tosoni, Antonio Mirijello, Stefania De Simone, Benedetta Baldari, Luigi Cipolloni and Raffaele La Russa
Neutropenic Enterocolitis and Sepsis: Towards the Definition of a Pathologic Profile
Reprinted from: *Medicina* **2021**, *57*, 638, doi:10.3390/medicina57060638 45

Francesco Perrotta and Marco Paolo Perrini
Successful Treatment of *Klebsiella pneumoniae* NDM Sepsis and Intestinal Decolonization with Ceftazidime/Avibactam Plus Aztreonam Combination in a Patient with TTP Complicated by SARS-CoV-2 Nosocomial Infection
Reprinted from: *Medicina* **2021**, *57*, 424, doi:10.3390/medicina57050424 55

Rita Murri, Sara Lardo, Alessio De Luca, Brunella Posteraro, Riccardo Torelli, Giulia De Angelis, Francesca Giovannenze, Francesco Taccari, Lucia Pavan, Lucia Parroni, Maurizio Sanguinetti and Massimo Fantoni
Post-Prescription Audit Plus Beta-D-Glucan Assessment Decrease Echinocandin Use in People with Suspected Invasive Candidiasis
Reprinted from: *Medicina* **2021**, *57*, 656, doi:10.3390/medicina57070656 63

Marcello Covino, Antonella Gallo, Massimo Montalto, Giuseppe De Matteis, Maria Livia Burzo, Benedetta Simeoni, Rita Murri, Marcello Candelli, Veronica Ojetti and Francesco Franceschi
The Role of Early Procalcitonin Determination in the Emergency Department in Adults Hospitalized with Fever
Reprinted from: *Medicina* **2021**, *57*, 179, doi:10.3390/medicina57020179 73

Emanuela Sozio, Alessio Bertini, Giacomo Bertolino, Francesco Sbrana, Andrea Ripoli, Fabio Carfagna, Alessandro Giacinta, Bruno Viaggi, Simone Meini, Lorenzo Ghiadoni and Carlo Tascini
Recognition in Emergency Department of Septic Patients at Higher Risk of Death: Beware of Patients without Fever
Reprinted from: *Medicina* 2021, 57, 612, doi:10.3390/medicina57060612 81

Alberto Tosoni, Anthony Cossari, Mattia Paratore, Michele Impagnatiello, Giovanna Passaro, Carla Vincenza Vallone, Vincenzo Zaccone, Antonio Gasbarrini, Giovanni Addolorato, Salvatore De Cosmo, Antonio Mirijello and on behalf of the Internal Medicine Sepsis Study Group
Delta-Procalcitonin and Vitamin D Can Predict Mortality of Internal Medicine Patients with Microbiological Identified Sepsis
Reprinted from: *Medicina* 2021, 57, 331, doi:10.3390/medicina57040331 89

Andrea Piccioni, Michele Cosimo Santoro, Tommaso de Cunzo, Gianluca Tullo, Sara Cicchinelli, Angela Saviano, Federico Valletta, Marco Maria Pascale, Marcello Candelli, Marcello Covino and Francesco Franceschi
Presepsin as Early Marker of Sepsis in Emergency Department: A Narrative Review
Reprinted from: *Medicina* 2021, 57, 770, doi:10.3390/medicina57080770 97

Andrea Piccioni, Angela Saviano, Sara Cicchinelli, Federico Valletta, Michele Cosimo Santoro, Tommaso de Cunzo, Christian Zanza, Yaroslava Longhitano, Gianluca Tullo, Pietro Tilli, Marcello Candelli, Marcello Covino and Francesco Franceschi
Proadrenomedullin in Sepsis and Septic Shock: A Role in the Emergency Department
Reprinted from: *Medicina* 2021, 57, 920, doi:10.3390/medicina57090920 109

Silvia Spoto, Domenica Marika Lupoi, Emanuele Valeriani, Marta Fogolari, Luciana Locorriere, Giuseppina Beretta Anguissola, Giulia Battifoglia, Damiano Caputo, Alessandro Coppola, Sebastiano Costantino, Massimo Ciccozzi and Silvia Angeletti
Diagnostic Accuracy and Prognostic Value of Neutrophil-to-Lymphocyte and Platelet-to-Lymphocyte Ratios in Septic Patients outside the Intensive Care Unit
Reprinted from: *Medicina* 2021, 57, 811, doi:10.3390/medicina57080811 117

Antonio Mirijello and Alberto Tosoni
Sepsis: New Challenges and Future Perspectives for an Evolving Disease—Precision Medicine Is the Way!
Reprinted from: *Medicina* 2021, 57, 1109, doi:10.3390/medicina57101109 129

About the Editors

Antonio Mirijello

He received his MD degree cum laude at the Catholic University of Rome, then attended the Internal Medicine residency program and a master-degree in Echography. He worked as Internal Medicine consultant at "A. Gemelli" University Hospital, Rome (IT). Since 2015, he has worked at IRCCS Casa Sollievo della Sofferenza, San Giovanni Rotondo (IT) - Chief: Dr. Salvatore De Cosmo. He collaborates with the Alcohol Use Disorders Unit directed by Professor Giovanni Addolorato.

His scientific production includes more than 120 publications in peer reviewed journals. His main research interests involve the treatment of alcohol addiction, the metabolic aspects of the alcohol addicted patients and the alcohol liver disease. He is a reviewer for several scientific peer reviewed journals. In 2008, he received the Young Investigators Award from the Italian Society of Internal Medicine (SIMI). He founded, in 2013, the Internal Medicine Sepsis Study Group.

Alberto Tosoni

Internal Medicine Specialist since 2018, he is now Consultant for Internal Medicine and Gastroenterology Department at Gemelli Hospital, Rome.

He spent part of his residency in Oxford (in 2015 at the John Ratcliffe Hospital) and Tel Aviv (in 2017 at the Hasharon Medical Hospital).

He has obtained two Master's degrees in 2018 and 2019, respectively, in Internal Ultrasound and Antibiotic Stewardship.

Since March 2020, he has held the role of COVID-19 Department Team Leader. He managed patients affected by SARS-CoV-2 infection, leading a multidisciplinary doctors team, managing over 500 hospitalized patients with moderate-to-severe respiratory failure due to COVID-19.

His research activities are mainly focused on management of sepsis in non-intensive care units, with numerous publications in peer-reviewed international journals. He is a member of the Internal Medicine Sepsis Study Group. He is also interested in alcohol-related diseases, leadership training for doctors and artificial intelligence in medicine.

Since 2019, he is also an active member of the European Federation of Internal Medicine - Early Career Subcommittee.

Preface to "New Strategies for Treatment of Sepsis"

Sepsis represents an emerging and one of the deadliest diseases worldwide, accounting for millions of preventable deaths every year, being the cause, directly or indirectly, of about half of all hospital deaths.

Until a decade ago, sepsis was managed almost exclusively by intensivists. Consequently, most of the literature on this topic derives from studies conducted in Intensive Care Units (ICUs). However, in recent years, there has been a progressive increase in admissions of septic patients to non-ICU wards. The characteristics of the septic population have gradually changed—being constantly older, more co-morbid and chronic—as well as the early management of sepsis and septic shock. As a consequence, there is the need for literature data derived both from intensive and non-intensive departments, in order to fill the gap of knowledge and for confirmatory purposes.

Being a time-dependent disease, sepsis requires a prompt recognition and a standardized approach for optimal treatment. In general medicine wards, the main limitations to this purpose are represented by the unfavorable proportion between patients and staff and by the lack of constant monitoring of vital functions.

We are still far from a full knowledge of the mechanisms underlying the development and progression of sepsis. It is in this context that, in the last few years, new scenarios have been opening for sepsis management, including the use of new diagnostic tools with less invasive approaches, the growing role of artificial intelligence, the development of better antibiotic therapy strategies and the optimization of involved health resourses.

This book aims to collect and disseminate the knowledge of different specialists involved in the management of septic patients, particularly non-intensivists physicians.

Antonio Mirijello, Alberto Tosoni
Editors

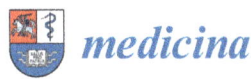

Editorial

New Strategies for Treatment of Sepsis

Antonio Mirijello [1,*], Alberto Tosoni [2,*] and on behalf of the Internal Medicine Sepsis Study Group [†]

1. Internal Medicine Unit, Department of Medical Sciences, IRCCS Casa Sollievo della Sofferenza, 71013 San Giovanni Rotondo, Italy
2. Department of Internal Medicine and Gastroenterology, Fondazione Policlinico Universitario "A. Gemelli" IRCCS, 00168 Rome, Italy
* Correspondence: a.mirijello@operapadrepio.it (A.M.); alberto.tosoni@policlinicogemelli.it (A.T.); Tel.: +39-0882-410-600 (A.M.); +39-06-3015-1 (A.T.)
† The Internal Medicine Sepsis Study Group: Stefano Carughi, Maria Maddalena D'Errico, Salvatore De Cosmo, Angela de Matthaeis, Michele Inglese, Antonio Pio Greco, Pamela Piscitelli, Leonardo Sacco (IRCCS Casa Sollievo della Sofferenza, San Giovanni Rotondo), Tommaso Dionisi, Michele Impagnatiello, Giovanna Passaro, Mattia Paratore (Fondazione Policlinico Universitario "A. Gemelli" IRCCS, Rome), Carla Vincenza Vallone (Azienda Ospedaliera Universitaria San Giovanni di Dio e Ruggi D'Aragona, Salerno), Vincenzo Zaccone (Azienda Ospedaliera Universitaria Ospedali Riuniti, Ancona).

Received: 2 October 2020; Accepted: 9 October 2020; Published: 10 October 2020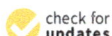

Abstract: Sepsis represents a major global health concern and is one of the most feared complications for hospitalized patients, being the cause, directly or indirectly, of about half of all hospital deaths. According to the last definition, sepsis is a life-threatening organ dysfunction caused by a dysregulated host response to infection and defined septic shock as a subset of sepsis in which underlying circulatory and cellular/metabolic abnormalities are profound enough to significantly increase mortality. Sepsis is a time-dependent disease and requires a prompt recognition and a standardized treatment. The Special Issue "New Strategies for Treatment of Sepsis" has been thought to connect the experience of physicians involved in the diagnosis, management, and treatment of sepsis at every stage of disease, from emergency departments to general and intensive wards. The focus will be pointed on new approaches to this syndrome, such as early recognition based on clinical features and biomarkers, management in non-ICUs, non-invasive treatment strategies, including non-antimicrobial agents, and, of course, invasive approaches. This Special Issue will highlight the many different facets of sepsis, seen through the eyes of different specialists. We hope to spread the knowledge of a new blueprint for treatment.

Keywords: internal medicine; intensive care; emergency department; organ dysfunction; immunomodulation; micronutrients; antimicrobial stewardship

---

Sepsis represents a major global health concern [1] and is one of the most feared complications for hospitalized patients, being the cause, directly or indirectly, of about half of all hospital deaths [2].

The definition of sepsis has changed during the years, with progressive attempts to provide a more defined picture of its real nature: a time-dependent syndrome, requiring early recognition and effective treatment. Thus, the last consensus conference defined sepsis as a life-threatening organ dysfunction caused by a dysregulated host response to infection and defined septic shock as a subset of sepsis in which underlying circulatory and cellular/metabolic abnormalities are profound enough to significantly increase mortality [3].

Although, in the last few decades, sepsis was managed quite exclusively by intensivists within intensive care units (ICUs), in recent years, there has been a progressive increase in admissions of septic patients to non-ICU wards, in particular internal medicine wards [4]. This change is effected for several reasons. First, patients have become progressively older and sicker (e.g., affected by multiple chronic diseases), often giving fewer chances to benefit from intensive treatments. Moreover, the early recognition and management of sepsis and septic shock has significantly improved, positively impacting on the prognosis of these patients. As a consequence, there is a growing collection of literature data derived from studies conducted in non-ICU settings, adding useful information for the management of sepsis with less invasive strategies, filling gaps of knowledge for non-intensivists and/or confirming previously acquired know-hows.

Being a time-dependent disease, sepsis requires a prompt recognition and a standardized approach for an optimal treatment. In general medicine wards, the main limitations to this purpose are represented by the absence of classical signs/symptoms of infection (e.g., fever) [5], the unfavorable proportion of patients vs. staff, and an environment with no advanced monitoring tools [4].

At present, there are still several unmet needs that should be addressed. The comprehension of mechanisms underlying the development and progression of sepsis, the use of new diagnostic tools [6] for a better and less invasive approach, including artificial intelligence, and the development of antimicrobial strategies in order to effectively fight antimicrobial resistance represent only a few of these.

On the other hand, returning to the most recent definition of sepsis, it still remains very generic and impractical. An organ dysfunction caused by a dysregulated host response to infection, for example, is a phrase that can well describe even severe forms of COVID-19 [7,8]. In this regard, this is only one of the many faces with which sepsis can manifest itself and is one of the many different pathophysiological mechanisms via which organ failure can develop. This is the reason why one of the objectives of this Special Issue is to carry out personalized medicine in the field of sepsis, based on the ability to identify its different manifesting typologies. Given all the variables involved (site and type of infection, microbial etiology, host comorbidity, genetic predisposition, released cytokines, hospital care setting, etc.), defining a specific, tailor-made treatment remains hard issue, however desirable.

The Special Issue "New Strategies for Treatment of Sepsis" has been thought to connect the experience of physicians involved in the diagnosis, management, and treatment of sepsis at every stage of disease, from emergency departments to general and intensive wards. The focus will be pointed on new approaches to this syndrome, such as early recognition based on clinical features and biomarkers, management in non-ICUs, non-invasive treatment strategies, including non-antimicrobial agents, and, of course, invasive approaches.

This Special Issue will highlight the many different facets of sepsis, seen through the eyes of different specialists. We hope to spread the knowledge of a new blueprint for treatment.

Author Contributions: A.M. and A.T. equally worked on the conceptualization, writing, review, and editing of the paper. Members of the Internal Medicine Sepsis Study Group participated in the writing and revision process. All authors have read and agreed to the published version of the manuscript.

Funding: This research received no external funding.

Conflicts of Interest: The authors declare no conflict of interest.

References

1. Reinhart, K.; Daniels, R.; Kissoon, N.; Machado, F.R.; Schachter, R.D.; Finfer, S. Recognizing sepsis as a global health priority—A WHO resolution. *N. Engl. J. Med.* **2017**, *377*, 414–417. [CrossRef] [PubMed]
2. Rudd, K.E.; Johnson, S.C.; Agesa, K.M.; Shackelford, K.A.; Tsoi, D.; Kievlan, D.R.; Colombara, D.V.; Ikuta, K.S.; Kissoon, N.; Finfer, S.; et al. Global, regional, and national sepsis incidence and mortality, 1990–2017: Analysis for the Global Burden of Disease Study. *Lancet* **2020**, *395*, 200–211. [CrossRef]
3. Singer, M.; Deutschman, C.S.; Seymour, C.W.; Shankar-Hari, M.; Annane, D.; Bauer, M.; Bellomo, R.; Bernard, G.R.; Chiche, J.D.; Coopersmith, C.M.; et al. The third international consensus definitions for sepsis and septic shock (Sepsis-3). *JAMA* **2016**, *315*, 801–810. [CrossRef] [PubMed]

4. Zaccone, V.; Tosoni, A.; Passaro, G.; Vallone, C.V.; Impagnatiello, M.; Li Puma, D.D.; De Cosmo, S.; Landolfi, R.; Mirijello, A.; Internal Medicine Sepsis Study Group. Sepsis in Internal Medicine wards: Current knowledge, uncertainties and new approaches for management optimization. *Ann. Med.* **2017**, *49*, 582–592. [CrossRef] [PubMed]
5. Mirijello, A.; Tosoni, A.; Zaccone, V.; Impagnatiello, M.; Passaro, G.; Vallone, C.V.; Cossari, A.; Ventura, G.; Gambassi, G.; De Cosmo, S.; et al. MEDS score and vitamin D status are independent predictors of mortality in a cohort of Internal Medicine patients with microbiological identified sepsis. *Eur. Rev. Med Pharmacol. Sci.* **2019**, *23*, 4033–4043. [CrossRef] [PubMed]
6. Tosoni, A.; Paratore, M.; Piscitelli, P.; Addolorato, G.; De Cosmo, S.; Mirijello, A.; Internal Medicine Sepsis Study Group. The use of procalcitonin for the management of sepsis in Internal Medicine wards: Current evidence. *Panminerva Med.* **2020**, *62*, 54–62. [CrossRef] [PubMed]
7. Wiersinga, W.J.; Rhodes, A.; Cheng, A.C.; Peacock, S.J.; Prescott, H.C. Pathophysiology, Transmission, Diagnosis, and Treatment of Coronavirus Disease 2019 (COVID-19): A Review. *JAMA* **2020**, *324*, 782–793. [CrossRef] [PubMed]
8. Lin, H.Y. The severe COVID-19: A sepsis induced by viral infection? And its immunomodulatory therapy. *Chin. J. Traumatol.* **2020**, *23*, 190–195. [CrossRef] [PubMed]

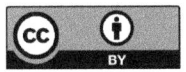

© 2020 by the authors. Licensee MDPI, Basel, Switzerland. This article is an open access article distributed under the terms and conditions of the Creative Commons Attribution (CC BY) license (http://creativecommons.org/licenses/by/4.0/).

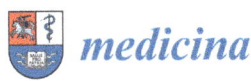

Review

Micronutrients in Sepsis and COVID-19: A Narrative Review on What We Have Learned and What We Want to Know in Future Trials

Matteo Rossetti [1], Gennaro Martucci [1], Christina Starchl [2] and Karin Amrein [2,*]

1 Department of Anesthesia and Intensive Care, IRCCS-ISMETT (Istituto Mediterraneo per i Trapianti e Terapie ad Alta Specializzazione), 90133 Palermo, Italy; mrossetti@ismett.edu (M.R.); gmartucci@ismett.edu (G.M.)
2 Division of Endocrinology and Diabetology, Department of Internal Medicine, Medical University of Graz, Auenbrugger Platz 15, 8036 Graz, Austria; christina.starchl@stud.medunigraz.at
* Correspondence: karin.amrein@medunigraz.at; Tel.: +43-316-3858-2383; Fax: +43-316-3851-3428

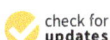

Citation: Rossetti, M.; Martucci, G.; Starchl, C.; Amrein, K. Micronutrients in Sepsis and COVID-19: A Narrative Review on What We Have Learned and What We Want to Know in Future Trials. *Medicina* 2021, 57, 419. https://doi.org/10.3390/medicina57050419

Academic Editors: Antonio Mirijello and Alberto Tosoni

Received: 27 March 2021
Accepted: 21 April 2021
Published: 26 April 2021

Publisher's Note: MDPI stays neutral with regard to jurisdictional claims in published maps and institutional affiliations.

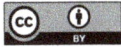

Copyright: © 2021 by the authors. Licensee MDPI, Basel, Switzerland. This article is an open access article distributed under the terms and conditions of the Creative Commons Attribution (CC BY) license (https://creativecommons.org/licenses/by/4.0/).

Abstract: Sepsis remains the leading cause of mortality in hospitalized patients, contributing to 1 in every 2–3 deaths. From a pathophysiological view, in the recent definition, sepsis has been defined as the result of a complex interaction between host response and the infecting organism, resulting in life-threatening organ dysfunction, depending on microcirculatory derangement, cellular hypoxia/dysoxia driven by hypotension and, potentially, death. The high energy expenditure driven by a high metabolic state induced by the host response may rapidly lead to micronutrient depletion. This deficiency can result in alterations in normal energy homeostasis, free radical damage, and immune system derangement. In critically ill patients, micronutrients are still relegated to an ancillary role in the whole treatment, and always put in a second-line place or, frequently, neglected. Only some micronutrients have attracted the attention of a wider audience, and some trials, even large ones, have tested their use, with controversial results. The present review will address this topic, including the recent advancement in the study of vitamin D and protocols based on vitamin C and other micronutrients, to explore an update in the setting of sepsis, gain some new insights applicable to COVID-19 patients, and to contribute to a pathophysiological definition of the potential role of micronutrients that will be helpful in future dedicated trials.

Keywords: vitamin D; vitamin C; zinc; thiamine; nutrition; critically ill patients; infections; mitochondria; shock

1. Introduction

In the USA alone, apart from COVID-19, sepsis affects around 1.5 million people annually [1]. Based on the most recent epidemiological trends, incidence of sepsis is growing [2], with an incidence that is more than 5-fold greater in the elderly population [3]. In a trend analysis conducted from 1993 to 2003, the percentage of severe sepsis cases requiring hospitalization increased from 25% to 44% [4]. In-hospital sepsis mortality has been estimated up to 140% higher compared to annual estimates of mortality due to other causes [5].

Sepsis remains the leading cause of mortality in hospitalized patients, contributing to 1 in every 2–3 deaths [6]. It is the result of a complex interaction between host response and the infecting organism, resulting in life-threatening organ dysfunction, depending on microcirculatory derangement, cellular hypoxia/dysoxia driven by hypotension and, potentially, leading to death. All these processes are finely regulated by merging pathways involving a number of cells and mediators.

Standard care for septic patients still involves the first-hour bundle, with the explicit intention of beginning resuscitation and management immediately. Mainstays of treatment are still lactate monitoring, early diagnosis/treatment using cultures and broad-spectrum antibiotics, as well as adequate hemodynamic support to guarantee adequate end-organ perfusion [7]. However, the high energy expenditure driven by a high metabolic state induced by the host response can rapidly lead to micronutrient depletion [8]. This deficiency can result in alterations in normal energy homeostasis, free radical damage, and immune system derangement [6]. In the critically ill septic patient, the adjunctive administration of vitamins and micronutrients, especially in defective scenarios, could lead to a better energy expenditure homeostasis [9]. Moreover, vitamins, and generally micronutrients, despite being neglected for years in the critically ill population, may represent a missing tool in the regulation of processes involved in sepsis, due to their ubiquitous presence and action, the involvement in several biochemical reactions as a cofactor and, in some cases, with indirect genomic and non-genomic effects on the cells involved in the inflammation pathways.

This review will address the topic, including the recent advancement in the study of some micronutrients, including vitamin D, vitamin C, thiamine, and zinc. These are the micronutrients for which, despite controversies, there is some evidence and associations between the disease severity in critically ill patients and their deficiency. In other cases, they have been tested as supplementation in clinical studies.

The field of micronutrients has been entered into clinical studies recently and suffers from methodology biases in clinical studies, since the exploration of such a topic was mainly relegated to pre-clinical interest. However, with its potential for fine-tuning the regulation of biochemical processes and the high evidence of association between disease severity and their deficiency, it is worthy of consideration by clinicians.

In this light, we will give an overview of the actions of micronutrients and their involvement in sepsis and in COVID-19, which has several clinical features in common with severe sepsis.

2. Vitamin D

Initially discovered and studied as a major regulator of calcium metabolism, vitamin D also plays an essential role as an immunomodulatory hormone [10] and in several biological activities interfering with the innate and adaptive immune system, with a role even in liver transplant recipients regarding graft function and sepsis incidence [11]. This is also proven by the fact that vitamin D receptors are expressed by immune cells such as lymphocytes, monocytes, macrophages, and dendritic cells [12].

2.1. Physiology and Requirements

There are two forms of native vitamin D. Vitamin D_2 is synthesized from ergosterol and can be found in yeast and sun-dried mushrooms. Vitamin D_3 is synthesized endogenously from 7-dehydrocholesterol in sun-exposed skin. Both D_2 and D_3 are metabolized by CYP2R1 (vitamin D-25 hydroxylase) [12] in the liver to 25-hydroxyvitaminD [25(OH)D], which is further metabolized by CYP27B1 to the active form 1,25-dihydroxyvitaminD [1,25(OH)$_2$D] [12], which exerts its endocrine and immune effects by binding to the vitamin D receptor (VDR) in the nucleus [13]. 1,25OHD is usually only needed in advanced renal dysfunction and rare conditions, including hypoparathyroidism.

The main site of conversion of 25(OH)D is the kidneys. Evidence shows that circulating levels of 25(OH)D maintained in the range of 40–60 ng/mL are associated with the lowest risk of several types of cancer, and cardiovascular and autoimmune diseases [14]. In order to maintain the blood levels in the range of 20–40 ng/mL, with minimal sun exposure, an adult would require the ingestion of 4000–6000 IU daily [15]; however, daily intakes using standard enteral/parenteral nutrition formulas rarely exceed 500 IU daily.

2.2. Vitamin D and Immunity

Vitamin D has a plausible link with response to infection. Macrophages and monocytes express CYP27B1 as a response to cytokines and IFN-γ. This enzyme converts 25(OH)D in the active form 1,25(OH)2D25, which is able to enhance macrophage and monocyte activity by the stimulation of the production of cathelicidin (LL-37), which acts by destabilizing microbial membranes [16]. Furthermore, it exerts antiviral effects by disrupting viral envelopes and altering the viability of host target cells.

In a mouse model, Horiuchi et al. found a low expression of the inflammatory molecule iTXB$_2$ in mice receiving oral 1,25(OH)$_2$D and intraperitoneal LPS compared to controls who were not receiving the vitamin D metabolite. A significant reduction in mortality was noticed [17].

As known, this modulation process is widely seen in clinical scenarios such as sarcoidosis and tuberculosis, explaining why, for example, some patients affected with granulomatous disorders develop hypercalcemia and hypercalciuria [18]. The upregulation of CYP27B1 also plays a role in regulating lymphocyte activity (reduces Th1 and Th17 activity and stimulates Th2 and Treg). Moreover, 1,25(OH)$_2$D modulates tolerance in antigen-presenting cells (APC) by decreasing the expression of major histocompatibility complex class II (MHC-II) [19]. This leads to a decrease in IL-12 production and an increase in IL-10, with tolerogenic effects [20].

Even endothelial function is influenced by vitamin D. Several experimental studies have shown that it can modulate vascular permeability via multiple genomic and extra-genomic pathways. For example, 1,25(OH)$_2$D is a transcriptional factor for endothelial nitric oxide synthase (eNOS), able to cause an upregulation of the gene expression augmenting nitric oxide production [21].

This is a potential role that may be interesting for the prevention and treatment of patients with severe cases of COVID-19, given that microangiopathy, coagulopathy, and thrombosis are frequent in COVID-19, and vitamin D deficiency is associated with a prothrombophilic profile, potentially reversible with vitamin D supplementation [22]. In fact, high dose vitamin D supplementation has been associated with reduced in vitro thrombin generation and decreased clot density.

These effects use non-genomic pathways including adenylyl cyclase/cyclic adenosine monophosphate (AC/cAMP) and inositol triphosphate/diacilgycerole (IP$_3$/DAG), which lead to an augmentation of intracellular calcium concentration [23].

Multiple studies have reported vitamin D effects also on gut integrity and intestinal homeostasis, showing an ability to alleviate intestinal damage from bacterial lipopolysaccaride [24]. Moreover, vitamin D can increase the expression of epithelial membrane junction proteins, crucial when facing bacterial translocation events.

Vitamin D's role in modulating adaptive immunity was originally observed on clonal human T-cell-expressing VDR [25]. It seems that resting T cells do not express VDR, while peripheral T cells do, making them a target of 1,25(OH)$_2$D produced by macrophages and monocytes involved in the inflammatory response [25]. Vitamin D promotes a shift from Th1 and Th17 to Th2 and Treg immunity by enhancing Th2 cytokine expression while inhibiting Th1. This leads to the suppression of an uncontested proinflammatory state [25,26], even playing a potential role in protection from autoimmune diseases. This role in modulating inflammation is also evident in vitamin-D-deficient individuals, where CD4/CD8 ratios decrease as an indicator of immune activation [27], while the administration of 5000–10,000 IUs of D$_3$ can increase CD4/CD8 ratio [28,29].

2.3. Vitamin D in the Critically Ill: The Septic Patient

In a large study involving more than 3000 critically ill patients, vitamin D deficiency was a significant predictor of sepsis and carried a 1.6-fold increase in mortality [30]. Several observational studies have reported a connection between low levels of 25(OH)D and the incidence of sepsis; data also support the link between low serum vitamin D levels and the increase in morbidity and mortality in septic, critically ill patients. The reasons seem to be related to the effects of 1,25(OH)2D on the expression of pro-inflammatory cytokines of T_H1(IL-2, IFN-γ, TNF-α) and T_H17 (IL-17, IL-12) [31–33].The role of vascular reactivity is under debate: lower levels of vitamin D$_3$ are associated with worse outcomes, but vitamin D may, at the same time, exert non-genomic actions on endothelial cells to prevent extravascular leakage, and it may be reduced in its plasmatic levels by the vascular leakage itself due to systemic inflammation [34]. Vitamin D's effects seem to encompass not only the modulation of the proinflammatory status, but also the local pathogen's control: Youssef and colleagues showed how the concentration of 50,000–90,000 IU/mL of D_3 was able to inhibit the growth of or even kill strains of *Staphylococcus aureus*, *Klebsiella pneumoniae*, *Escherichia coli*, and *Streptococcus pyogenes* [35]. As a direct antimicrobial role becomes better understood, especially considering the modulating effect exerted by $1,25(OH)_2D$ after LPS exposure, strong evidence connects vitamin D metabolites to a decrease in pro-inflammatory status, e.g., in yeast-induced sepsis [36]. In addition to basic biological research, some observational studies have explored vitamin D's role in the clinical setting. One observational study pointed to a connection between vitamin D plasma concentrations and respiratory infection [37], where Ginde et al. observed an inverse relationship between 25(OH)D levels and the incidence of upper respiratory infections (URI), data corroborated by Sabetta and colleagues' study, in which 25(OH)D levels greater than 38 ng/mL were associated with a 2-fold decrease in URI incidence [38]. In the critically ill population, several studies have revealed a high prevalence of poor vitamin D status [39]: in a single-center study, the prevalence of 25(OH)D < 24 ng/mL was 79% [40], though lacking any association with mortality or hospital-acquired infections. In contrast, a retrospective study of 437 ICU patients showed a significant correlation between low vitamin D levels and 25(OH)D < 20 ng/mL and mortality [41]. In a study of 70 patients divided into three groups, Jeng et al. found vitamin D insufficiency in 100% of critically ill patients admitted with sepsis in the ICU (group 1) and in 92% when considering the non-septic ICU group (group 2), compared with 66.5% in the control group of normal healthy individuals (group 3) [42]. In a case-control cohort study of 36 ventilated patients admitted to the ICU, the group receiving a high-dose intramuscular injection of vitamin D obtained a significant reduction of ventilation days and length of stay.

A summary of the potential positive effects of vitamin D in sepsis is presented in Figure 1.

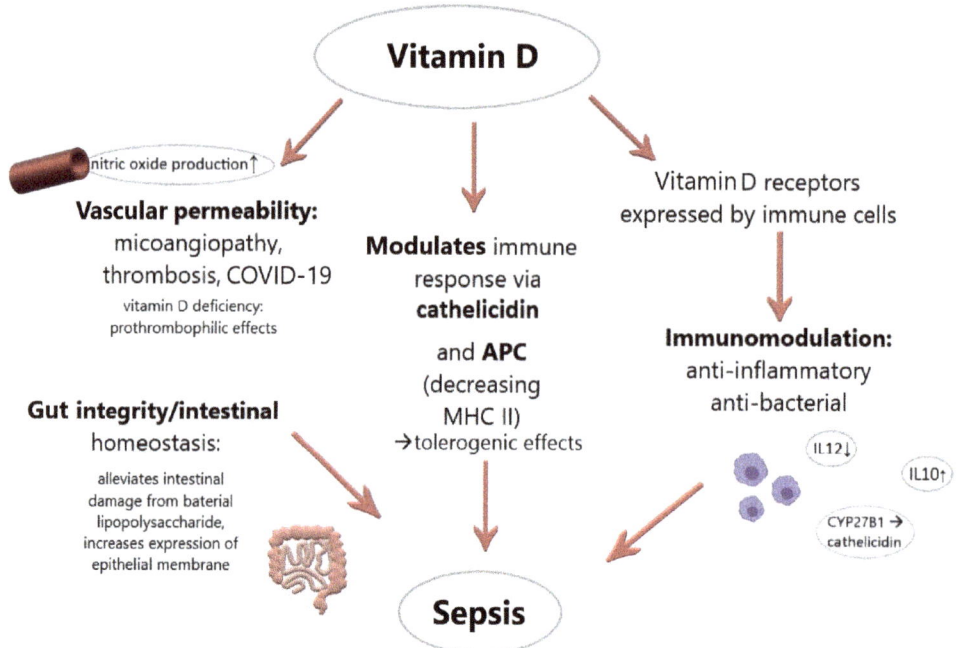

Figure 1. Summary of potential implications of vitamin D during sepsis. (APC: antigen-presenting cell; MCH II: major histocompatibility complex, class II; IL-12: interleukin 12; IL-10: interleukin 10).

3. Vitamin C

3.1. Physiology and Requirements

Involved in several biosynthetic and metabolic processes, vitamin C is essential for collagen and carnitine [43], and neurotransmitter synthesis [44] plays an antioxidant role [45], acting as an immunomodulatory agent [46] (Figure 2). The level considered normal in plasma [47], about 50 μmol/L, according to the EU food safety authority, can be achieved by an intake of 90 mg/day for men and 80 mg/day for women. This is the plausible solution, at a population level, to avoid scurvy, but it has been not demonstrated that it is a sufficient intake in case of viral infections of other processes with a high level of antioxidant consumptions. The overt vitamin C deficiency can be diagnosed by a plasma level below 11 μmol/L, but it is rarely checked in hospitalized patients, and even among the most severe patients, this feature is definitely neglected [47]. This happens despite the fact that we know that the level of vitamins decreases rapidly in sepsis, trauma, surgery, and, recently, in COVID-19 patients.

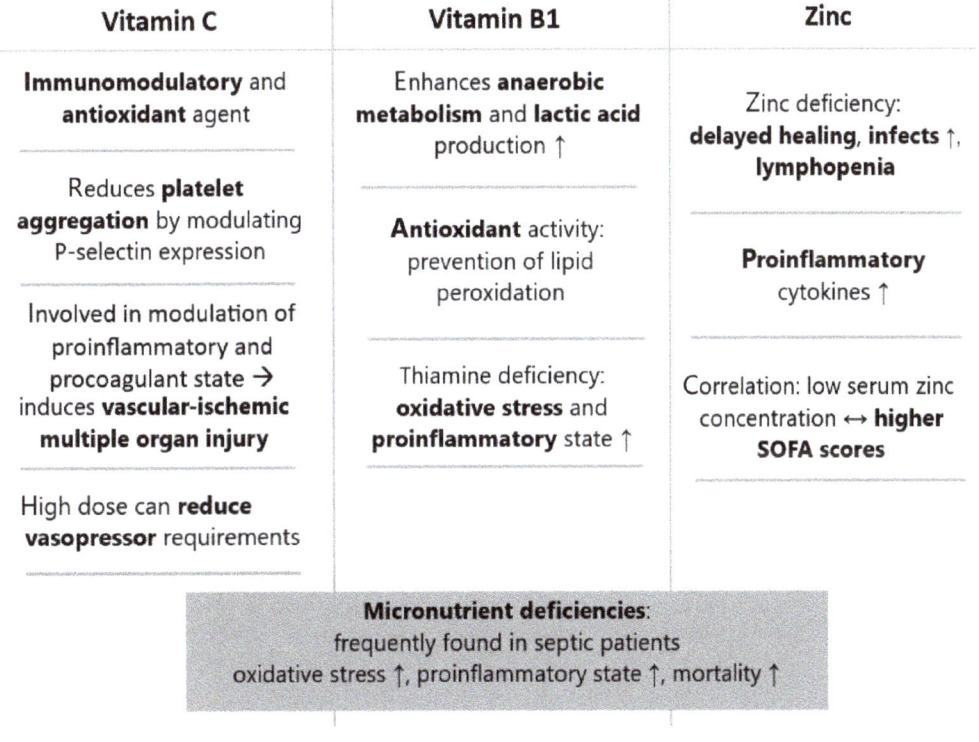

Figure 2. Effects of micronutrients on septic patients, other than vitamin D.

In septic patients, vitamin C is involved in the modulation of the proinflammatory and procoagulant state believed to induce vascular-ischemic induced multiple organ injury [48]. In addition, vitamin C seems to reduce platelet aggregation by modulating surface P-selectin expression [49], attenuate hypothalamic neuronal damage, and prevent immunosuppression, in addition to inducing endogenous vasopressor synthesis [50]. As with studies on vitamin D, several studies have found a reduction in vitamin-C-circulating levels in septic patients admitted to the ICU, and deficiency may be exacerbated by the reduction in cell uptake due to inflammatory cascade activation (TNF-α and IL-1β can down-regulate the ascorbate-specific transporter [51]). On the other hand, plasma concentration can lower (<10 micromol/L) in the first 24 h after septic onset, an event that is strongly associated with an increase in the severity of organ dysfunction and mortality.

3.2. Vitamin C in the Critically Ill Septic Patient

Within the ICU population, to achieve normal plasma concentration and counteract organ dysfunction, high dose administration is necessary (3 g/daily) for 72 h. This may reduce vasopressor requirements in septic shock and mortality in the ICU septic population [52], though more evidence will be needed. This hypothesis has a strong pathophysiological plausibility and relies mainly on a small and controversial before-after retrospective study [53]. Several RCTs were unable to demonstrate a reduction in mortality through the use of vitamin C, potentially due to several limitations, such as heterogeneous populations or too severe patients and a lack of early administration [54]. The principal criticism is the use of such a therapy in cases of advanced severe septic shock, at least in light of mortality as an outcome, since, as demonstrated for vitamin D, the action of micronutrients on severely ill patients may be less relevant, likely because the severity of the organ failure is the result of several metabolic pathways that cannot easily be improved upon.

Another relevant topic on vitamin C administration is related to the pharmacokinetic aspect. In fact, being a water-soluble vitamin, it is rapidly excreted if not used. For this reason, due to its rapid use in the oxidative process, the main results were reached with repeated administration every 6 h. In the largest trial of intravenous vitamin C in sepsis-associated ARDS, the CITRIS-ALI trial [55], patients were given placebo or vitamin C at a dose of 50 mg/kg every 6 h for 4 days. This means about an average dose of 3.5 g every 6 h in adults. Looking at the stated primary study outcomes, vitamin C did not improve markers of inflammation, vascular injury, or organ dysfunction. However, there were statistically significant benefits in three clinically relevant outcomes: mortality ($p = 0.03$), duration of ICU-free days ($p = 0.03$), and hospital-free days ($p = 0.04$). As a matter of fact, examining the data, during the 4-day vitamin C administration, mortality was 81% lower in the vitamin C group, but after the cessation of study drug administration, there was no difference between the two trial groups. This study, as well as other similar negative studies, poses a relevant question about seeking proper evidence in critically ill patients, when the research objectives just apparently, contrast with the clinical effects.

4. Other Micronutrients

4.1. Thiamine (Vitamin B1)

Thiamine is a cofactor for several enzymes involved in aerobic carbohydrate metabolism, maintenance of cellular redox homeostasis, and synthesis of adenosine triphosphate [56] (Figure 2). In particular, thiamine is needed to convert pyruvate into acetyl-CoA, allowing entry into the citric acid cycle and aerobic metabolism. The human body has limited storage abilities within skeletal muscle, heart, kidney, and brain [57], and due to its quick turnover, without supplementation, deficiency can develop in just two weeks, with a clinical spectrum ranging from cardiac beriberi to Wernicke's encephalopathy [58].

In septic patients, thiamine deficiency is commonly found, with a prevalence of 20% to 71%: 20% of septic patients and 71% of those presenting with septic shock exhibit thiamine deficiency (<9 nmol/L) [59,60] (normal range of value is considered to be within 33–99 ng/mL). Several mechanisms have been identified to explain the association between thiamine deficiency and sepsis, though it remains unclear whether the deficiency can contribute as a cause of sepsis or if it is just a consequence. What is clear is that by decreasing pyruvate dehydrogenase activity (needed to convert pyruvate in acetyl-CoA to enter the citric acid cycle), thiamine deficiency can increase anaerobic metabolism and lactic acid production, possibly worsening sepsis-related consumption of endogenous antioxidants, a hallmark of septic multi-organ damage [61]. Moreover, its antioxidant activity is manifested through the prevention of lipid peroxidation and oleic acid oxidation. Therefore, in De Andrade and colleagues' murine model, thiamine deficiency was associated with oxidative stress and a proinflammatory state [62]. The clinical consequence is, however, unclear: in a large randomized clinical study, the administration of thiamine in ICU patients considered to be thiamine deficient did not improve mortality or ICU stay, but was associated with a lower rate in progression to renal replacement therapy [63,64]. In a small observational study, Marik et al. suggested that the combination of hydrocortisone (50 mg every 6 h for 4 days), vitamin C (1.5 mg every 6 h for 4 days), and thiamine (200 mg every 12 h for 4 days) significantly improved outcomes in patients with sepsis and septic shock [65].

4.2. Zinc

Zinc homeostasis may be fundamental in the organism's reaction to sepsis. As an essential trace element, it works as a co-factor for several enzymes and its deficiency leads to delayed wound healing, lymphopenia, and a high incidence of infection [66]. Concentrating on the immune system, zinc is crucial for T-cell maturation and differentiation [67] and protects against the premature apoptosis of immature T cells, which can lead to altered Th1/Th2 ratios and, eventually, to total T-cell count decrease [68]. On the cellular level, zinc serves as a second messenger and is involved in the development of pro-inflammatory cytokines by monocytes [69] presentation, of major histocompatibility complex type II by dendritic cells [70], and proliferation of T cells [71] via IL-2 stimulation. As part of the acute phase reaction in sepsis, zinc deficiency is linked to an increase in TNF-α and IL-6, and to explain this phenomenon, some authors have proposed a model of redistribution of zinc mediated by cytokines [72], and a reduced concentration of serum zinc has been found in septic patients admitted to ICUs for no alimentary reason [73] (Figure 2). A series of studies has found that exposure to LPS and pro-inflammatory cytokines such as IL-6 led to an upregulation of the protein ZIP14 in the liver [74], where it serves as a zinc transporter and is essential for the phosphorylation of c-Met during liver regeneration [75]. In a murine model, ZIP14 ko mice exposed to LPS did not show hypozincemia, but developed hypoglycemia as a mark of hepatic glycemic dysregulation [75]. Where the ZIP14 protein can be upregulated, by contrast, hypozincemia begins within 9 hours [76], and the redistribution of zinc in the liver has been associated with lower degrees of accumulation of superoxide anion and necrotic cell death in the organ [77], suggesting a possible protective role of zinc in acute phase liver dysfunction. On the other hand, a decrease in serum zinc concentration can lead to a downregulation of lymphopoiesis and an upregulation of myelopoiesis, showing a sort of reprogramming of the immune response with a shift from adaptive-based to innately-predominant during hypozincemia [78]. Despite the unclear, but potential, physiological role of zinc redistribution, its serum reduction could lead to higher levels of proinflammatory cytokines, higher oxidative stress, lipid peroxidation, and damage to DNA [79]. Though zinc's role is largely an unexplored path, several studies have shown a correlation between low serum zinc concentration and higher SOFA scores [80], and sepsis non-survivors had much lower zinc concentrations than patients with favorable outcomes [81].

Data regarding a potential beneficial role of zinc supplementation in septic patients still fail to reach statistical significance, though a possible role might be played by albumin, which is the main zinc serum transporter and one of the most important negative acute phase proteins [82,83]. For this reason, more evidence is needed to implement zinc administration in standard sepsis treatment and care, even as a possible biomarker in terms of morbidity and outcome.

5. COVID-19 and Micronutrients: What Is Known

SARS-CoV-2 infection resulting in COVID-19 has reached an unexpected, worldwide burden in terms of morbidity and mortality, with 5% of patients hospitalized among all those who tested positive and 20% of those hospitalized developing a severe illness [84]. The most common clinical presentation includes fever (70–90%), dry cough (60–86%), shortness of breath (53–80%), fatigue (38%), myalgias (15–44%), nausea/vomiting or diarrhea (15–39%), headache, weakness (25%), and rhinorrhea (7%). In some cases, anosmia/ageusia can be the presenting symptom (3%). Common laboratory findings include lymphopenia

(83%), elevated inflammatory markers like erythrocyte sedimentation rate (ESR), C-reactive protein (CRP), ferritin, IL-1, and IL-6. Chest X-rays often reveal bilateral infiltrates with ground glass opacities [85]. A study of 20,133 hospitalized patients in the UK found that 17.1% had been admitted to high-dependency units or ICUs [86], prompting an exhausting effort by the health system to counteract the pandemic. Impaired function of the heart, brain, liver, lung, kidney, and coagulation systems have been observed, so that approximately 17–35% of hospitalized patients are currently treated in the ICU, due to hypoxemic respiratory failure in the most common scenario. Interestingly, in the case of COVID-19, the clinical picture of the severe cases requiring ICU admission is characterized by multi-organ failure, with many tracts very similar to those of severe sepsis. Therefore, the mechanisms of disease also seem to have some similarity since in COVID-19 as well in severe sepsis and septic shock, the cause of multi-organ failure is not due to a "cytopathic" effect of the bacteria or the virus, but mainly due to the host's response to the infection.

COVID-19 therapy, especially when treating ICU patients, is strictly supportive, including mechanical ventilation, extracorporeal life support systems such as veno-venous ECMO and antibiotic therapy in the case of bacterial over-infection. Non-specific anti-viral therapy has been proven to be effective in ICU patients. There might be a role, though, for micronutrient supplementation in deficient patients. In the current scenario of limited health resources, it would be important to adopt any adjuvant treatment that may contribute to a better outcome if it is inexpensive and with few or unimportant side effects at tested doses.

5.1. Vitamin D and COVID-19

As already described above, vitamin D as an immunomodulatory agent has a strong rationale also in COVID-19. The risk of developing respiratory tract infections is reduced two-fold in adults with a higher serum concentration of 25(OH)D (>38 ng/mL) [38], and the role of 1,25(OH)$_2$D in exerting anti-viral activity and modulating immune response by stimulating cathelicidin release is well known. This leads to the suppression of proinflammatory cytokine release [87]. Furthermore, 1,25(OH)$_2$D specifically acts as a modulator of the renin-angiotensin pathway and is able to downregulate angiotensin-converting enzyme-2 expression, which is known to be the entry receptor for SARS-CoV-2 in cells [88]. Recently, the effect of a single dose of 200,000 IU of vitamin D$_3$ on hospital length of stay in patients with COVID-19 was tested, showing no effect between the vitamin D$_3$ and the placebo group for the primary or secondary end points [89]. This study is paradigmatic of how the basic science should be deeply known to start a clinical trial on the topic to avoid the risk of eventually misleading negative conclusions [90]. In fact, though a loading dose is imperative in acute settings to improve vitamin D levels rapidly, it is unphysiological to give only a loading dose not followed by a maintenance dose [91]. Despite the practical advantage, a single or annual dose has repeatedly been shown to be ineffective or even harmful for respiratory tract infections and musculoskeletal outcomes. Considering the population enrolled in the study, only 115 of 240 patients were vitamin D deficient at baseline (25OHD < 20 ng/mL), with no information on the proportion of patients with severe deficiency (25OHD < 12 ng/mL). Finally, symptom onset was 10 days before the intervention, so the infection likely took place well over two weeks before the intervention. This topic of the right intervention time returns in many studies approaching micronutrients because it is quite impossible that a single intervention can be the only reason for a change in prognosis when a wide intersection of different pathways has been started with superimposing circles.

5.2. Vitamin C and COVID-19

Vitamin C could exert many potentially beneficial roles in counteracting SARS-CoV-2 infection: antiviral, immunomodulatory, anti-inflammatory, and antioxidant effects coexist in molecular pharmacodynamics. In vitro studies have confirmed that vitamin C alone is able to suppress the replication of some viral species, such as herpes simplex-1, influenza

A, polyvirus type 1, and rhynovirus [92]. In vivo, vitamin C supplementation can reduce the incidence of postherpetic neuralgi [93] and the duration and severity of the common cold [94]. High-dose vitamin C treatment can also reduce symptoms in patients affected with acquired immune deficiency syndrome (AIDS), being able to ameliorate even the severity of opportunistic infections [95]. Vitamin C is also able to modulate the release of proinflammatory cytokines, and in mice models led to augmented release of interferon, thus being able to reduce lung inflammation in viral pneumonitis [96]. With regard to COVID-19, the combination of vitamin C and quercetin has shown promising synergic antiviral activity [97] and can lead to augmented endothelial repair in widespread microvascular and microvascular thrombosis with increased permeability [98]. In a Chinese trial, high IV dose vitamin C (10 g/day for moderate cases and 20 g/day for severe cases for 7–10 days) was able to shorten the hospital stay by 3–5 days in 50 patients [99]. In another randomized controlled pilot-trial in three hospitals in China on 56 critically ill COVID-19 patients, 24 g of vitamin C was not able to improve the primary outcome (invasive mechanical ventilation-free days in 28 days) and the 28-day mortality ($p = 0.27$), but it was able to improve the PaO_2/FiO_2 ratio in the treatment group on day 7 (229 vs. 151 mmHg, 95% CI 33–122; p value = 0.01) as well as reduce the value of IL-6 in the treatment group on day 7 ($p = 0.04$) [100]. Both of the reached positive outcomes were clinically relevant and should prompt further investigations on the topic.

6. Conclusions

Micronutrients contribute greatly to the human body's homeostasis and metabolism. For decades, they have been considered an ancillary concern in critically ill patients. However, with the current need for a new increase in survival for critically ill patients, they should enter any clinical consideration in daily practice. As another side of the coin, research on this topic should consider not only mortality, since in severely ill patients the outcome is too often confounded by concomitant factors; but reliable and clinically sensitive surrogate outcomes, including the functional recovery of daily activities, should be explored in the coming years.

Author Contributions: Conceptualization, G.M. and K.A.; methodology, M.R. and C.S.; writing—original draft preparation, M.R.; writing—review and editing, G.M., C.S., and K.A. All authors have read and agreed to the published version of the manuscript.

Funding: This research received no external funding.

Institutional Review Board Statement: Not applicable.

Informed Consent Statement: Not applicable.

Data Availability Statement: Not applicable.

Acknowledgments: We acknowledge the contribution of our editor, Warren Blumberg.

Conflicts of Interest: The authors declare no conflict of interest.

References

1. Adrie, C.; Alberti, C.; Chaix-Couturier, C.; Azoulay, E.; De Lassence, A.; Cohen, Y.; Meshaka, P.; Cheval, C.; Thuong, M.; Troche, G.; et al. Epidemiology and economic evaluation of severe sepsis in France: Age, severity, infection site, and place of acquisition as determinants of workload and cost. *J. Crit. Care* **2005**, *20*, 46–58. [CrossRef] [PubMed]
2. Stoller, J.; Halpin, L.; Weis, M.; Aplin, B.; Qu, W.; Georgescu, C.; Nazzal, M. Epidemiology of severe sepsis: 2008-2012. *J. Crit. Care* **2016**, *31*, 58–62. [CrossRef] [PubMed]
3. Angus, D.C.; Linde-Zwible, W.T.; Lidicker, J.; Clermont, G.; Carcillo, J.; Pinsky, M.R. Epidemiology of severe sepsis in the Unites States: Analysis of incidence, outcome, and associated costs of care. *Crit. Care Med.* **2001**, *29*, 1303–1310. [CrossRef]
4. Dombrovskiy, V.Y.; Martin, A.A.; Sunderram, J.; Paz, H. Rapid increase in hospitalization and mortality rates for severe sepsis in the United States: A trend analysis from 1993 to 2003. *Crit. Care Med.* **2007**, *35*, 1244–1250. [CrossRef]
5. Epstein, L.; Dantes, R.; Magill, S.; Fiore, A. Varying estimates of sepsis mortality using death certificates and administrative codes–Unites States, 1999–2014. *MMWR Morb. Mortal. Wkly. Rep.* **2016**, *65*, 342–345. [CrossRef]

6. Belsky, J.B.; Wira, C.R.; Jacob, V.; Sather, J.E.; Lee, P.J. A review of micronutrients in sepsis: The role of thiamine, l-carnitine, vitamin C, selenium and vitamin D. *Nutr. Res. Rev.* **2018**, *31*, 281–290. [CrossRef]
7. Martucci, G.; Tuzzolino, F.; Arcadipane, A.; Pieber, T.R.; Schnedl, C.; Urbanic Purkart, T.; Treiber, G.; Amrein, K. The effect of high-dose cholecalciferol on bioavailable vitamin D levels in critically ill patients: A post hoc analysis of the VITdAL-ICU trial. *Intensive Care Med.* **2017**, *43*, 1732–1734. [CrossRef]
8. L'Her, E.; Sebert, P. A global approach to energy metabolism in an experimental model of sepsis. *Am. J. Respir. Crit. Care Med.* **2001**, *164*, 1444–1447. [CrossRef]
9. Amrein, K.; Oudemans-van Straaten, H.M.; Berger, M.M. Vitamin therapy in critically ill patients: Focus on thiamine, vitamin C, and vitamin D. *Intensive Care Med.* **2018**, *44*, 1940–1944. [CrossRef]
10. Prietl, B.; Treiber, G.; Pieber, T.R.; Amrein, K. Vitamin D and immune function. *Nutrients* **2013**, *5*, 2502–2521. [CrossRef]
11. Martucci, G.; Volpes, R.; Panarello, G.; Tuzzolino, F.; Di Carlo, D.; Ricotta, C.; Gruttadauria, S.; Conaldi, P.G.; Luca, A.; Amrein, K.; et al. Vitamin D levels in liver transplantation recipients and early postoperative outcomes: Prospective observational DLiverX study. *Clin. Nutr.* **2020**, *40*, 2355–2363. [CrossRef]
12. Charoenngam, N.; Shirvani, A.; Holick, M.F. Vitamin D for skeletal and non-skeletal health: What we should know. *J. Clin. Orthop. Trauma* **2019**, *10*, 1082–1093. [CrossRef]
13. Haussler, M.R.; Haussler, C.A.; Jurutka, P.W.; Thompson, P.D.; Hsieh, J.C.; Remus, L.S.; Selznick, S.H.; Whitfield, G.K. The vitamin D hormone and its nuclear receptor: Molecular actions and disease states. *J. Endocrinol.* **1997**, *154*, S57–S73.
14. Amrein, K.; Scherkl, M.; Hoffmann, M.; Neuwersch-Sommeregger, S.; Köstenberger, M.; Tmava Berisha, A.; Martucci, G.; Pilz, S.; Malle, O. Vitamin D deficiency 2.0: An update on the current status worldwide. *Eur J Clin Nutr.* **2020**, *74*, 1498–1513. [CrossRef]
15. Holick, M.F.; Binkley, N.C.; Bischoff-Ferrari, H.A.; Gordon, C.M.; Hanley, D.A.; Heaney, R.P.; Murad, M.H.; Weaver, C.M.; Endocrine, S. Evaluation, treatment, and prevention of vitamin D deficiency: An Endocrine Society clinical practice guideline. *J. Clin. Endocrinol. Metab.* **2011**, *96*, 1911–1930. [CrossRef]
16. Herr, C.; Greulich, T.; Koczulla, R.A.; Meyer, S.; Zakharkina, T.; Branscheidt, M.; Eschmann, R.; Bals, R. The role of vitamin D in pulmonary disease: COPD, asthma, infection, and cancer. *Respir. Res.* **2011**, *12*, 31. [CrossRef]
17. Horiuchi, H.; Nagata, I.; Komoriya, K. Protective effect of vitamin D3 analogues on endotoxin shock in mice. *Agents Actions* **1991**, *33*, 343–348. [CrossRef]
18. Papapoulos, S.E.; Clemens, T.L.; Fraher, L.J.; Lewin, I.G.; Sandler, L.M.; O'Riordan, J.L. 1, 25-dihydroxycholecalciferol in the pathogenesis of the hypercalcaemia of sarcoidosis. *Lancet* **1979**, *1*, 627–630. [CrossRef]
19. Adorini, L.; Penna, G. Induction of tolerogenic dendritic cells by vitamin D receptor agonists. *Handb. Exp. Pharmacol.* **2009**, *188*, 251–273.
20. Urry, Z.; Xystrakis, E.; Richards, D.F.; McDonald, J.; Sattar, Z.; Cousins, D.J.; Corrigan, C.J.; Hickman, E.; Brown, Z.; Hawrylowicz, C.M. Ligation of TLR9 induced on human IL-10-secreting Tregs by 1alpha,25-dihydroxyvitamin D3 abrogates regulatory function. *J. Clin. Investig.* **2009**, *119*, 387–398.
21. Andrukhova, O.; Slavic, S.; Zeitz, U.; Riesen, S.C.; Heppelmann, M.S.; Ambrisko, T.D.; Markovic, M.; Kuebler, W.M.; Erben, R.G. Vitamin D is a regulator of endothelial nitric oxide synthase and arterial stiffness in mice. *Mol. Endocrinol.* **2014**, *28*, 53–64. [CrossRef]
22. Kowalewski, M.; Fina, D.; Słomka, A.; Raffa, G.M.; Martucci, G.; Lo Coco, V.; De Piero, M.E.; Ranucci, M.; Suwalski, P.; Lorusso, R. COVID-19 and ECMO: The interplay between coagulation and inflammation-a narrative review. *Crit Care* **2020**, *24*, 205. [CrossRef]
23. Molinari, C.; Uberti, F.; Grossini, E.; Vacca, G.; Carda, S.; Invernizzi, M.; Cisari, C. 1α,25-Dihydroxycholecalciferol Induces Nitric Oxide Production in Cultured Endothelial Cells. *Cell. Physiol. Biochem.* **2011**, *27*, 661–668. [CrossRef]
24. Lee, C.; Lau, E.; Chusilp, S.; Filler, R.; Li, B.; Zhu, H.; Yamoto, M.; Pierro, A. Protective effects of vitamin D against injury in intestinal epithelium. *Pediatr. Surg. Int.* **2019**, *35*, 1395–1401. [CrossRef]
25. Cantorna, M.T.; Snyder, L.; Lin, Y.D.; Yang, L. Vitamin D and 1,25(OH)2D regulation of T cells. *Nutrients* **2015**, *7*, 3011–3021. [CrossRef]
26. Mocanu, V.; Oboroceanu, T.; Zugun-Eloae, F. Current status in vitamin D and regulatory T cells-immunological implications. *Med. Surg. J.* **2013**, *117*, 965–973.
27. Mao, X.; Hu, B.; Zhou, Z.; Xing, X.; Wu, Y.; Gao, J.; He, Y.; Hu, Y.; Cheng, Q.; Gong, Q. Vitamin D levels correlate with lymphocyte subsets in elderly patients with age-related diseases. *Sci. Rep.* **2018**, *8*, 7708. [CrossRef]
28. Eckard, A.R.; O'Riordan, M.A.; Rosebush, J.C.; Lee, S.T.; Habib, J.G.; Ruff, J.H.; Labbato, D.; Daniels, J.E.; Uribe-Leitz, M.; Tangpricha, V.; et al. Vitamin D supplementation decreases immune activation and exhaustion in HIV-1-infected youth. *Antivir. Ther.* **2018**, *23*, 315–324. [CrossRef]
29. Stallings, V.A.; Schall, J.I.; Hediger, M.L.; Zemel, B.S.; Tuluc, F.; Dougherty, K.A.; Samuel, J.L.; Rutstein, R.M. High-dose vitamin D3 supplementation in children and young adults with HIV: A randomized, placebo-controlled trial. *Pediatr. Infect. Dis. J.* **2015**, *34*, e32–e40. [CrossRef]
30. Moromizato, T.; Litonjua, A.A.; Braun, A.B.; Gibbons, F.K.; Giovannucci, E.; Christopher, K.B. Association of low serum 25-hydroxyvitamin D levels and sepsis in the critically ill. *Crit Care Med.* **2014**, *42*, 97–107. [CrossRef]
31. Lemire, J.M.; Archer, D.C.; Beck, L.; Spiegelberg, H.L. Immunosuppressive actions of 1,25-dihydroxyvitamin D3: Preferential inhibition of Th1 functions. *J. Nutr.* **1995**, *125*, 1704S–1708S.

32. Boonstra, A.; Barrat, F.J.; Crain, C.; Heath, V.L.; Savelkoul, H.F.J.; O'Garra, A. 1α,25-Dihydroxyvitamin D3 Has a Direct Effect on Naive CD4+ T Cells to Enhance the Development of Th2 Cells. *J. Immunol.* 2001, *167*, 4974. [CrossRef]
33. Tang, J.; Zhou, R.; Luger, D.; Zhu, W.; Silver, P.B.; Grajewski, R.S.; Su, S.B.; Chan, C.C.; Adorini, L.; Caspi, R.R. Calcitriol suppresses antiretinal autoimmunity through inhibitory effects on the Th17 effector response. *J. Immunol.* 2009, *182*, 4624–4632. [CrossRef] [PubMed]
34. Rübsamen, D.; Kunze, M.M.; Buderus, V.; Brauß, T.F.; Bajer, M.M.; Brüne, B.; Schmid, T. Inflammatory conditions induce IRES-dependent translation of cyp24a1. *PLoS ONE* 2014, *9*, e85314. [CrossRef]
35. Youssef, D.A.; Miller, C.W.; El-Abbassi, A.M.; Cutchins, D.C.; Cutchins, C.; Grant, W.B.; Peiris, A.N. Antimicrobial implications of vitamin D. *Dermato-endocrinology* 2011, *3*, 220–229. [CrossRef] [PubMed]
36. Khoo, A.L.; Chai, L.Y.; Koenen, H.J.; Kullberg, B.J.; Joosten, I.; van der Ven, A.J.; Netea, M.G. 1,25-dihydroxyvitamin D3 modulates cytokine production induced by Candida albicans: Impact of seasonal variation of immune responses. *J. Infect. Dis.* 2011, *203*, 122–130. [CrossRef] [PubMed]
37. Ginde, A.A.; Mansbach, J.M.; Camargo, C.A., Jr. Association between serum 25-hydroxyvitamin D level and upper respiratory tract infection in the Third National Health and Nutrition Examination Survey. *Arch. Intern. Med.* 2009, *169*, 384–390. [CrossRef]
38. Martineau, A.R.; Jolliffe, D.A.; Hooper, R.L.; Greenberg, L.; Aloia, J.F.; Bergman, P.; Dubnov-Raz, G.; Esposito, S.; Ganmaa, D.; Ginde, A.A.; et al. Vitamin D supplementation to prevent acute respiratory tract infections: Systematic review and meta-analysis of individual participant data. *BMJ* 2017, *356*, i6583. [CrossRef]
39. Amrein, K.; Zajic, P.; Schnedl, C.; Waltensdorfer, A.; Fruhwald, S.; Holl, A.; Purkart, T.; Wünsch, G.; Valentin, T.; Grisold, A.; et al. Vitamin D status and its association with season, hospital and sepsis mortality in critical illness. *Crit. Care* 2014, *18*, R47. [CrossRef]
40. Lucidarme, O.; Messai, E.; Mazzoni, T.; Arcade, M.; du Cheyron, D. Incidence and risk factors of vitamin D deficiency in critically ill patients: Results from a prospective observational study. *Intensive Care Med* 2010, *36*, 1609–1611. [CrossRef]
41. Venkatram, S.; Chilimuri, S.; Adrish, M.; Salako, A.; Patel, M.; Diaz-Fuentes, G. Vitamin D deficiency is associated with mortality in the medical intensive care unit. *Crit. Care* 2011, *15*, R292. [CrossRef] [PubMed]
42. Jeng, L.; Yamshchikov, A.V.; Judd, S.E.; Blumberg, H.M.; Martin, G.S.; Ziegler, T.R.; Tangpricha, V. Alterations in vitamin D status and anti-microbial peptide levels in patients in the intensive care unit with sepsis. *J. Transl. Med.* 2009, *7*, 28. [CrossRef]
43. Hulse, J.D.; Ellis, S.; Henderson, L.M. Carnitine biosynthesis: β hydroxylation of trimethyllysine by an α-keto glutarate dependent mitochondrial dioxygenase. *J. Biol. Chem.* 1978, *253*, 1654–1659. [CrossRef]
44. Harrison, F.; May, J. Vitamin C function in the brain: Vital role of the ascorbate transporter (SVCT2). *Free Radic. Biol. Med.* 2009, *46*, 719–730. [CrossRef] [PubMed]
45. Mandl, J.; Szarka, A.; Banhegyi, G. Vitamin C: Update on physiology and pharmacology. *Br. J. Pharmacol.* 2009, *157*, 1097–1110. [CrossRef] [PubMed]
46. Carr, A.; Maggini, S. Vitamin C and immune function. *Nutrients* 2017, *9*, 1211. [CrossRef] [PubMed]
47. European Food Safety Authority Panel on Dietetic Products, Nutrition and Allergies. Scientific opinion on dietary reference values for vitamin C. *EFSA J.* 2013, *11*, 3418.
48. Fisher, B.J.; Seropian, I.M.; Kraskauskas, D.; Thakkar, J.N.; Voelkel, N.F.; Fowler, A.A.; Natarajan, R. Ascorbic acid attenuates lipopolysaccharide-induced acute lung injury. *Crit Care Med* 2011, *39*, 1454–1460. [CrossRef] [PubMed]
49. Secor, D.; Swarbreck, S.; Ellis, C.G.; Sharpe, M.D.; Tyml, K. Ascorbate reduces mouse platelet aggregation and surface P-selectin expression in an ex vivo model of sepsis. *Microcirculation* 2013, *20*, 502–510. [CrossRef]
50. Carr, A.C.; Shaw, G.M.; Natarajan, R. Ascorbate-dependent vasopressor synthesis: A rationale for vitamin C administration in severe sepsis and septic shock? *Crit. Care* 2015, *19*, 1–8. [CrossRef]
51. Seno, T.; Inoue, N.; Matsui, K.; Ejiri, J.; Hirata, K.I.; Kawashima, S.; Yokoyama, M. Functional expression of sodium-dependent vitamin C transporter 2 in human endothelial cells. *J. Vasc. Res.* 2004, *41*, 345–351. [CrossRef]
52. Khalili, H.; Zabet, M.H.; Mohammadi, M.; Ramezani, M. Effect of high-dose ascorbic acid on vasopressor requirement in septic shock. *J. Res. Pharm. Pract.* 2016, *5*, 94–100. [CrossRef]
53. Fowler, A.A.; Nursing, M.R.I.C.U.; Syed, A.A.; Knowlson, S.; Sculthorpe, R.; Farthing, D.; Dewilde, C.; A Farthing, C.; Larus, T.L.; Martin, E.; et al. Phase I safety trial of intravenous ascorbic acid in patients with severe sepsis. *J. Transl. Med.* 2014, *12*, 32. [CrossRef] [PubMed]
54. Zhang, M.; Jativa, D.F. Vitamin C supplementation in the critically ill: A systematic review and meta-analysis. *SAGE Open Med.* 2018, *6*, 2050312118807615. [CrossRef] [PubMed]
55. Fowler, A.A., 3rd; Truwit, J.D.; Hite, R.D.; Morris, P.E.; DeWilde, C.; Priday, A.; Fisher, B.; Thacker, L.R., 2nd; Natarajan, R.; Brophy, D.F.; et al. Effect of Vitamin C Infusion on Organ Failure and Biomarkers of Inflammation and Vascular Injury in Patients with Sepsis and Severe Acute Respiratory Failure: The CITRIS-ALI Randomized Clinical Trial. *JAMA* 2019, *322*, 1261–1270. [CrossRef]
56. Manzanares, W.; Hardy, G. Thiamine supplementation in the critically ill. *Curr. Opin. Clin. Nutr. Metab. Care* 2011, *14*, 610–617. [CrossRef] [PubMed]
57. Ariaey-Nejad, M.R.; Balaghi, M.; Baker, E.M.; Sauberlich, H.E. Thiamin metabolism in man. *Am. J. Clin. Nutr.* 1970, *23*, 764–778. [CrossRef]
58. DiNicolantonio, J.J.; Niazi, A.K.; Lavie, C.J.; O'Keefe, J.H.; Ventura, H.O. Thiamine supplementation for the treatment of heart failure: A review of the literature. *Congest Heart Fail* 2013, *19*, 214–222. [CrossRef]

59. Donnino, M.W.; Carney, E.; Cocchi, M.N.; Barbash, I.; Chase, M.; Joyce, N.; Chou, P.P.; Ngo, L. Thiamine deficiency in critically ill patients with sepsis. *J. Crit. Care* **2010**, *25*, 576–581. [CrossRef]
60. Costa, N.A.; Gut, A.L.; de Souza Dorna, M.; Pimentel, J.A.C.; Cozzolino, S.M.F.; Azevedo, P.S.; Henrique Fernandes, A.A.; Mamede Zornoff, L.A.; Ruppde Paiva, S.A.; Minicucci, M.F.; et al. Serum thiamine concentration and oxidative stress as predictors of mortality in patients with septic shock. *J. Crit. Care* **2014**, *29*, 249–252. [CrossRef]
61. Goode, H.F.; Cowley, H.C.; Walker, B.E.; Howdle, P.D.; Webster, N.R. Decreased antioxidant status and increased lipid peroxidation in patients with septic shock and secondary organ dysfunction. *Crit. Care Med.* **1995**, *23*, 646–651. [CrossRef]
62. De Andrade, J.A.A.; Gayer, C.R.M.; Nogueira, N.P.D.A.; Paes, M.C.; Bastos, V.L.F.C.; Neto, J.D.C.B.; Alves, S.C.; Coelho, R.M.; Da Cunha, M.G.A.T.; Gomes, R.N.; et al. The effect of thiamine deficiency on inflammation, oxidative stress and cellular migration in an experimental model of sepsis. *J. Inflamm.* **2014**, *11*, 11. [CrossRef]
63. Donnino, M.W.; Andersen, L.W.; Chase, M.; Berg, K.M.; Tidswell, M.; Giberson, T.; Wolfe, R.; Moskowitz, A.; Smithline, H.; Ngo, L.; et al. Randomized, double-blind, placebo-controlled trial of thiamine as a metabolic resuscitator in septic shock: A pilot study. *Crit. Care Med.* **2016**, *44*, 360–367. [CrossRef] [PubMed]
64. Moskowitz, A.; Andersen, L.W.; Cocchi, M.N.; Karlsson, M.; Patel, P.V.; Donnino, M.W. Thiamine as a renal protective agent in septic shock: A secondary analysis of a randomized, double-blind, placebo-controlled trial. *Ann. Am. Thorac. Soc.* **2017**, *14*, 737–741. [CrossRef] [PubMed]
65. Marik, P.E.; Khangoora, V.; Rivera, R.; Hooper, M.H.; Catravas, J. Hydrocortisone, vitamin C and thiamine for the treatment of severe sepsis and septic shock: A retrospective before-after study. *Chest* **2016**, *151*, 1229–1238. [CrossRef] [PubMed]
66. King, L.E.; Frentzel, J.W.; Mann, J.J.; Fraker, P.J. Chronic zinc deficiency in mice disrupted T cell lymphopoiesis and erythropoiesis while B cell lymphopoiesis and myelopoiesis were maintained. *J. Am. Coll. Nutr.* **2005**, *24*, 494–502. [CrossRef] [PubMed]
67. Incefy, G.S.; Mertelsmann, R.; Yata, K.; Dardenne, M.; Bach, J.F.; Good, R.A. Induction of differentiation in human marrow T cell precursors by the synthetic serum thymic factor, FTS. *Clin. Exp. Immunol.* **1980**, *40*, 396–406.
68. Prasad, A.S. Effects of zinc deficiency on Th1 and Th2 cytokine shifts. *J. Infect. Dis.* **2000**, *182*, S62–S68. [CrossRef] [PubMed]
69. Haase, H.; Ober-Blöbaum, J.L.; Engelhardt, G.; Hebel, S.; Heit, A.; Heine, H.; Rink, L. Zinc signals are essential for lipopolysaccharide-induced signal transduction in monocytes. *J. Immunol.* **2008**, *181*, 6491–6502. [CrossRef]
70. Kitamura, H.; Morikawa, H.; Kamon, H.; Iguchi, M.; Hojyo, S.; Fukada, T.; Yamashita, S.; Kaisho, T.; Akira, S.; Murakami, M.; et al. Toll-like receptor–mediated regulation of zinc homeostasis influences dendritic cell function. *Nat. Immunol.* **2006**, *7*, 971. [CrossRef]
71. Kaltenberg, J.; Plum, L.M.; Ober-Blöbaum, J.L.; Hönscheid, A.; Rink, L.; Haase, H. Zinc signals promote IL-2-dependent proliferation of T cells. *Eur. J. Immunol.* **2010**, *40*, 1496–1503. [CrossRef]
72. Gaetke, L.M.; McClain, C.J.; Talwalkar, R.T.; Shedlofsky, S.I. Effects of endotoxin on zinc metabolism in human volunteers. *Am. J. Physiol. Endocrinol. Metab.* **1997**, *272*, E952–E956. [CrossRef]
73. Besecker, B.Y.; Exline, M.C.; Hollyfield, J.; Phillips, G.; DiSilvestro, R.A.; Wewers, M.D.; Knoell, D.L. A comparison of zinc metabolism, inflammation, and disease severity in critically ill infected and noninfected adults early after intensive care unit admission123. *Am. J. Clin. Nutr.* **2011**, *93*, 1356–1364. [CrossRef] [PubMed]
74. Huber, K.L.; Cousins, R.J. Metallothionein expression in rat bone marrow is dependent on dietary zinc but not dependent on interleukin-1 or interleukin-6. *J. Nutr.* **1993**, *123*, 642–648. [CrossRef] [PubMed]
75. Aydemir, T.B.; Chang, S.M.; Guthrie, G.J.; Maki, A.B.; Ryu, M.S.; Karabiyik, A.; Cousins, R.J. Zinc transporter ZIP14 functions in hepatic zinc, iron and glucose homeostasis during the innate immune response (endotoxemia). *PLoS ONE* **2012**, *7*, e48679.
76. Wessels, I.; Cousins, R.J. Zinc dyshomeostasis during polymicrobial sepsis in mice involves zinc transporter Zip14 and can be overcome by zinc supplementation. *Am. J. Physiol. Gastrointest. Liver Physiol.* **2015**, *309*, G768–G778. [CrossRef] [PubMed]
77. Zhou, Z.; Wang, L.; Song, Z.; Saari, J.T.; McClain, C.J.; Kang, Y.J. Abrogation of nuclear factor-κB activation is involved in zinc inhibition of lipopolysaccharide-induced tumor necrosis factor-α production and liver injury. *Am. J. Pathol.* **2004**, *164*, 1547–1556. [CrossRef]
78. Fraker, P.J.; King, L.E. Reprogramming of the immune system during zinc deficiency. *Annu. Rev. Nutr.* **2004**, *24*, 277–298. [CrossRef]
79. Song, Y.; Chung, C.S.; Bruno, R.S.; Traber, M.G.; Brown, K.H.; King, J.C.; Ho, E. Dietary zinc restriction and repletion affects DNA integrity in healthy men. *Am. J. Clin. Nutr.* **2009**, *90*, 321–328. [CrossRef]
80. Cander, B.; Dundar, Z.D.; Gul, M.; Girisgin, S. Prognostic value of serum zinc levels in critically ill patients. *J. Crit. Care* **2011**, *26*, 42–46. [CrossRef]
81. Hoeger, J.; Simon, T.-P.; Beeker, T.; Marx, G.; Haase, H.; Schuerholz, T. Persistent low serum zinc is associated with recurrent sepsis in critically ill patients—A pilot study. *PLoS ONE* **2017**, *12*, e0176069. [CrossRef]
82. Foote, J.W.; Delves, H.T. Albumin bound and alpha 2-macroglobulin bound zinc concentrations in the sera of healthy adults. *J. Clin. Pathol.* **1984**, *37*, 1050–1054. [CrossRef]
83. Castell, J.V.; Gómez-Lechón, M.J.; David, M.; Andus, T.; Geiger, T.; Trullenque, R.; Fabra, R.; Heinrich, P.C. Interleukin-6 is the major regulator of acute phase protein synthesis in adult human hepatocytes. *FEBS Lett.* **1989**, *242*, 237–239. [CrossRef]
84. Wiersinga, W.J.; Rhodes, A.; Cheng, A.C.; Peacock, S.J.; Prescott, H.C. Pathophysiology, Transmission, Diagnosis, and Treatment of Coronavirus Disease 2019 (COVID-19): A Review. *JAMA* **2020**, *324*, 782–793. [CrossRef]

85. Xu, Z.; Shi, L.; Wang, Y.; Zhang, J.; Huang, L.; Zhang, C.; Liu, S.; Zhao, P.; Liu, H.; Zhu, L.; et al. Pathologicalfindings of COVID-19 associated with acute respiratory distress syndrome. *Lancet Respir. Med.* **2020**, *8*, 420–422. [CrossRef]
86. Docherty, A.B.; Harrison, E.M.; Green, C.A.; Hardwick, H.E.; Pius, R.; Norman, L.; Holden, K.A.; Read, J.M.; Donderlinger, F.; Carson, G.; et al. ISARIC4C investigators. Features of 20 133 UK patients in hospital with COVID-19 using the ISARIC WHO Clinical Characterisation Protocol: Prospective observational cohortstudy. *BMJ* **2020**, *369*, m1985. [CrossRef] [PubMed]
87. Matthay, M.A.; Zemans, R.L. The acute respiratory distress syndrome: Pathogenesis and treatment. *Annu. Rev. Pathol.* **2011**, *6*, 147–163. [CrossRef] [PubMed]
88. Cui, C.; Xu, P.; Li, G.; Qiao, Y.; Han, W.; Geng, C.; Liao, D.; Yang, M.; Chen, D.; Jiang, P. Vitamin Dreceptor activation regulates microglia polarization and oxidative stress in spontaneously hypertensive rats and angiotensin II-exposed microglial cells: Role of renin-angiotensin system. *Redox Biol.* **2019**, *26*, 101295. [CrossRef] [PubMed]
89. Murai, I.H.; Fernandes, A.L.; Sales, L.P.; Pinto, A.J.; Goessler, K.F.; Duran, C.S.C.; Silva, C.B.R.; Franco, A.S.; Macedo, M.B.; Dalmolin, H.H.H.; et al. Effect of a single dose of vitamin D on hospital length of stay in patients with moderate to severe COVID-19. *JAMA* 2021, Online ahead of print. [CrossRef]
90. Rubin, R. Sorting out whether vitamin D deficiency raises COVID-19 risk. *JAMA* **2021**, *325*, 329–330. [CrossRef] [PubMed]
91. Amrein, K.; Parekh, D.; Westphal, S.; Preiser, J.-C.; Berghold, A.; Riedl, R.; Eller, P.; Schellongowski, P.; Thickett, D.; Meybohm, P. Effect of high-dose vitamin D3 on 28-day mortality in adult critically ill patients with severe vitamin D deficiency: A study protocol of a multicentre, placebo-controlled double-blind phase III RCT (the VITDALIZE study). *BMJ Open* **2019**, *9*, e031083. [CrossRef]
92. Furuya, A.; Uozaki, M.; Yamasaki, H.; Arakawa, T.; Arita, M.; Koyama, A. Antiviral effects of ascorbic and dehydroascorbic acids in vitro. *Int J Mol Med.* **1998**, *22*, 541–545.
93. Chen, J.; Chang, C.; Feng, P.; Chu, C.; So, E.; Hu, M. Plasma vitamin C is lower in postherpetic neuralgia patients and administration of vitamin C reduces spontaneous pain but not brush-evoked pain. *Clin. J. Pain* **2009**, *25*, 562–569. [CrossRef] [PubMed]
94. Hemilä, H.; Chalker, E. Vitamin C for preventing and treating the common cold. *Cochrane Database Syst. Rev.* **2013**. [CrossRef] [PubMed]
95. Cathcart, R. Vitamin C in the treatment of acquired immune deficiency syndrome (AIDS). *Med. Hypotheses* **1984**, *14*, 423–433. [CrossRef]
96. Kim, H.; Jang, M.; Kim, Y.; Choi, J.; Jeon, J.; Kim, J.; Hwang, Y.; Kang, J.S.; Lee, W.J. Red ginseng and vitamin C increase immune cell activity and decrease lung inflammation induced by influenza A virus/H1N1 infection. *J. Pharm. Pharmacol.* **2016**, *68*, 406–420. [CrossRef]
97. Colunga Biancatelli, R.; Berrill, M.; Catravas, J.; Marik, P. Quercetin and vitamin C: An experimental, synergistic therapy for the prevention and treatment of SARS-CoV-2 related disease (COVID-19). *Front. Immunol.* **2020**. [CrossRef] [PubMed]
98. Pons, S.; Fodil, S.; Azoulay, E.; Zafrani, L. The vascular endothe- lium: The cornerstone of organ dysfunction in severe SARS-CoV-2 infection. *Crit. Care* **2020**. [CrossRef]
99. Zhang, J.; Rao, X.; Li, Y.; Zhu, Y.; Liu, F.; Guo, G.; Luo, G.; Meng, Z.; De Backer, D.; Xiang, H.; et al. Pilot trial of high-dose vitamin C in critically ill COVID-19 patients. *Ann. Intensive Care* **2021**, *11*, 5. [CrossRef]
100. Bilezikian, J.P.; Bikle, D.; Hewison, M.; Lazaretti-Castro, M.; Formenti, A.M.; Gupta, A.; Madhavan, M.V.; Nair, N.; Babalyan, V.; Hutchings, N.; et al. Mechanisms in endocrinology: Vitamin D and COVID-19. *Eur. J. Endocrinol.* **2020**, *183*, R133–R147. [CrossRef]

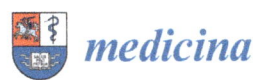

Article

Usefulness of Antioxidants as Adjuvant Therapy for Septic Shock: A Randomized Clinical Trial

Alfredo Aisa-Alvarez [1,†], María Elena Soto [1,2,†], Verónica Guarner-Lans [3], Gilberto Camarena-Alejo [1], Juvenal Franco-Granillo [1], Enrique A. Martínez-Rodríguez [1], Ricardo Gamboa Ávila [3], Linaloe Manzano Pech [4] and Israel Pérez-Torres [4,*]

1. Critical Care Department, American British Cowdray (ABC) Medical Center, I.A.P. ABC Sur 136 No. 116 Col. las Américas, Mexico City 01120, Mexico; alfredoaisaa@gmail.com (A.A.-A.); mesoto50@hotmail.com (M.E.S.); drcamarena@gmail.com (G.C.-A.); jfranco@abchospital.com (J.F.-G.); enrique_timc@hotmail.com (E.A.M.-R.)
2. Immunology Department Instituto Nacional de Cardiología Ignacio Chávez. Juan Badiano 1, Sección XVI, Tlalpan, Mexico City 14080, Mexico
3. Physiology Department Instituto Nacional de Cardiología Ignacio Chávez. Juan Badiano 1, Sección XVI, Tlalpan, Mexico City 14080, Mexico; gualanv@yahoo.com (V.G.-L.); rgamboaa_2000@yahoo.com (R.G.Á.)
4. Cardiovascular Biomedicine Department Instituto Nacional de Cardiología Ignacio Chávez. Juan Badiano 1, Sección XVI, Tlalpan, Mexico City 14080, Mexico; loe_mana@hotmail.com
* Correspondence: pertorisr@yahoo.com.mx; Tel.: +52-5573-2911 (ext. 25203); Fax: +52-5573-0926
† The authors Alfredo Aisa-Álvarez and María E Soto share the first authorship.

Received: 15 October 2020; Accepted: 13 November 2020; Published: 17 November 2020

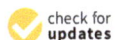

Abstract: *Background and objectives:* Oxidative stress (OS) participates in the pathophysiology of septic shock, which leads to multiple organ failure (MOF), ischemia-reperfusion injury, and acute respiratory distress syndrome. Therefore, antioxidants have been proposed as therapy. Here, we evaluated the effect of antioxidant treatments in patients with septic shock with MOF and determined levels OS before and after treatment. This study was a randomized, controlled, triple-masked, and with parallel assignment clinical trial with a control group without treatment. *Materials and Methods:* It included 97 patients of either sex with septic shock. 5 treatments were used each in an independent group of 18 patients. Group 1 received vitamin C (Vit C), group 2 vitamin E (Vit E), group 3 n-acetylcysteine (NAC), group 4 melatonin (MT), and group 5 served as control. All antioxidants were administered orally or through a nasogastric tube for five days as an adjuvant to the standard therapy. *Results:* The results showed that all patients presented MOF due to sepsis upon admission and that the treatment decreased it ($p = 0.007$). The antioxidant treatment with NAC increased the total antioxidant capacity ($p < 0.05$). The patients that received Vit C had decreased levels of the nitrate and nitrite ratio ($p < 0.01$) and C-reactive protein levels ($p = 0.04$). Procalcitonin levels were reduced by Vit E ($p = 0.04$), NAC ($p = 0.001$), and MT ($p = 0.04$). Lipid-peroxidation was reduced in patients that received MT ($p = 0.04$). *Conclusions:* In conclusion, antioxidant therapy associated with standard therapy reduces MOF, OS, and inflammation in patients with septic shock.

Keywords: shock septic; antioxidant therapy; oxidative stress; multiple organ failure

1. Introduction

Damage caused by oxidative stress (OS) participates in the pathophysiology of serious diseases including multiple organ failure (MOF) due to sepsis. Sepsis is caused by bacteria, fungi, and viruses, or by a combination of them [1]. Sepsis and septic shock are the largest cause of mortality worldwide in intensive care units (ICU) [2] and MOF constitutes a high cost to health systems [3].

Studies in animal models and in patients with septic shock have shown an imbalance between the production of reactive oxygen (ROS) and nitrogen (RNS) species and antioxidant defenses [4]. ROS are generated by phagocytic cells, by the increased activity of enzymes such as NAD(P)H oxidase, xanthine oxidase and inducible nitric oxide (iNOS) and by increased inflammatory mediators through the activation of nuclear factor κB (NFκB) [5]. Mitochondrial damage caused by OS is a component of the pathophysiology of MOF secondary to sepsis [6].

Antioxidants such as N-acetylcysteine (NAC), melatonin (MT), vitamins (A, C and E), enzyme cofactors (selenium and zinc), and endogenous compounds (ubiquinone, α lipoic acid, bilirubin, albumin, ferritin, and quercetin) may inhibit ROS and RNS, counteracting their effects [7]. NAC has anti-inflammatory and antioxidant properties [8]. Its antioxidant capacity is due to the replenishment of glutathione (GSH) deposits and to the sequestration of ROS [9]. NAC improves hemodynamic variables, cardiac indexes, oxygenation and compliance of lung statics [10], hepatosplenic flow, and liver function in septic shock. Thus, NAC could decrease MOF [11] and reduce the levels of IL-8, soluble α receptor tumor necrosis factor p55 [12], IL-6, and ICAM-1 [13]. It reduces mechanical ventilation length, number of days in the ICU, and mortality [14].

Vitamin C (Vit C) can reduce the production of nitric oxide by the iNOS pathway and it may decrease vasoconstriction and loss of vascular permeability [15]. Decreased Vit C levels are related to the severity of MOF and mortality [16]. In some clinical studies, therapy with Vit C decreased sequential organ failure assessment (SOFA) scores, procalcitonin (PCT), C-reactive protein (CRP), and thrombomodulin, leading to a lower mortality rate [17]. Several studies have shown that vitamin E (Vit E) is an important lipophilic antioxidant in cell membranes, protecting them from lipid peroxidation (LPO) [18]. It has also been reported that the administration of Vit E in combination with simvastatin inactivates NAD(P)H oxidase, a source of ROS, in patients with sepsis that have decreased levels of Vit E and O_2^- overproduction [19].

Melatonin (MT) lowers OS both in plasma and intracellular membranes due to its hydrophilic and lipophilic properties. MT possesses ROS sequestration properties, thus protecting cell membrane lipids, cytosol proteins, and nuclear and mitochondrial DNA [20].

There is a marked increase in ROS and a decrease in endogenous antioxidant defenses in critically ill patients with sepsis [21]. However, the usefulness of different antioxidants has not yet been evaluated through clinical randomized trials. Thus, the aim of this study was to evaluate the antioxidant effect of Vit C, Vit E, NAC, and MT in patients with septic shock determining the SOFA score and measuring antioxidant markers in plasma.

2. Material and Methods

2.1. Study Population

This was a controlled, randomized, and triple masked clinical trial that included 97 patients of either sex with septic shock. It was run in 2 ICUs in Mexico City. Patients were admitted to the ICU with a primary diagnosis of septic shock. Diagnostic criteria for septic shock were based on the Sepsis-3 consensus [22], and patients had to fulfill the criteria within a maximum of 24 h prior to enrollment. Data were collected upon admission to the ICU. In addition, other patients met selection criteria during their stay in intensive care, and they were then randomized. Patients had to have an acute increase of at least 2 points in the SOFA score [23], lactate level greater than 2 mmol/L, and they had to be dependent on a vasopressor for at least 2 h before the time of enrollment. Exclusion occurred when patients were younger than 18 years, when they were not able to grant an informed consent or refused to be included, if they were pregnant or breastfeeding or if they were under chronic use (last 6th months) or recent use of steroids, statins or antioxidants. Patients were also excluded if there was any contraindication for the use of Vit C, Vit E, NAC, or MT.

Ethical approval was obtained from the local ethics committee 24 the April of the 2018 (INcar PT-18-076; ABC-18-19). A written informed consent for enrollment or consent to continue and use patient data was obtained from each patient or their legal surrogate. The protocol was registered (TRIAL REGISTRATION: ClinicalTrials.gov Identifier: NCT 03557229).

2.2. Randomization, Masking, and Drug Administration

A total of five treatments were used each in an independent group of 18 patients. Group 1 received Vit C, group 2 Vit E, group 3 NAC, group 4 MT and group 5 control (this group did not receive any type of antioxidant therapy).The control group did not receive treatment since the treating physician did not agree for the patient to receive any antioxidant. However, the patients agreed that samples could be processed. All antioxidants were administered orally or through a nasogastric tube during 5 days in addition to the standard therapy. The random allocation sequence for the administration of the antioxidants was generated at the coordinating center, using a computer-generated random program (Figure 1). Blinding was maintained by the investigational pharmacy at each institution. Researchers were also blinded from the onset of the study until the analysis of the outcomes.

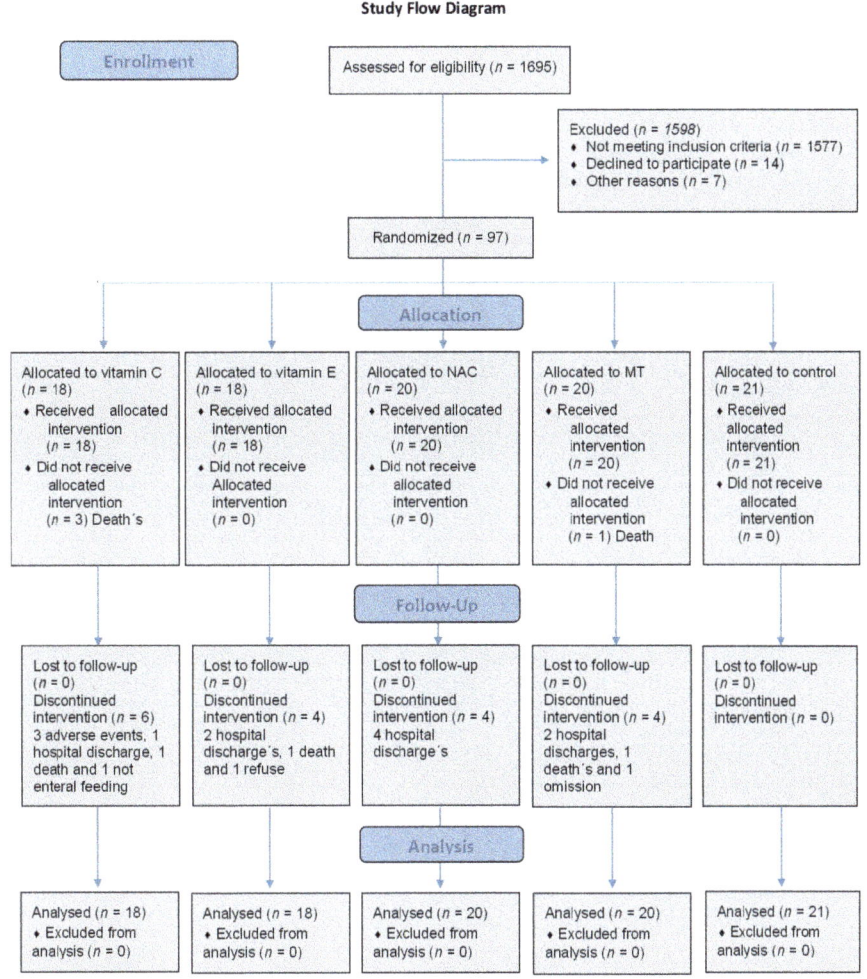

Figure 1. Flow diagram of the study. Abbreviations: Vit C = vitamin C, Vit E = vitamin E, NAC = n-acetylcysteine, MT = melatonin.

All antioxidants were orally administered or applied through a nasogastric tube for 5 days. Tablets of 600 mg every 12 h of NAC were used. Further, 50 mg of MT in capsules of 5 mg were given to patients once a day, and 1 mg Vit C tablets were administered every 6 h. Vit E capsules of 400 UI were given every 8 h. The doses of antioxidants were chosen according to what has been reported in the literature [24–27]. All data entry was monitored at the coordinating center, with site visits for source data verification. Also, patients were equally distributed, and all patients were analyzed. For patients receiving Vit C ($n = 18$), there were 3 deaths. For patients receiving Vit E ($n = 18$) there were 3 deaths. For patients receiving NAC ($n = 20$), there were 2 deaths, and for those receiving MT ($n = 20$), there were 4 deaths. Finally, in the control group ($n = 21$), there were 5 deaths.

2.3. Standard Therapy at the ICU

Patients were treated according to the recommendation of the International Guidelines for Management of Sepsis and Septic Shock. For the evaluation of the outcome, the SOFA scores for 5 days were the primary result. Additionally, 14 pre-specified laboratory results were determined, including plasma OS markers such as nitrate/nitrite (NO_3^-/NO_2^-) ratio, LPO, glutathione (GSH) levels, total antioxidant capacity (TAC), carbonylation and Vit C levels at 48 h. Other secondary outcomes were measured on day 28 including mortality due to any cause, ventilator-free days, ICU-free days, and hospital-free days. Ventilator-free days were defined as the number of days a patient was extubated from mechanical ventilation, after ICU admission. When reintubation was required the days without intubation were subtracted from the total days. If the patient died in the hospital, a value of zero was assigned to post-extubation. ICU-free days began the moment the patient was transferred out of the ICU to day 28. Hospital- and ICU-free days were calculated similarly.

2.4. Study Measurements and Procedures

To evaluate the organ dysfunction, the SOFA score (neurologic, respiratory, hemodynamic, hepatic, and hematologic) was calculated on admission and during the days of treatment. The CRP and the PCT determinations were performed on admission, before the beginning of the antioxidant therapy, and during the next 7 days.

2.5. Sampling for the Determination of Oxidative Stress and Antioxidant State

The measurement of OS markers was done before the beginning of the antioxidant therapy and 48 h after its initiation.

2.6. Sample Obtainment and Storage

Blood samples were obtained from each patient that entered the draw, before initiation of the treatment and 48 h after its administration. The blood samples were centrifuged for 20 min at $936\times g$ and 4 °C. The plasma of the samples was placed in 3 or 4 aliquots and stored at −30 °C.

2.7. Oxidative Stress Markers in Plasma

2.7.1. NO_3^-/NO_2^- Ratio

The NO_3^- was reduced to NO_2^- by the nitrate reductase enzyme reaction. 100 µL of plasma previously deproteinization with 0.5 N, NaOH and 10%, $ZnSO_4$ were mixed and the supernatant was incubated for 30 min at 37 °C in presence of nitrate reductase (5 units). At the end of the incubation period, 200 µL of sulfanilamide 1% and 200 µL of N-naphthyl-ethyldiamine 0.1% were added and the total volume was adjusted to 1 mL. The absorbance was measured at 540 nm [28].

2.7.2. LPO Levels

Briefly, 50 µL CH3-OH with 4% butylated hydroxytoluene plus phosphate buffer pH 7.4 was added to 100 µL of plasma. It was incubated and centrifuged at 4000 rpm in room temperature for 2 min. Then, the n-butanol phase was extracted, and absorbance was measured at 532 nm [28].

2.7.3. GSH Concentration

Briefly, 800 µL of phosphate buffer 50 mM, pH 7.3, plus 100 µL of Ellman reactive (5,5' dithiobis 2-nitrobenzoic) 1M were added to 100 µL of plasma prior to deproteinization with 20% trichloroacetic acid (v/v). It was incubated at room temperature and absorbance was read at 412 nm [28].

2.7.4. Evaluation of TAC

Briefly, 100 µL of plasma were suspended in 1.5 mL of a reaction mixture prepared as follows: 300 mM acetate buffer pH 3.6, 20 mM hexahydrate of ferric chloride, and 10 mM of 2,4,6-Tris-2-pyridil-s-triazine dissolved in 40 mM HCl. These reactive were added in a relation of 10:1:1 v/v, respectively. After mixing, samples were incubated at 37 °C for 15 min in the dark. The absorbance was measured at 593 nm [28].

2.7.5. Carbonylation Protein Concentration

Briefly, 100 µL of plasma were added to 500 µL of HCl 2.5 N in parallel with another sample with 500 µL of 2, 4-dinitrophenylhydrazine (DNPH) and incubated. At the end of the incubation period, they were centrifuged at 15,000× g for 5 min. The supernatant was discarded. Two washings were performed. The mixture was incubated again at 37 °C for 30 min. Absorbance was read in a spectrophotometer at 370 nm, using bi-distilled water as blank and a molar absorption coefficient of 22,000 M^{-1} cm^{-1} [28].

2.7.6. Vitamin C Levels

Briefly, 100 µL of 20% trichloroacetic acid were added to 100 µL of plasma and centrifuged at 5000 rpm for 5 min. Then, 200 µL of Folin-Ciocalteu reagent 0.20 mM was added to the supernatant. The mixture was incubated for 10 min. The absorbance was measured at 760 nm [28].

2.8. Statistical Analysis

Based on a SD of 2.9 of the SOFA score, the study was estimated to require 55 patients (11 per group) to have 84% power (2-sided with an $\alpha = 0.05$) and 160 (32 per group) for 100% power. In accordance with these calculations, our study enrolled 97 patients to allow for a 10% of dropouts, providing a statistical power of 99%, with an $\alpha = 0.05$. Testing was 2-sided. Effects are reported with a point estimate and 95% CIs in addition to p values.

Group comparisons were made using χ^2 tests for equal proportions, t tests for normally distributed data, Kruskal–Wallis and Wilcoxon rank sum tests otherwise, with results presented as frequencies with percentages, means with SDs, and medians with minimum and maximum, respectively.

The primary end point of the SOFA score and the secondary end points CRP and PCT were analyzed with a mixed linear model and fit to repeated-measures analysis of variance. The model included 1 between-participant factor (group (Vit C, Vit E, NAC, MT, no treatment [control])), 1 within-participant factor (time (0, 1, 2, 3, 4, and 5 days)), and the interaction between group and time, testing the hypothesis that differences between treatment groups are the same over time. Because of a potential for type I error caused by multiple comparisons, findings for analyses of secondary end points should be interpreted as exploratory. Statistical analysis was performed with Stata version 15.1.

3. Results

3.1. Characteristics of the Patients

From July 2018 to November 2019 a total of 1695 eligible patients were identified, of whom 1598 were excluded (reasons listed in Figure 1). Ninety-seven patients were randomized, with 18 assigned to each antioxidant and 21 to the control group. Of all patients included, none was lost in the follow up. Baseline demographic data (age, gender, etc.) were similar between the groups (Table 1).

Table 1. General characteristics of the patients during hospital stay.

Characteristics	Vit C (n = 18)	Vit E (n = 18)	NAC (n = 20)	MT (n = 20)	C (n = 21)
Age (median, min–max)	62 (22–95)	65.5 (22–91)	67.5 (18–95)	62.5 (46–95)	76 (51–89)
Weight kg (median, min–max)	71 (33–112)	71.5 (40–120)	69.5 (39–95)	67 (50–106)	68 (50–105)
BM weight/height^2 (median, min–max)	25.4 (14.7–40.4)	25 (15.1–41.4)	22.45 (16.5–0.3)	25.35 (17.3–52)	25.4 (19.6–58)
Gender (%)					
Men	6 (6.19)	12 (12.37)	11 (11.34)	10 (10.31)	10 (10.31)
Women	12 (12.37)	6 (6.19)	9 (9.28)	10 (10.31)	11 (11.34)
Chronic health condition (%)					
Diabetes Mellitus	4 (4.12)	4 (4.12)	3 (3.09)	5 (5.15)	6 (6.19)
Hypertension	6 (6.19)	8 (8.25)	9 (9.28)	7 (7.22)	11 (11.34)
Cancer	5 (5.15)	9 (9.28)	7 (7.22)	7 (7.22)	11 (11.34)
Chronic renal failure	1 (1.03)	2 (2.03)	4 (4.12)	3 (3.09)	2 (2.06)
Admission source (%)					
Emergency department	9 (9.28)	12 (13.37)	10 (10.31)	14 (14.43)	9 (9.28)
Operating room	4 (4.12)	2 (2.06)	3 (3.09)	2 (2.06)	4 (4.12)
Inpatient ward transfer	3 (3.09)	4 (4.12)	7 (7.22)	4 (4.12)	7 (7.22)
Other	2 (2.06)	0	0	0	1 (1.03)
Primary site of infection (%)					
Pulmonary	7 (7.37)	9 (9.97)	9 (9.97)	8 (8.42)	6 (6.32)
Gastrointestinal	7 (7.37)	3 (3.16)	4 (4.21)	3 (3.16)	9 (9.97)
Urinary	2 (2.11)	2 (2.11)	5 (5.26)	5 (5.26)	3 (3.16)
CNS	0	2 (2.11)	0	0	1 (1.05)
Blood	0	1 (1.05)	0	2 (2.11)	0
Physiological variables 24 h before randomization (median, min–max)					
White blood cell count × 10^3/μL	11 (5.1–39.9)	10.8 (0.4–25.4)	8.6 (0–32.5)	11.7 (5.2–29.6)	12 (0.9–49.8)
Platelet count × 10^3/μL	256 (7–409)	158 (10–363)	155 (22–470)	187.5 (29–543)	225 (24–436)
Lactate (mmol/L)	1.65 (0–4.8)	2.1 (0.82–10.5)	1.74 (0.99–7.8)	2.27 (1–17)	2.52 (1.1–12.4)
Serum creatinine (mg/dL)	0.9 (0.5–5.5)	1.35 (0.5–3.8)	0.92 (0.5–6.6)	1.27 (0.57–6.6)	1.2 (0.5–5.2)
Bilirubin (mg/dL)	0.75 (0.23–3.5)	1.05 (0.35–4.4)	0.80 (0.2–4)	1.03 (0.17–3.7)	1.15 (0.2–13.6)
PaO$_2$/FiO$_2$ (mmHg)	168.5 (61–408)	215 (39–271)	146 (71–367)	197 (57–261)	197 (131–560)
C reactive protein (mg/dL)	18.33 (1.9–1.4)	20.12 (0.5–47)	13.34 (0.02–6.7)	21.75 (1.35–6.7)	20.25 (1.36–5.3)
Procalcitonin (ng/dL)	1.46 (0.16–321)	2.92 (0.08–109)	2.35 (0.06–95.5)	2.32 (0.22–38.7)	8.25 (0.08–100)
Intervention before randomization (%)					
Mechanical ventilation	11 (11.58)	9 (9.47)	14 (14.47)	12 (12.63)	16 (16.84)
Vasopressors	9 (9.38)	7 (7.29)	12 (12.50)	9 (9.38)	11 (11.46)
Norepinephrine	0	1 (1.04)	0	0	0
Vasopressin	8 (8.33)	10 (10.42)	8 (8.33)	11 (11.46)	10 (10.42)
Norepinephrine plus vasopressin					
Inotropes					
Dobutamine	0	0	0	0	1 (1.04)
Levosimendan	0	5 (5.21)	1 (1.04)	3 (3.13)	5 (5.21)
Dopamine	1 (1.04)	0	0	1 (1.04)	0
Renal replacement Therapy	1 (1.04)	2 (2.08)	2 (2.08)	1 (1.04)	3 (3.13)
Corticosteroid use before randomization during the study (%)	6 (6.19)	11 (11.34)	9 (9.28)	8 (8.25)	10 (10.31)
SAPS II (median, min–max)	38 (16–62)	40 (24–73)	38.5 (12–97)	41.5 (13–73)	40 (18–79)
APACHE III (median, min–max)	13.5 (5–47)	19 (11–33)	14.5 (5–46)	17 (6–39)	15 (5–38)
SOFA score (median, min–max)	8.5 (3–16)	8.5 (5–14)	8.5 (1–17)	8 (3–14)	8 (1–16)
Time from ICU admission to randomization hours (median, min–max)	5 (1.5–70)	6 (1–17)	3 (1–140)	9 (3–48)	-

The data presented in this table are on admission to intensive care. Several patients met the inclusion criteria several hours or days after admission to the intensive care unit and all patients used vasopressors since it was an inclusion criterion. Abbreviations: Vit C: vitamin C; Vit E: vitamin E; NAC: n-acetylcysteine; MT: melatonin; (min–mx): minimum–maximum; BMI: body mass index; CNS: central nervous system; SAPS II: Simplified Acute Physiology Score; APACHE, Acute Physiology and Chronic Health Evaluation; SOFA, Sequential Organ Failure Assessment; ICU: intensive care unit.

3.2. Treatments

Treatments were given for a median of five days. The median of adherence in the 4 different groups of treatment was 100%. There was no difference between groups in the time from meeting eligibility criteria to the first dose, the time receiving the treatment, and the adherence.

Primary Outcome

Patients receiving MT and Vit C showed a significant decrease in SOFA score (−1.27 (95% CI −2.21 to −0.34); $p = 0.007$ for MT and −1.94 (95% CI −2.95 to −0.93); $p < 0.001$ for Vit C) (Figure 2).

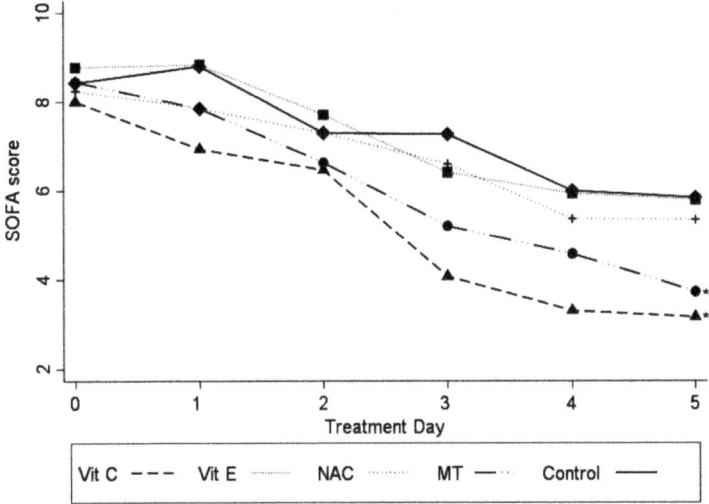

Figure 2. SOFA score variations in patients with the different antioxidant treatments. Abbreviations: SOFA = sequential organ failure assessment, Vit C = vitamin C, Vit E = vitamin E, NAC = n-acetylcysteine, MT = melatonin, Const = constant. Marginal approximation model considering the control group as a base: Vit C −1.94 (−2.95 to −0.94); $p < 0.001$); Vit E −0.14 (−1.10 to 0.81; $p = 0.77$); NAC −0.62 (−1.55 to 0.30; $p = 0.18$); MT −1.27 (−2.21 to −0.34; $p = 0.007$); Const 7.46 (6.78 to 8.13). * $p \leq 0.007$.

The LPO levels were significantly reduced in patients treated with MT ($p = 0.04$) and there was a significant decrease in NO_3^-/NO_2^- levels in patients with lung infection treated with Vit C ($p < 0.01$), Table 2.

Patients receiving Vit C had a significant decrease in CRP levels on the different days of treatment ($p \leq 0.05$), as shown in Figure 3.

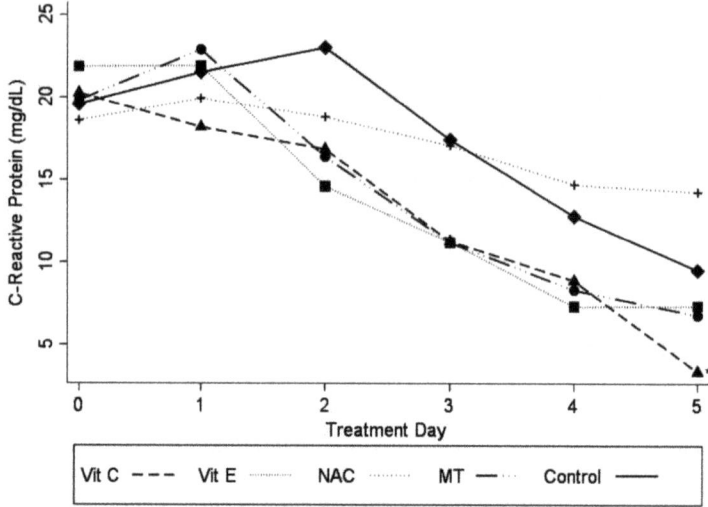

Figure 3. Variations in CRP levels in plasma of patients in receiving the different antioxidant treatments. Abbreviations: CRP = C-reactive protein, Vit C = vitamin C, Vit E = vitamin E, NAC: n-acetylcysteíne, MT = melatonin, Cons = constant. Marginal approximation model considering the control group as a base: Vit C −3.82 (−7.49 to −0.15; $p \leq 0.05$); Vit E −2.97 (−6.54 to 6.01; $p = 0.103$); NAC −2.41 (−3.74 to 3.25; $p = 0.892$); MT −2.30 (−5.88 to 1.27; $p = 0.207$); Cons 17.9 (15.45 to 20.36) * $p \leq 0.05$.

PCT levels were significantly decreased in patients receiving Vit E, NAC, and MT ($p < 0.05$), as shown in Figure 4. Carbonylation levels tended to be reduced before treatment and Vit E tended to decrease its level after treatment ($p = 0.07$) without there being a statistically significant difference.

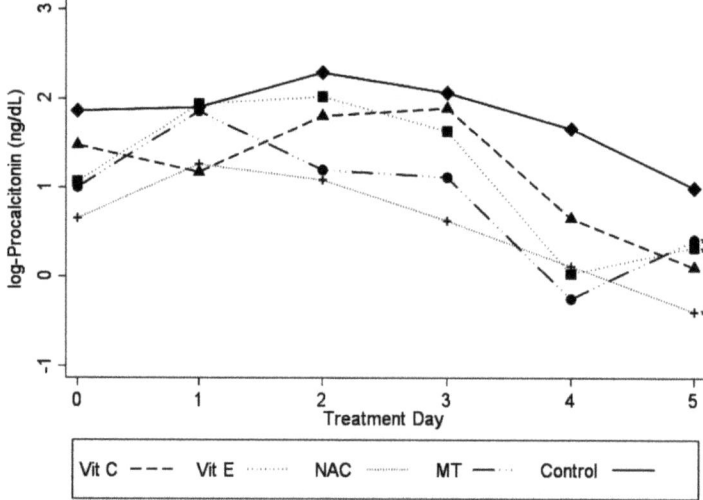

Figure 4. Log PCT concentration in the plasma from patients of the experimental groups with the different antioxidant treatments. Abbreviations: Log PCT = logarithm of procalcitonin, Vit C = vitamin C, Vit E = vitamin E, NAC = n-acetylcysteíne, MT = melatonin. Marginal approximation model considering the control group as a base: Vit C −0.43 (−1.03 to 0.15; $p = 0.149$); Vit E −0.59 (−1.18 to −0.006; $p \leq 0.05$); NAC −0.92 (−1.48 to −0.35; $p = 0.001$); MT −0.57 (−1.15 to 0.006; $p = 0.05$); Cons 1.46 (1.05 to 1.86); * $p \leq 0.05$.

Regarding the secondary outcomes, 13 patients (13.68%) required renal replacement therapy, 63 (65.63%) needed mechanical ventilation and 17 (17.89%) died. There was no statistically significant difference in days free of renal replacement therapy, mechanical ventilation, ICU stay length, or hospitalization at 28 days. There was also no statistically significant difference in intrahospital mortality.

Table 2. Oxidative stress markers before and after 48 h of antioxidant therapy.

Lipid Peroxidation (nM MDA/mL of Plasma)	Pre	Post	p
Vit C (n = 18)	3.44 (0.52–19.62)	2.81 (0.23–8.70)	0.14
Vit E (n = 18)	4.33 (1.25–15.25)	3.24 (0.38–12.07)	0.17
NAC (n = 20)	3.46 (0.23–9.49)	3.46 (0.38–11.01)	0.77
MT (n = 20)	2.13 (0.23–11.68)	2.42 (0.23–7.11)	**0.04**
Control (n = 21)	3.44 (0.52–9.49)	3.90 (0.23–9.10)	0.75
$NO_3 + NO_2$ (μM/mL of plasma)	Pre	Post	p
Vit C (n = 18)	2.10 (0.98–2.73)	1.49 (0.03–2.57)	**<0.01**
Vit E (n = 18)	1.79 (0.53–3.81)	2.00 (0.76–5.65)	0.36
NAC (n = 20)	2.43 (0.80–7.02)	2.15 (0.01–8.16)	0.81
MT (n = 20)	1.72 (0.67–4.77)	1.32 (0.03–7.42)	0.19
Control (n = 21)	2.25 (0.28–2.76)	2.24 (0.01–7.22)	0.97
Total antioxidant capacity (nM/mL of plasma)	Pre	Post	p
Vit C (n = 18)	2226.2 (747.6–3053.4)	2050.9 (966.6–2551.8)	0.11
Vit E (n = 18)	2148.4 (886.3–3287.6)	2223.1 (618.3–3841.9)	0.90
NAC (n = 20)	1453.6 (621.5–2351.4)	1951 (812.6–3528.7)	**0.05**
MT (n = 20)	1999 (561.3–2519.2)	1747.5 (456.5–2745.6)	0.59
Control (n = 21)	2451.6 (1600–3467.1)	2064.7 (312.4–3501)	0.42
Carbonylation (ng/mL of plasma)	Pre	Post	p
Vit C (n = 18)	48.85 (10.90–114.53)	44.76 (12.72–98.17)	0.59
Vit E (n = 18)	52.26 (27.27–137.25)	42.723 (21.36–89.53)	0.07
NAC (n = 20)	40.22 (22.27–89.99)	41.13 (22.72–93.17)	0.47
MT (n = 20)	74.76 (8.63–181.34)	62.721 (29.99–142.25)	0.40
Control (n = 21)	46.359 (9.99–106.80)	44.08 (26.36–111.80)	0.28
GSH concentration (nM/mL of plasma)	Pre	Post	p
Vit C (n = 18)	0.10 (0.01–0.24)	0.08 (0.01–0.20)	0.50
Vit E (n = 18)	0.05 (0.00–0.30)	0.07 (0.00–0.32)	0.38
NAC (n = 20)	0.08 (0.00–0.54)	0.10 (0.009–0.57)	0.14
MT (n = 20)	0.07 (0.00–0.32)	0.07 (0.010–0.51)	0.64
Control (n = 21)	0.06 (0.03–0.20)	0.05 (0.01–0.16)	0.15
Vit C (μM/mL of plasma)	Pre	Post	p
Vit C (n = 18)	0.17 (0.04–0.87)	0.27 (0.06–0.99)	**<0.01**
Vit E (n = 18)	0.27 (0.08–0.99)	0.26 (0.12–0.79)	0.58
NAC (n = 20)	0.21 (0.09–0.61)	0.18 (0.00–0.96)	1.00
MT (n = 20)	0.21 (0.04–0.56)	0.21 (0.04–0.43)	0.83
Control (n = 21)	0.22 (0.08–0.77)	0.19 (0.07–0.64)	**0.02**

Abbreviations: Pre: pre-treatment; Post: post-treatment; Vit C: vitamin C; Vit E: vitamin E; NAC: n-acetylcysteine; MT: melatonin. All values are expressed as median (minimum-maximum). Wilcoxon matched pairs signed rank tests. The bold in the table is to highlight the results with statistical change.

3.3. Undesired Side Effects

A patient receiving Vit C presented abdominal pain and another patient underwent a skin rash. Only one patient who received MT reported drowsiness. No adverse events were reported in patients with NAC or Vit E.

4. Discussion

Treatment with antioxidants as an adjuvant in the standard management of patients with sepsis and/or septic shock has been suggested [29,30]. We studied critically ill patients with septic shock, regardless of the etiology and site of infection. All patients had initial low levels of Vit C. This was related with the severity of organ failure and mortality [17]. The decrease in Vit C levels confirms the reported hypovitaminosis (<0.23 µM ascorbic ac/mL) in septic shock [31]. This condition may be due to augmented metabolic demand since intestinal absorption was not compromised in the patients in our study [32]. Vit C restored the normal values of this vitamin, and organ function was improved. The best result was found in subjects with pneumonia which showed a statistically significant difference. This finding is in agreement with previous results [33,34]. The combined use of Vit C, thiamine, and steroids has recently been suggested. It is still necessary to compare if the use of Vit C alone has worse effects than the combinations [35]. In patients with septic shock, the administration of Vit C and MT improved the organ dysfunction assessed by the SOFA score. This finding could be associated to a decrease in the NO_3^-/NO_2^- ratio and LPO levels.

The Vitamin C infusion for treatment in sepsis induced acute lung injury (CITRIS-ALI) study in patients with acute respiratory distress syndrome, and organ failure showed no improvement with Vit C [36]. The median time before starting treatment with Vit C was of 5 h in this study, and markers such as CRP were significantly decreased, as in another previous study [37]. The possible difference between the findings of this study and our results could be related to the fact that, in the CITRIS-ALI study, they started the therapy with Vit C later than we did.

The VITAMINS trial showed no significant difference in the SOFA score, or in days without ventilation. However, the use of Vit C lowered mortality [38]. In that same study, CRP levels were not decreased, which was probably due to the late administration of Vit C in advanced stages of sepsis before developing acute respiratory distress syndrome (ARDS) [37]. In contrast, we found a decrease in the levels of NO_3^-/NO_2^- which is relevant, since Vit C inhibits the production of superoxide and peroxynitrite, thus preventing abundant NO synthesis, inhibiting mRNA expression and decreasing pathological vasoconstriction [16]. These effects might underlie the clinical benefits of the treatment. A shorter time of use of vasopressors and decreased intrahospital mortality was found in patient receiving Vit C [39].

This is the first study in which the use of MT has been tested in humans with septic shock. Recently MT has been applied in subjects with COVID 19 and it had a high safety profile limiting the disease. Experimental and clinical studies are required to confirm this hypothesis [40]. MT possesses free radical scavenging properties thus protecting cell membrane lipids, cytosol proteins, and nuclear and mitochondrial DNA [29]. In our findings, LPO was significantly decreased in the group of patients who received MT. This result resembled the findings in Galley's study [29]. MT has beneficial effects in experimental cells, plants, and animals. However, its mechanisms of action remain unknown. The effects of MT might be related to its detoxifying ability, thus protecting molecules from the destructive effects of OS in ischemia/reperfusion (stroke, heart attack), ionizing radiation and drug toxicity. In sepsis, the protective effects of MT are associated with the inhibition of the apoptotic processes and the reduction of OS [41].

Production of ROS was increased in an animal model of septic shock [42]. This coincides with a lowering of the TAC and a reduction of the activity of superoxide dismutase and GSH peroxidase [43]. MT reversed morphological damage and increased the activities of antioxidant enzymes [44–46]. Therefore, research through blinded clinical trials and multicenter studies with adequate amounts of MT are needed to determine the potential of MT as an antioxidant treatment [47]. In this clinical trial, we found a reduction of LPO and a potentially benefic effect of MT in organ dysfunction. Its use as an adjuvant in septic shock reduces inflammation and oxidation in animal models with respiratory damage induced by infection. MT has positive physiological actions and could be effective and safe for patients with septic shock of any etiology, including those infected with SARS-CoV-2 [7].

The use of NAC improved the antioxidant capacity and tended to increase GSH, although the difference was not statistically significant. This confirms its antioxidant effect through the replacement of GSH deposits [12]. NAC decreased organ failure, confirming previous findings [14]. Other antioxidants such as polyphenols, β-glucan, and antioxidants targeting mitochondria, selenium salts, and selenium organ compounds are effective for improving OS in sepsis. The study of their pathophysiological implications justifies the combined therapy with antioxidants and standard treatments.

Vit E tended to decrease LPO and carbonylation. This vitamin protects cell membranes from LPO, ending the chain reaction. It is also an O_2^- and OH sequestrant [48].

In summary, antioxidants benefit subjects with septic shock. Septic shock is triggered by bacterial stimuli, fungi, or viruses. In this medical condition, it is necessary to regulate inflammation and other mechanisms that lead to OS [48]. In Figure 5, we show the mechanisms involved in the oxidative stress mismatch, the role they play during the induction of damage, and we describe the role of antioxidant systems and enzyme cofactors in the management of sepsis.

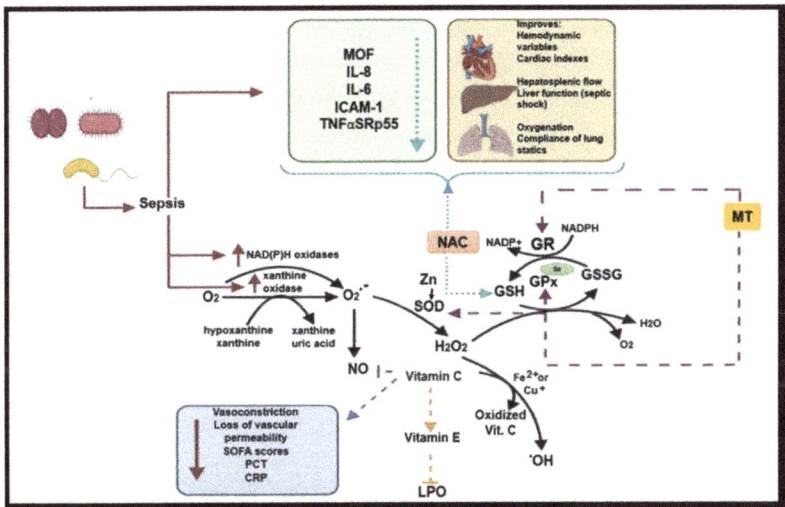

Figure 5. Role of antioxidant systems and enzyme cofactors in the management sepsis and ROS formation. Abbreviations: O_2^- = superoxide anion, NO = nitric oxide, Zn = zinc, SOD = superoxide dismutase, H_2O_2 = hydrogen peroxide, OH = hydroxyl radical, NAC = N-acetylcysteine, MT = melatonin, GSH = glutathione, GSSG = oxidized glutathione, GR = glutathione reductase, GPx = glutathione peroxidase, TNFαSRp55 = soluble α receptor tumor necrosis factor p55, MOF = multiple organ failure, LPO = lipoperoxidation, CRP = C reactive protein, SOFA = sequential organ failure assessment.

5. Conclusions

Adding antioxidants to standard therapy regulates inflammation in patients with septic shock. In pulmonary sepsis, replacement therapy with Vit C increases its serum levels, and decreases the levels of CRP, PCT, and NO_3^-/NO_2^-. MT decreases LPO and the SOFA score. NAC reduces LPO and improves the antioxidant capacity. Vit E tends to decrease LPO. Each antioxidant has beneficial effect. Thus, they might be combined in clinical trials in patients with septic shock.

6. Limitations

The absorption may be altered by the enteral route of administration. However, we found increases of Vit C levels in serum. The present trial is underpowered to detect differences in mortality and in outcomes between groups because the sample size was calculated for differences in OS.

Author Contributions: A.A.-A., I.P.-T., and M.E.S. designed the study and wrote the manuscript. V.G.-L. revised the manuscript; A.A.-A., G.C.-A., J.F.-G., and E.A.M.-R. treated and recruited the patients in the intensive care unit and collected all of the results, including the pretreatment and post treatment dates; I.P.-T., A.A.-A., L.M.P., V.G.-L., and R.G.Á. made the laboratory determination; L.M.P. designed the graphical abstract and A.A.-A. designed the tables and figures; A.A.-A. and M.E.S. performed and planned the statistical analysis. All authors have read and agreed to the published version of the manuscript.

Funding: This research received funding of American British Cowdray (ABC) Medical Center, I.A.P.

Acknowledgments: We thank the Pharmacist Omar Gonzalez Marcos and the nursing staff and the central laboratory and mixing laboratories of the ABC hospital for their unconditional support to this project.

Conflicts of Interest: The authors declare no conflict of interest.

References

1. Timsit, J.F.; Perner, A.; Bakker, J.; Bassetti, M.; Benoit, D.; Cecconi, M.; Curtis, J.R.; Doig, G.S.; Herridge, M.; Jaber, S.; et al. Year in review in intensive care Medicine 2014: III. Severe infections, septic shock, healthcare-associated infections, highly resistant bacteria, invasive fungal infections, severe viral infections, Ebola virus disease and paediatrics. *Intensive. Care Med.* **2015**, *41*, 575–588. [CrossRef] [PubMed]
2. Marshall, J.C.; Vincent, J.L.; Guyatt, G.; Angus, D.C.; Abraham, E.; Bernard, G.; Bombardier, C.; Calandra, T.; Jørgensen, H.S.; Sylvester, R.; et al. Outcome measures for clinical research in sepsis: A report of the 2nd Cambridge Colloquium of the International Sepsis Forum. *Crit. Care Med.* **2005**, *33*, 1708–1716. [CrossRef] [PubMed]
3. Angus, D.C.; Linde-Zwirble, W.T.; Lidicker, J.; Clermont, G.; Carcillo, J.; Pinsky, M.R. Epidemiology of severe sepsis in the United States: Analysis of incidence, outcome, and associated costs of care. *Crit. Care Med.* **2001**, *29*, 1303–1310. [CrossRef]
4. Pisoschi, A.M.; Pop, A. The role of antioxidants in the chemistry of oxidative stress: A review. *Eur. J. Med. Chem.* **2015**, *97*, 55–74. [CrossRef]
5. Galley, H.F. Oxidative stress and mitochondrial dysfunction in sepsis. *Br. J. Anaesth.* **2011**, *107*, 57–64. [CrossRef] [PubMed]
6. Crouser, E.D. Mitochondrial dysfunction in septic shock and multiple organ dysfunction syndrome. *Mitochondrion* **2004**, *4*, 729–741. [CrossRef] [PubMed]
7. Soto, M.E.; Guarner-Lans, V.; Soria-Castro, E.; Manzano-Pech, L.; Pérez-Torres, I. Is Antioxidant Therapy a Useful Complementary Measure for Covid-19 Treatment? An Algorithm for Its Application. *Medicina* **2020**, *56*, 386. [CrossRef] [PubMed]
8. Chertoff, J. N-Acetylcysteine's role in sepsis and potential benefit in patients with microcirculatory derangements. *J. Intensive Care Med.* **2018**, *33*, 87–96. [CrossRef]
9. Rushworth, G.F.; Megson, I.L. Existing and potential therapeutic uses for N-acetylcysteine: The need for conversion to intracellular glutathione for antioxidant benefits. *Pharmacol. Ther.* **2014**, *141*, 150–159. [CrossRef]
10. Rank, N.; Michel, C.; Haertel, C.; Lenhart, A.; Welte, M.; Meier-Hellmann, A.; Spies, C. N-acetylcysteine increases liver blood flow and improves liver function in septic shock patients: Results of a prospective, randomized, double-blind study. *Crit. Care Med.* **2000**, *28*, 3799–3807. [CrossRef]
11. Spapen, H.D.; Diltoer, M.W.; Nguyen, D.N.; Hendrickx, I.; Huyghens, L.P. Effects of N-acetylcysteine on microalbuminuria and organ failure in acute severe sepsis: Results of a pilot study. *Chest* **2005**, *127*, 1413–1419. [CrossRef] [PubMed]
12. Cazzola, M.; Calzetta, L.; Facciolo, F.; Rogliani, P.; Matera, M.G. Pharmacological investigation on the anti-oxidant and anti-inflammatory activity of N-acetylcysteine in an ex vivo model of COPD exacerbation. *Respir. Res.* **2017**, *18*, 26. [CrossRef] [PubMed]

32. Evans-Olders, R.; Eintracht, S.; Hoffer, L.J. Metabolic origin of hypovitaminosis C in acutely hospitalized patients. *Nutrition* **2010**, *26*, 1070–1074. [CrossRef] [PubMed]
33. Ferreira, F.L.; Bota, D.P.; Bross, A.; Mélot, C.; Vincent, J.L. Serial evaluation of the SOFA score to predict outcome in critically ill patients. *JAMA* **2001**, *286*, 1754–1758. [CrossRef] [PubMed]
34. Joo, Y.M.; Chae, M.K.; Hwang, S.Y.; Jin, S.C.; Lee, T.R.; Cha, W.C.; Jo, I.J.; Sim, M.S.; Song, K.J.; Jeong, Y.K.; et al. Impact of timely antibiotic administration on outcomes in patients with severe sepsis and septic shock in the emergency department. *Clin. Exp. Emerg. Med.* **2014**, *1*, 35–40. [CrossRef]
35. Hwang, S.Y.; Park, J.E.; Jo, I.J.; Kim, S.; Chung, S.P.; Kong, T.; Shin, J.; Lee, H.J.; You, K.M.; Jo, Y.H.; et al. Combination therapy of vitamin C and thiamine for septic shock in a multicentre, double-blind, randomized, controlled study (ATESS): Study protocol for a randomized controlled trial. *Trials* **2019**, *20*, 420. [CrossRef]
36. Mitchell, A.B.; Ryan, T.E.; Gillion, A.R.; Wells, L.D.; Muthiah, M.P. Vitamin C and thiamine for sepsis and septic shock. *Am. J. Med.* **2020**, *133*, 635–638. [CrossRef]
37. Boretti, A.; Banik, B.K. Intravenous vitamin C for reduction of cytokines storm in acute respiratory distress syndrome. *PharmaNutrition* **2020**, *12*, 100190. [CrossRef]
38. Fujii, T.; Luethi, N.; Young, P.J.; Frei, D.R.; Eastwood, G.M.; French, C.J.; Deane, A.M.; Shehabi, Y.; Hajjar, L.A.; Oliveira, G.; et al. Effect of vitamin C, hydrocortisone, and thiamine vs hydrocortisone alone on time alive and free of vasopressor support among patients with septic shock: The Vitamins Randomized Clinical Trial. *JAMA* **2020**, *323*, 423–431. [CrossRef]
39. Marik, P.E.; Khangoora, V.; Rivera, R. Hydrocortisone, vitamin C and thiamine for the treatment of severe sepsis and septic shock: A retrospective before-after study. *Chest* **2017**, *151*, 1229–1238. [CrossRef]
40. Anderson, G.; Reiter, R.J. Melatonin: Roles in influenza, Covid-19, and other viral infections. *Rev. Med. Virol.* **2020**, *30*, e2109. [CrossRef]
41. Carrillo-Vico, A.; Lardone, P.J.; Naji, L.; Fernández-Santos, J.M.; Martín-Lacave, I.; Guerrero, J.M.; Calvo, J.R. Beneficial pleiotropic actions of melatonin in an experimental model of septic shock in mice: Regulation of pro-/anti-inflammatory cytokine network, protection against oxidative damage and anti-apoptotic effects. *J. Pineal Res.* **2005**, *39*, 400–408. [CrossRef] [PubMed]
42. Wu, C.C.; Chiao, C.W.; Hsiao, G.; Chen, A.; Yen, M.H. Melatonin prevents endotoxin-induced circulatory failure in rats. *J. Pineal Res.* **2001**, *30*, 147–156. [CrossRef] [PubMed]
43. D'Amato, L.A.; Mistraletti, G.; Longhi, D.; Piva, I.R.; Marrazzo, F.; Villa, C.; Tozzi, M.; Paroni, R.; Finati, E.; Lapichino, G. Melatonin blood values and total antioxidant capacity in critically ill patients. *Crit. Care* **2014**, *18*, P436.
44. Wang, H.; Wei, W.; Shen, Y.X.; Dong, C.; Zhang, L.L.; Wang, N.P.; Yue, L.; Xu, S.-Y. Protective effect of melatonin against liver injury in mice induced by Bacillus Calmette-Guerin plus lipopolysaccharide. *World J. Gastroenterol.* **2004**, *10*, 2690–2696. [CrossRef] [PubMed]
45. Li, V.G.; Musumeci, T.; Pignatello, R.; Murabito, P.; Barbagallo, I.; Carbone, C.; Gullo, A.; Puglisi, G. Antioxidant potential of different melatonin-loaded nanomedicines in an experimental model of sepsis. *Exp. Biol. Med.* **2012**, *237*, 670–677.
46. Sánchez-Barceló, E.J.; Mediavilla, M.D.; Tan, D.X.; Reiter, R.J. Clinical uses of melatonin: Evaluation of human trials. *Curr. Med. Chem.* **2010**, *17*, 2070–2095. [CrossRef]
47. Lassnigg, A.; Punz, A.; Barker, R.; Keznickl, P.; Manhart, N.; Roth, E.; Hiesmayr, M. Influence of intravenous vitamin E supplementation in cardiac surgery on oxidative stress: A double-blinded, randomized, controlled study. *Br. J. Anaesth.* **2003**, *90*, 148–154. [CrossRef]
48. Prauchner, C.A. Oxidative stress in sepsis: Pathophysiological implications justifying antioxidant co-therapy. *Burns* **2017**, *43*, 471–485. [CrossRef]

Publisher's Note: MDPI stays neutral with regard to jurisdictional claims in published maps and institutional affiliations.

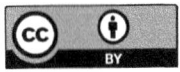

© 2020 by the authors. Licensee MDPI, Basel, Switzerland. This article is an open access article distributed under the terms and conditions of the Creative Commons Attribution (CC BY) license (http://creativecommons.org/licenses/by/4.0/).

13. Paterson, R.L.; Galley, H.F.; Webster, N.R. The effect of N-acetylcysteine on nuclear factor-kappa B activatio interleukin-6, interleukin-8, and intercellular adhesion molecule-1 expression in patients with seps Crit. Care Med. **2003**, *31*, 2574–2578. [CrossRef]
14. Kim, J.C.; Hong, S.W.; Shim, J.K.; Yoo, K.J.; Chun, D.H.; Kwak, Y.L. Effect of N-acetylcysteine on pulmonar function in patients undergoing off-pump coronary artery bypass surgery. *Acta Anaesthesiol. Scand.* **2011**, *5* 452–459. [CrossRef] [PubMed]
15. Berger, M.M.; Oudemans-van, S.H.M. Vitamin C supplementation in the critically ill patient. *Curr. Opi Clin. Nutr. Metab. Care* **2015**, *18*, 193–201. [CrossRef]
16. Spoelstra-de Man, A.M.E.; De Grooth, H.J.; Elbers, P.W.G.; Oudemans-van Straaten, H.M. Response Adjuvant vitamin C in cardiac arrest patients undergoing renal replacement therapy: An appeal for a high high-dose. *Crit. Care* **2018**, *22*, 350. [CrossRef]
17. Fowler, A.A.; Syed, A.A.; Knowlson, S.; Sculthorpe, R.; Farthing, D.; DeWilde, C.; Farthing, C.A.; Larus, T.] Martin, E.; Brophy, D.F.; et al. Phase I safety trial of intravenous ascorbic acid in patients with severe seps *J. Transl. Med.* **2014**, *12*, 32. [CrossRef]
18. Traber, M.G.; Atkinson, J. Vitamin E, antioxidant and nothing more. *Free. Radic. Biol. Med.* **2007**, *43*, 4–1 [CrossRef]
19. Durant, R.; Klouche, K.; Delbosc, S.; Morena, M.; Amigues, L.; Beraud, J.J.; Canaud, B.; Cristol, J.P. Superoxid anion overproduction in sepsis: Effects of vitamin E and simvastatin. *Shock* **2004**, *22*, 34–39. [CrossRef]
20. Galley, H.F.; Lowes, D.A.; Allen, L.; Cameron, G.; Aucott, L.S.; Webster, N.R. Melatonin as a potential therap for sepsis: A phase I dose escalation study and an ex vivo whole blood model under conditions of seps *J. Pineal Res.* **2014**, *56*, 427–438. [CrossRef]
21. Berger, M.M.; Chioléro, R.L. Antioxidant supplementation in sepsis and systemic inflammatory respons syndrome. *Crit. Care Med.* **2007**, *35*, S584–S590. [CrossRef] [PubMed]
22. Shankar-Hari, M.; Phillips, G.S.; Levy, M.L.; Seymour, C.W.; Liu, V.X.; Deutschman, C.S.; Angus, D.C Rubenfeld, G.D.; Singer, M. Sepsis definitions task force. Developing a new definition and assessing ne clinical criteria for septic shock: For the third international consensus definitions for sepsis and septic shoc (Sepsis-3). *JAMA* **2016**, *315*, 775–787. [CrossRef] [PubMed]
23. Lambden, S.; Laterre, P.F.; Levy, M.M.; Francois, B. The SOFA score-development, utility, and challenges accurate assessment in clinical trials. *Crit. Care* **2019**, *23*, 374. [CrossRef] [PubMed]
24. Mohamed, Z.U.; Prasannan, P.; Moni, M.; Edathadathil, F.; Prasanna, P.; Menon, A.; Nair, S.; Greeshma, C.] Sathyapalan, D.T.; Menon, V.; et al. Vitamin C therapy for routine care in septic shock (ViCTOR) tria Effect of intravenous vitamin C, thiamine, and hydrocortisone administration on inpatient mortality amon patients with septic shock. *Indian. J. Crit. Care. Med.* **2020**, *8*, 653–661.
25. Fowler, A.A.; Truwit, J.D.; Hite, R.D.; Morris, P.E.; DeWilde, C.; Priday, A.; Fisher, B.; Thacker, L.F Natarajan, R.; Brophy, D.F.; et al. Effect of vitamin c infusion on organ failure and biomarkers of inflammatio and vascular injury in patients with sepsis and severe acute respiratory failure: The CITRIS-ALI randomize clinical trial. *JAMA* **2019**, *322*, 1261–1270. [CrossRef]
26. Lowes, D.A.; Almawash, A.M.; Webster, N.R.; Reid, V.L.; Galley, H.F. Melatonin and structurally simila compounds have differing effects on inflammation and mitochondrial function in endothelial cells unde conditions mimicking sepsis. *Br. J. Anaesth.* **2011**, *107*, 193–201. [CrossRef]
27. Howe, K.P.; Clochesy, J.M.; Goldstein, L.S.; Owen, H. Mechanical ventilation antioxidant trial. *Am. Crit. Care* **2015**, *24*, 440–445. [CrossRef]
28. Soto, M.E.; Manzano-Pech, L.G.; Guarner-Lans, V.; Díaz-Galindo, J.A.; Vásquez, X.; Castrejón-Tellez, V Gamboa, R.; Huesca, C.; Fuentevilla-Alvárez, G.; Pérez-Torres, I. Oxidant/antioxidant profile in the thoraci aneurysm of patients with the Loeys-Dietz syndrome. *Oxidative Med. Cell. Longev.* **2020**, *2020*, 5392454 [CrossRef]
29. Zhang, R.; Wang, X.; Ni, L.; Di, X.; Ma, B.; Niu, S.; Liu, C.; Reiter, R.J. COVID-19: Melatonin as a potentia adjuvant treatment. *Life Sci.* **2020**, *250*, 117583. [CrossRef]
30. Marik, P.E. Hydrocortisone, ascorbic acid and thiamine (HAT Therapy) for the treatment of sepsis. Focus on ascorbic acid. *Nutrients* **2018**, *10*, 1762. [CrossRef]
31. Carr, A.C.; Rosengrave, P.C.; Bayer, S.; Chambers, S.; Mehrtens, J.; Shaw, G.M. Hypovitaminosis C and vitamin C deficiency in critically ill patients despite recommended enteral and parenteral intakes. *Crit. Care* **2017**, *21*, 300. [CrossRef] [PubMed]

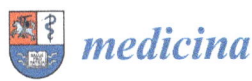

Review
Immune Modulation in Critically Ill Septic Patients

Salvatore Lucio Cutuli [1,*], Simone Carelli [1], Domenico Luca Grieco [1] and Gennaro De Pascale [1,2]

1. Dipartimento di Scienze dell' Emergenza, Anestesiologiche e della Rianimazione, Fondazione Policlinico Universitario A. Gemelli IRCCS, 00168 Rome, Italy; simonecarelli.sc@gmail.com (S.C.); dlgrieco@outlook.it (D.L.G.); gennaro.depascalemd@gmail.com (G.D.P.)
2. Facoltà di Medicina e Chirurgia "A. Gemelli", Università Cattolica del Sacro Cuore, 00168 Rome, Italy
* Correspondence: sl.cutuli@gmail.com; Tel.: +06-3015-9906

Abstract: Sepsis is triggered by infection-induced immune alteration and may be theoretically improved by pharmacological and extracorporeal immune modulating therapies. Pharmacological immune modulation may have long lasting clinical effects, that may even worsen patient-related outcomes. On the other hand, extracorporeal immune modulation allows short-term removal of inflammatory mediators from the bloodstream. Although such therapies have been widely used in clinical practice, the role of immune modulation in critically ill septic patients remains unclear and little evidence supports the role of immune modulation in this clinical context. Accordingly, further research should be carried out by an evidence-based and personalized approach in order to improve the management of critically ill septic patients.

Keywords: sepsis; septic shock; infection; extracorporeal immune modulation; blood purification; renal replacement therapy

1. Introduction

Sepsis [1] represents an acute syndrome of major interest for intensive care physicians because of significant incidence and severe clinical outcomes [2]. Pathophysiology of sepsis originates from a non-physiological, non-protective, non-adaptive inflammatory response to microbiological threats [1]. Identification and control of the source of infection [2] as well as timely and appropriate antibiotic therapy [3] were shown as the most effective interventions that may improve sepsis-induced organ dysfunction. Accordingly, a pathophysiological approach to sepsis is strongly advocated. In the light of this view, immune modulation by pharmacological and extracorporeal blood purification therapies (EBPT) represents a complementary therapy for sepsis and many studies have been conducted with the aim to find a role for such an intervention in this field. In this paper, we clarified the rationale and the role of immune modulation in critically ill septic patients.

2. Immune Alteration in Sepsis

2.1. Pathophysiology of Immune Alteration in Sepsis

Sepsis is a life-threatening organ dysfunction, which is caused by dysregulated host response to infection [1]. Sepsis is an old disease [4] and seminal research hypothesized a causative link between the pathogenicity of specific microorganisms and the severity of this syndrome. However, recent research, most of which was based on molecular assessment of human inflammatory genes, has described the pivotal role of host response in the development of sepsis-associated organ dysfunction and consequent clinical outcomes [5,6]. Specifically, sepsis results from host-pathogen interactions that occur when microorganisms invade sterile organs of the body as well as when microbiota are altered by concurrent conditions (e.g., drug and diet) that shift symbiosis to dysbiosis [7,8]. In some patients, this process results in an exaggerated, uncontrolled, and self-sustaining systemic inflammatory response that causes metabolic derangements and organ dysfunction [6].

Immune response to pathogen invasion is initiated by the recognition of highly conserved pathogen-associated molecular patterns (PAMPs) and danger-associated molecular patterns (DAMPs), which belong to microorganisms and injured tissues of the host, respectively. These molecules are recognized by specific receptors (e.g., Toll-like Receptors) that activate multiple intracellular pathways. Specifically, the activation of selective receptors induces the phosphorylation of mitogen-activated protein kinases (MAPKs), Janus kinases (JAKs), or signal transducers and activators of transcription (STATs) [9]. These molecular pathways induce the expression of specific genes, which codify for inflammatory (e.g., cytokines) and metabolic molecules (e.g., hormones) that orient host response to deal with microbial threats. Moreover, PAMPs e DAMPs trigger further cellular (e.g., neutrophil release of toxic agent) and non-cellular (e.g., complement activation) responses that magnify immune response to pathogen invasion [10]. Among PAMPs, lipopolysaccharide (LPS), a molecule of the outer membrane of the Gram negative bacteria, has been found to induce a dose-dependent activation of the inflammatory system [11]. Among DAMPs, nuclear and cytosolic factors as well as hyaluronan and heparan sulfate of the extracellular matrix are potent activators of the immune system response [12]. On the other hand, a growing body of evidence supports the role of microbiota as organs that may influence immune system response to infection and induce tolerance towards specific molecules (e.g., endotoxins) [13–15], which may have an impact on patient-related clinical outcomes.

The physiological inflammatory response to pathogen invasion of the body implies immune activation and immune suppression, while sepsis occurs when the balance between these pathways is lost [9]. Traditionally, immune activation was considered as the early stage of inflammation, which is triggered by innate pathways of response. Many cytokines have been identified as immune-activating molecules and include tumor necrosis factor-α (TNF-α), several interleukins (e.g., IL-1β, IL-2, IL-6, IL-8), and interferon-γ (IFN-γ). On the other hand, immune suppression was considered the late stage of inflammation, which was intended to extinguish immune activation when the pathogen threat is solved. This stage is mediated by the release of specific molecules like IL-10 and is pathologically exaggerated when chronic critical illness occurs [16].

2.2. Immune Alteration-Induced Organ Dysfunction in Sepsis

In the last few years, an increasing body of evidence has demonstrated that immune activation and immune suppression happen concurrently and cause organ dysfunction, and the severity of which may be evaluated by the Sequential Organ Failure Assessment (SOFA) score [17] (Table 1). The SOFA score has been demonstrated important to synthetize and report sepsis-associated organ dysfunction as well as to provide prognostication for this patient population [18]. Moreover, a simplified version of the SOFA score, namely the quick SOFA (qSOFA) [1], has been identified as an effective tool to identify patients with suspected infection outside the ICU, at risk of poor clinical outcomes. The qSOFA has such an important diagnostic implication when at least two of the following clinical criteria are present: respiratory rate of 22/minute or greater, altered mentation and systolic blood pressure of 100 mmHg or less [19].

Table 1. The Sequential Organ Failure Assessment (SOFA) Score.

Systems	Score				
	0	1	2	3	4
Respiration, PaO$_2$/FiO$_2$ ratio, mmHg (kPa)	≥400 (53.3)	<400 (53.3)	<300 (40)	<200 (26.7) with respiratory support	<100 (13.3) with respiratory support
Coagulation, Platelet count, cells × 10^3/mm^3	≥150	<150	<100	<50	<20
Hepatic, Bilirubin, mg/dL (µg/L)	≤1.2 (20)	1.2–1.9 (20–32)	2–5.9 (33–101)	6–11.9 (102–204)	≥12 (204)
Cardiovascular MAP, mmHg Catecholamines, µg/kg/min for at least 1 h.	≥70 -	<70 -	- Dopamine < 5 Dobutamine (any)	- Dopamine 5.1–15 or epinephrine ≤ 0.1 or norepinephrine ≤ 0.1	- Dopamine > 15 or epinephrine > 0.1 or norepinephrine > 0.1
Central Nervous System, Glasgow Coma Score	15	13–14	10–12	6–9	<6
Renal Creatinine, mg/dL (µmol/L) Diuresis, mL/day	<1.2 (110)	1.2–1.9 (110–170)	2–3.4 (171–299)	3.5–4.9 (300–440) <500	≥5 (440) <200

Abbreviations: FiO$_2$, fraction of inspired oxygen; MAP, mean arterial pressure; PaO$_2$, partial pressure of oxygen.

3. Immune Modulation in Sepsis

3.1. Rationale of Immune Modulation in Sepsis

Immune alteration represents the main pathological pathway that causes and sustains sepsis. Accordingly, immune modulation has appeared as a promising adjuvant therapy in patients who suffer from such disease. Immune modulation may be carried out by specific interventions with the aim to mitigate both pro- and anti-inflammatory bursts, thus allowing for an appropriate and protective response to microbial threat. Immune modulation should be considered as a complementary therapy and should be used with the aim of limiting infection-induced inflammatory alteration by the time appropriate etiologic therapies (e.g., source infection control and antibiotics) are delivered to the patient [2].

3.2. Indirect Immune Modulation in Sepsis

In order to limit immune alteration caused by host response to infection, the microbiological threat must be identified and treated. Such an approach implies the identification of both source (organ or system) and agent (bacterium, virus, parasite or fungus) that cause infection. The source of infection must be determined by clinical assessment (e.g., symptoms) of the patient and possibly confirmed by radiological examination (e.g., Ultra-Sound Scan, chest X-Ray, or CT-scan) [2]. The identification of the source of infection may guide the decision to withdraw samples from specific organs (e.g., cerebrospinal fluid from the central nervous system) that will be tested to identify the agent responsible for infection. In this context, blood samples should always be withdrawn and sent for microbiological examination in order to identify systemic diffusion of the microorganism, which may be associated with the risk of delivering infection to other sites [2]. The identification of the microbiological threats offers the possibility to target antimicrobial therapy to the etiologic cause of infection and deliver an appropriate treatment [2]. Moreover, identifying the source offers the possibility to control the progression of infection at a local level by surgery (e.g., intestinal resection after organ perforation) or interventional radiology (e.g., drainage of an abscess) [2].

3.3. Direct Immune Modulation in Sepsis

3.3.1. Pharmacologic Immune Modulation in Sepsis

Many different drugs have been tested with the aim to provide immune modulation in patients with sepsis (Table 2).

Table 2. Immune modulating strategies in critically ill septic patients.

Immune Modulating Strategies in Sepsis

• Pharmacological
    - Interferon-γ
    - Granulocyte-macrophage colony-stimulating factor
    - Interleukin 7
    - Anti-C5a
    - Recombinant human soluble thrombomodulin
    - Recombinant human-activated protein C
    - Intravenous Immunoglobulin
    - Glucocorticoids
    - Neutrophil elastase inhibitors
    - Programmed cell death protein 1/programmed death ligand
    - Heme oxygenase inducers
 	
• Extracorporeal blood purification therapies
    Non selective:
    - Acrylonitrile-69 Surface-Treated (AN69-ST)
    - Oxiris®
    - Hemofeel®
    - Cytosorb®
    - *Seraph®-100*
    - Coupled Plasma Filtration and Adsorption
    - High cut-off membranes
    Selective:
    - Toraymyxin®

The pathophysiological hypothesis beyond the administration of immune modulating drugs in patients with sepsis relies on the concept of smoothing both hyper- and hypo-inflammation via synthetic analogues of cytokines that are intended to hold such features. As an example, IFN-γ and the granulocyte-macrophage colony-stimulating factor (GM-CSF) have been investigated in order to provide immune modulation due to pleiotropic effects on innate inflammation. The administration of these drugs has shown controversial efficacy and no significant adverse events [20,21]. However, the administration of these drugs was conducted under specific clinical criteria that did not take into account any immune system biomarker (C-reactive protein, cytokines), which may have hampered the results of trials. Specifically, GM-CSF has been demonstrated as effective to improve immune suppression in other clinical contexts and provide some benefit on attenuating lung remodeling in patients with pulmonary fibrosis [22] or immunosuppressive T-regulatory cells replication in cancer vaccine therapy [23]. Moreover, the administration of cytokine analogues like IL-7 have shown significant anti-apoptotic and lymphopoietic effects on T-cells, which may reverse sepsis-associated lymphocyte depletion. Recombinant IL-7 has been described to improve survival in animal models of bacterial and fungal sepsis [24,25], although no definitive clinical evidence supports its use in daily clinical practice.

Recently, complement manipulation may play a role in the development of sepsis-associated immune alteration. Specifically, C5a activity has been demonstrated as crucial in the development of inflammatory mediated tissue damage and its inhibition via selective antibodies was demonstrated effective to mitigate sepsis severity in animal models [26]. However, no definitive clinical data support the use of this therapy in daily clinical life. On top of that, an increasing amount of evidence has shown the interaction between complement and coagulative systems [27]. The latter is frequently altered in patients with sepsis and many drugs have been tested with the aim to improve coagulative dysfunction. However, the administration of recombinant human soluble thrombomodulin [28] as well as activated protein C [29] did not show any benefit on 28-day mortality of critically ill patients with sepsis.

In the last decades, the administration of intravenous immunoglobulins (IVIg) has been increasing in patients with sepsis and such therapy appears characterized by multiple mechanisms of action that include pathogen recognition and killing, toxin scavenging, inflammatory genes-reduced transcription, and anti-apoptosis effects on immune cells [30]. Both polyclonal and monoclonal IgG as well as IgM-enriched polyclonal antibodies have been tested as adjuvant therapies. However, no significant benefits on patient-related outcomes have been observed in clinical trials [31]. As a result, current guidelines [2] do not recommend the use of IVIg in patients with sepsis. On the other hand, small sample sizes and the heterogeneity of IVIg formulations tested in clinical trials support the need for further investigations on the role of this adjuvant therapy in patients with sepsis [32].

Moreover, glucocorticoids are drugs with immune-modulating properties and mimic hormones that are released by adrenal glands when the organism in under stress [33]. Glucocorticoids exert long lasting immune suppressing effects by inhibiting cellular synthesis of pro-inflammatory cytokines [34]. Although the administration of Dexamethasone and Methylprednisolone may increase the risk of secondary infections [35] in patients with sepsis, Hydrocortisone appeared safe and effective to shorten shock duration, mechanical ventilation and ICU length of stay [36]. On the contrary, Methylprednisolone decreased treatment failure of patients with severe community-acquired pneumonia and high initial inflammatory response [37] while Dexamethasone was demonstrated effective to reduce 28-day mortality of patients with acute respiratory failure caused by Coronavirus Disease 19 (COVID-19) [38]. As a result, Hydrocortisone is recommended in patients with septic shock [2], Dexamethasone in patients with COVID-19, and Methylprednisolone, as a rescue therapy, in patients with severe community-acquired pneumonia [39].

Finally, many drugs have been tested with the aim to provide immune modulation via the interaction with ultra-specific pathways of inflammatory host response to infection. As an example, the administration of Sivelestat, a neutrophil elastase inhibitor, may play some role to improve the outcome of septic patients with acute respiratory distress syndrome and disseminated intravascular coagulation [40]. Moreover, sepsis-associated immune paralysis may be improved by the administration of immune checkpoints such as the programmed cell death protein 1/programmed death ligand (PD-1/PD-L) pathway inhibitor [41]. Furthermore, Heme oxygenase inducers promote oxidative conversion of Heme to carbon monoxide, iron, and biliverdin, thus playing pleiotropic modulation of inflammatory pathways involved in host response to infection [42]. In summary, neutrophil elastase inhibitors, PD-1/PD-L, and Heme oxygenase inducers represent promising immune modulating therapies in critically ill septic patients and ongoing clinical trials will shed light on their role in this population.

3.3.2. Extracorporeal Immune Modulation in Sepsis

Extracorporeal removal of PAMPs, DAMPs, and cytokines is considered the new frontier of immune modulation in patients with sepsis. Such interventions allow mediators removal from the bloodstream via specific characteristics of the internal surface of membranes. Moreover, their application in critically ill patients with sepsis appeared feasible and was made easy by the significant rate of acute kidney injury that required continuous renal replacement therapy (CRRT) [43]. Accordingly, EBPT allows selective and non-selective removal of mediators, thus providing short term immune modulation and preventing long-term immune complications that were associated with longer-lasting pharmacological interventions. In the light of this view, the last version of the Surviving Sepsis Campaign Guidelines [2] refers to EBPT as complementary treatments that should be applied with the aim to provide immune system control and multi-organ support by the time etiologic treatments will be delivered to the patient (e.g., control of source of infection and antibiotics).

EBPT are characterized by important features that should be considered when prescribing such interventions [44]. First, each device is characterized by a certain degree of biocompatibility, which refers to the level of complement and platelet activation that results from the interaction between blood and artificial surfaces [44]. Biocompatibility may influence the half-life of the device, condition its efficacy, and worsen inflammatory burst of the host. Although any device available in the market must adhere to specific requirements of the ISO10993, no clinical data exist on the comparison of different devices in terms of biocompatibility [44]. Moreover, EBPT may cause unintended removal of drugs or vitamins, which may have a non-favorable impact on patients' related clinical outcomes. Specifically, lowering antibiotic blood concentration by extracorporeal removal may worsen infection control and increase sepsis-associated inflammatory burst with consequent life-threatening complications [44]. Accordingly, antibiotic dosage should be adapted to any specific EBPT and a strict control of antibiotic blood level concentration is strongly advocated due to the lack of information about clearance characteristics of the majority of new membranes available in the market [44]. Third, EBPT imply a certain degree of heat dissipation to the environment, despite any device for such therapy being endowed by heaters. Heat dissipation may mask fever and cause hypothermia, thus increasing peripheral vasoconstriction [45] and risk of organ hypoperfusion as well as conditioning drug solubility in the bloodstream, enzymes function, and mediators removal at a membrane level. Moreover, hypothermia itself was associated with increased organ dysfunction and 28-day and in-hospital mortality in critically ill patients [46].

Main Application of Extracorporeal Immune Modulation in Critically Ill Septic Patients

Mediators removal via extracorporeal therapy may be selective or non-selective [44] (Table 2). Selective removal of mediators is allowed by specific interaction between soluble molecules and membrane characteristics.

- Non selective extracorporeal removal of inflammatory mediators

PAMPs and cytokines may be non-selectively removed by EBPT via:
- electrostatic interactions between soluble molecules and the internal surface of the membrane (adsorption);
- trans-membrane flux via gradient (diffusion via hemodialysis) and pressure (convection via hemofiltration) concentration, according to the cut-off of the device.

Electrostatic interactions regulate mediator removal of many different devices for EBPT. Specifically, acrylonitrile-69 surface-treated (AN69-ST, Baxter, IL, USA) and surface modified membranes (Oxiris®, Baxter, IL, USA) are devices for CRRT that are characterized by heparin-coated polymers of sodium methallylsulfonate and polyethyleneimine. They allow adsorption of both pro- and anti-inflammatory cytokines (tumor necrosis factor α, IL 6, IL 8, and interferon γ) as well as endotoxin (Oxiris®), both in vitro [47] and in patients with septic acute renal failure [48]. Moreover, EBPT with Oxiris® was associated with significant reduction of IL-6 blood level concentration in critically ill patients admitted to the ICU for COVID-19 [49,50].

Another EBPT which allows for CRRT and mediators removal by adsorption is Hemofeel® (Toray Medical Co Ltd., Tokyo, Japan), a device made by polymethylmethacrylate that was demonstrated as effective in the removal of IL-8 and IL-6 by in-vitro study [51].

However, no clinical evidence exists on the effect of such therapy on the outcome of critically ill patients with sepsis.

Among EBPT that allow mediators removal via adsorption, Cytosorb® represented a promising tool to deliver immune modulation in patients with sepsis. This cartridge is made by highly porous polystyrene divinylbenzene copolymer covered with a biocompatible polyvinylpyrrolidone coating and in-vitro studies demonstrated a certain degree of efficacy to remove pro- and anti-inflammatory cytokines [47]. However, a recently published randomized trial, which enrolled critically ill patients with sepsis, did not demonstrate any effect of Cytosorb® hemoperfusion compared with standard care on IL-6 blood level concentration and 60-day mortality [52].

Moreover, the Seraph®-100 is a sorbent made by polyethylene beads, whose internal surface contains heparin. Although in vitro studies have shown some efficacy of this EBPT on cytokines (TNF-α), bacteria (Staphylococcus Aureus) and viruses (Zika virus, Cytomegalovirus, Adenovirus and Severe Acute Respiratory Syndrome Coronavirus-2) by adsorption [53], no clinical evidence exists on the effect of such therapy on the outcome of critically ill patients with sepsis.

On the other hand, Coupled Plasma Filtration and Adsorption (CPFA) represents a hybrid EBPT which allows mediator removal via plasma filtration and adsorption by styrene resin. Although in vitro studies demonstrated a direct relationship between cytokines removal and volume of plasma cleared by such device, a recent randomized controlled trial was stopped because of futility. Furthermore, this trial observed a significant rate of clotting (48% of the treatments) despite anticoagulation with heparin [54].

Finally, immune modulation may be performed by trans-membrane removal of mediators via gradient (diffusion via haemodialysis) and pressure (convection via hemofiltration) concentration. However, only membranes with a large pore size (20 nm) [55], namely high cut-off membrane (HCO), have been demonstrated as effective to remove inflammatory mediators (the majority of which have a molecular weight above 60 kDa). Although convection appears more effective than diffusion for mediator removal, the significant albumin loss associated with the former is of concern [56]. Accordingly, diffusive modalities are preferred when HCO membranes are used. Immune modulating effect of EBPT via HCO membranes have been suggested by an increasing number of randomized controlled trials that demonstrated significant cytokines blood level reduction when this therapy was compared to conventional renal replacement therapy [56–60]. Despite such promising effect of HCO EBPT on mediator removal, this intervention has not been demonstrated effective on other patients' related clinical outcomes and its application in daily clinical practice is still a matter of debate.

- Selective extracorporeal removal of inflammatory mediators

To the best of our knowledge, endotoxin is the only PAMP that may be selectively removed via adsorption by Toraymyxin® (Toray Industries, Tokyo, Japan) hemoperfusion. Toraymyxin® is a cartridge made by polystyrene fibers and Polymyxin-B, a cationic antibiotic that is characterized by high affinity for endotoxin via ionic and hydrophobic bonds [47]. This device has been widely used in daily clinical practice [61,62], although randomized controlled trials carried out in this field have shown controversial results [63]. However, these trials enrolled patients with inhomogeneous characteristics mainly due to comorbidities, clinical severity, type of infection, timing, and protocol of EBPT provided that do not allow any final conclusion in this field. On the other hand, Toraymyxin® was demonstrated as effective to improve the outcome patients at high risk of mortality (above 30%) [64] and for whom endotoxin level did not exceed the capability of the cartridge to remove such a molecule [65]. Moreover, Toraymyxin® has shown immune modulating effect beyond endotoxin removal and very recently it was demonstrated effective as to improve immune suppression by allowing Monocyte Human Leukocyte Antigen-DR increase [66]. Finally, Toraymyxin® hemoperfusion was used in a cohort of critically ill patients admitted to the ICU for COVID-19 [67] who developed secondary bacterial infections and for whom blood endotoxin activity was deemed implicated in the pathophysiology of immune system alteration and organ dysfunction.

3.4. Filling the Gap of Immune Modulation in Sepsis

Immune modulation offers enticing perspectives of treatment for critically ill septic patients. However, the real application of this complementary treatment is still a matter of debate due to controversial results between laboratory and clinical trials. Sepsis is a clinical syndrome, which complex pathophysiology may be explained by the multifaced genetic (e.g., polymorphic inflammatory pathways) and epigenetic (e.g., comorbidities and clinical intervention applied) interplay that characterizes each single patient. Accordingly, a personalized approach to sepsis may address such a gap via the clinical application of biomarkers of single-cell transcriptomics [68], big data analysis [69], and machine-learning methods by specific models [70], in order to identify specific patient populations that may benefit more from some specific immune modulating intervention and help the design of future clinical trials.

4. Conclusions

Immune modulation represents a complementary therapy for critically ill patients with sepsis. Among immune modulating strategies, EBPT appear safe and timely targeted compared with longer lasting pharmacological therapies. However, little evidence supports the efficacy of immune modulation in critically ill patients with sepsis. Accordingly, immune modulation remains a matter of debate and further research, carried out by evidence-based and personalized approaches, is warranted in order to improve the management of critically ill septic patients.

Author Contributions: Conceptualization, S.L.C. and G.D.P.; S.L.C. and G.D.P.; methodology, S.L.C. and G.D.P.; data curation, S.C. and D.L.G.; writing—original draft preparation, S.L.C. and S.C.; writing—review and editing, S.L.C., S.C., D.L.G. and G.D.P.; supervision, S.L.C. and G.D.P.; All authors have read and agreed to the published version of the manuscript.

Funding: This research received no external funding.

Institutional Review Board Statement: Not applicable.

Informed Consent Statement: Not applicable.

Data Availability Statement: Not applicable.

Conflicts of Interest: The authors declare no conflict of interest with this paper.

References

1. Singer, M.; Deutschman, C.S.; Seymour, C.W.; Shankar-Hari, M.; Annane, D.; Bauer, M.; Bellomo, R.; Bernard, G.R.; Chiche, J.-D.; Coopersmith, C.M.; et al. The Third International Consensus Definitions for Sepsis and Septic Shock (Sepsis-3). *JAMA* **2016**, *315*, 801–810. [CrossRef]
2. Rhodes, A.; Evans, L.E.; Alhazzani, W.; Levy, M.M.; Antonelli, M.; Ferrer, R.; Kumar, A.; Sevransky, J.E.; Sprung, C.L.; Nunnally, M.E.; et al. Surviving Sepsis Campaign: International Guidelines for Management of Sepsis and Septic Shock: 2016. *Intensive Care Med.* **2017**, *43*, 304–377. [CrossRef]
3. Seymour, C.W.; Gesten, F.; Prescott, H.C.; Friedrich, M.E.; Iwashyna, T.J.; Phillips, G.S.; Lemeshow, S.; Osborn, T.; Terry, K.M.; Levy, M.M. Time to Treatment and Mortality during Mandated Emergency Care for Sepsis. *N. Engl. J. Med.* **2017**, *376*, 2235–2244. [CrossRef] [PubMed]
4. Cutuli, S.; De Pascale, G.; Antonelli, M. 'σήψις' yesterday, sepsis nowadays: What's changing? *J. Thorac. Dis.* **2017**, *9*, E166–E167. [CrossRef]
5. De Pascale, G.; Cutuli, S.; Pennisi, M.; Antonelli, M. The role of mannose-binding lectin in severe sepsis and septic shock. *Mediat. Inflamm.* **2013**, *2013*, 625803. [CrossRef] [PubMed]
6. Davenport, E.; Burnham, K.L.; Radhakrishnan, J.; Humburg, P.; Hutton, P.; Mills, T.C.; Rautanen, A.; Gordon, A.C.; Garrard, C.; Hill, A.V.S.; et al. Genomic landscape of the individual host response and outcomes in sepsis: A prospective cohort study. *Lancet Respir. Med.* **2016**, *4*, 259–271. [CrossRef]
7. Cutuli, S.L.; Carelli, S.; De Pascale, G. The gut in critically ill patients: How unrecognized "7th organ dysfunction" feeds sepsis. *Minerva Anestesiol.* **2020**, *86*, 595–597. [CrossRef]

8. Cutuli, S.L.; De Maio, F.; De Pascale, G.; Grieco, D.L.; Monzo, F.R.; Carelli, S.; Tanzarella, E.S.; Pintaudi, G.; Piervincenzi, E.; Cascarano, L.; et al. COVID-19 influences lung microbiota dynamics and favors the emergence of rare infectious diseases: A case report of Hafnia Alvei pneumonia. *J. Crit. Care* **2021**, *64*, 173–175. [CrossRef]
9. Hotchkiss, R.; Moldawer, L.; Opal, S.; Reinhart, K.; Turnbull, I.; Vincent, J. Sepsis and septic shock. *Nat. Rev. Dis. Primers* **2016**, *2*, 16045. [CrossRef]
10. Boomer, J.; Green, J.; Hotchkiss, R. The changing immune system in sepsis: Is individualized immuno-modulatory therapy the answer? *Virulence* **2014**, *5*, 45–56. [CrossRef] [PubMed]
11. Marshall, J.C.; Foster, D.M.; Vincent, J.; Cook, D.J.; Cohen, J.; Dellinger, R.P.; Opal, S.M.; Abraham, E.H.; Brett, S.J.; Smith, T.J.; et al. Diagnostic and Prognostic Implications of Endotoxemia in Critical Illness: Results of the MEDIC Study. *J. Infect. Dis.* **2004**, *190*, 527–534. [CrossRef] [PubMed]
12. Rubartelli, A.; Lotze, M.T. Inside, outside, upside down: Damage-associated molecular-pattern molecules (DAMPs) and redox. *Trends Immunol.* **2007**, *28*, 429–436. [CrossRef] [PubMed]
13. Binnie, A.; Tsang, J.L.; Hu, P.; Carrasqueiro, G.; Castelo-Branco, P.; Dos Santos, C.C. Epigenetics of Sepsis. *Crit. Care Med.* **2020**, *48*, 745–756. [CrossRef] [PubMed]
14. Wolff, N.S.; Hugenholtz, F.; Wiersinga, W.J. The emerging role of the microbiota in the ICU. *Crit. Care* **2018**, *22*, 78. [CrossRef]
15. Kitsios, G.D.; Morowitz, M.J.; Dickson, R.P.; Huffnagle, G.B.; McVerry, B.J.; Morris, A. Dysbiosis in the intensive care unit: Microbiome science coming to the bedside. *J. Crit. Care* **2017**, *38*, 84–91. [CrossRef]
16. Yadav, H.; Cartin-Ceba, R. Balance between Hyperinflammation and Immunosuppression in Sepsis. *Semin. Respir. Crit. Care Med.* **2016**, *37*, 042–050. [CrossRef]
17. Vincent, J.; Moreno, R.; Takala, J.; Willatts, S.; Mendonça, A.D.; Bruining, H.; Reinhart, C.K.; Suter, P.M.; Thijs, L.G. The SOFA (Sepsis-related Organ Failure Assessment) score to describe organ dysfunction/failure. On behalf of the Working Group on Sepsis-Related Problems of the European Society of Intensive Care Medicine. *Intensive Care Med.* **1996**, *22*, 707–710. [CrossRef]
18. Ferreira, F.L.; Bota, D.P.; Bross, A.; Mélot, C.; Vincent, J.-L. Serial Evaluation of the SOFA Score to Predict Outcome in Critically Ill Patients. *JAMA* **2001**, *286*, 1754–1758. [CrossRef]
19. Seymour, C.; Liu, V.; Iwashyna, T.; Brunkhorst, F.; Rea, T.; Scherag, A.; Rubenfeld, G.; Kahn, J.M.; Shankar-Hari, M.; Singer, M.; et al. Assessment of Clinical Criteria for Sepsis: For the Third International Consensus Definitions for Sepsis and Septic Shock (Sepsis-3). *JAMA* **2016**, *315*, 762–774. [CrossRef]
20. Mathias, B.; Szpila, B.E.; Moore, F.A.; Efron, P.A.; Moldawer, L.L. A Review of GM-CSF Therapy in Sepsis. *Medicine* **2015**, *94*, e2044. [CrossRef] [PubMed]
21. Döcke, W.; Randow, F.; Syrbe, U.; Krausch, D.; Asadullah, K.; Reinke, P.; Volk, H.-D.; Kox, W. Monocyte deactivation in septic patients: Restoration by IFN-gamma treatment. *Nat. Med.* **1997**, *3*, 678–681. [CrossRef]
22. Piguet, P.F.; Grau, G.E.; De Kossodo, S. Role of Granulocyte-Macrophage Colony-Stimulating Factor in Pulmonary Fibrosis Induced in Mice by Bleomycin. *Exp. Lung Res.* **1993**, *19*, 579–587. [CrossRef]
23. Serafini, P.; Carbley, R.; Noonan, K.A.; Tan, G.; Bronte, V.; Borrello, I. High-Dose Granulocyte-Macrophage Colony-Stimulating Factor-Producing Vaccines Impair the Immune Response through the Recruitment of Myeloid Suppressor Cells. *Cancer Res.* **2004**, *64*, 6337–6343. [CrossRef]
24. Shindo, Y.; Fuchs, A.G.; Davis, C.G.; Eitas, T.; Unsinger, J.; Burnham, C.-A.D.; Green, J.M.; Morre, M.; Bochicchio, G.V.; Hotchkiss, R.S. Interleukin 7 immunotherapy improves host immunity and survival in a two-hit model of Pseudomonas aeruginosa pneumonia. *J. Leukoc. Biol.* **2017**, *101*, 543–554. [CrossRef] [PubMed]
25. Unsinger, J.; Burnham, C.-A.D.; McDonough, J.; Morre, M.; Prakash, P.S.; Caldwell, C.C.; Dunne, W.M.; Hotchkiss, R.S. Interleukin-7 Ameliorates Immune Dysfunction and Improves Survival in a 2-Hit Model of Fungal Sepsis. *J. Infect. Dis.* **2012**, *206*, 606–616. [CrossRef]
26. Rittirsch, D.; Flierl, M.; Nadeau, B.; Day, D.; Huber-Lang, M.; Mackay, C.R.; Zetoune, F.S.; Gerard, N.P.; Cianflone, K.; Köhl, J.; et al. Functional roles for C5a receptors in sepsis. *Nat. Med.* **2008**, *14*, 551–557. [CrossRef] [PubMed]
27. Oncul, S.; Afshar-Kharghan, V. The interaction between the complement system and hemostatic factors. *Curr. Opin. Hematol.* **2020**, *27*, 341–352. [CrossRef]
28. Vincent, J.; Francois, B.; Zabolotskikh, I.; Daga, M.K.; Lascarrou, J.-B.; Kirov, M.Y.; Pettilä, V.; Wittebole, X.; Meziani, F.; Mercier, E.; et al. Effect of a Recombinant Human Soluble Thrombomodulin on Mortality in Patients with Sepsis-Associated Coagulopathy: The SCARLET Randomized Clinical Trial. *JAMA* **2019**, *321*, 1993–2002. [CrossRef]
29. Ranieri, V.M.; Thompson, B.T.; Barie, P.S.; Dhainaut, J.-F.; Douglas, I.S.; Finfer, S.; Gårdlund, B.; Marshall, J.C.; Rhodes, A.; Artigas, A.; et al. Drotrecogin Alfa (Activated) in Adults with Septic Shock. *N. Engl. J. Med.* **2012**, *366*, 2055–2064. [CrossRef] [PubMed]
30. Shankar-Hari, M.; Spencer, J.; Sewell, W.; Rowan, K.M.; Singer, M. Bench-to-bedside review: Immunoglobulin therapy for sepsis-biological plausibility from a critical care perspective. *Crit. Care* **2012**, *16*, 206–214. [CrossRef]
31. Alejandria, M.M.; Lansang MA, D.; Dans, L.F.; Mantaring, J.B., III. Intravenous immunoglobulin for treating sepsis, severe sepsis and septic shock. *Cochrane Database Syst. Rev.* **2013**, *2013*, CD001090. [CrossRef]
32. Laupland, K.B.; Kirkpatrick, A.W.; Delaney, A. Polyclonal intravenous immunoglobulin for the treatment of severe sepsis and septic shock in critically ill adults: A systematic review and meta-analysis. *Crit. Care Med.* **2007**, *35*, 2686–2692. [PubMed]
33. Peeters, B.; Langouche, L.; Berghe, G.V.D. Adrenocortical Stress Response during the Course of Critical Illness. *Compr. Physiol.* **2017**, *8*, 283–298. [CrossRef]

34. Heming, N.; Sivanandamoorthy, S.; Meng, P.; Bounab, R.; Annane, D. Immune Effects of Corticosteroids in Sepsis. *Front. Immunol.* **2018**, *9*, 1736. [CrossRef]
35. Gibbison, B.; López-López, J.A.; Higgins, J.P.T.; Miller, T.; Angelini, G.D.; Lightman, S.L.; Annane, D. Corticosteroids in septic shock: A systematic review and network meta-analysis. *Crit. Care* **2017**, *21*, 1–8. [CrossRef]
36. Rygård, S.L.; Butler, E.; Granholm, A.; Møller, M.H.; Cohen, J.; Finfer, S.; Perner, A.; Myburgh, J.; Venkatesh, B.; Delaney, A. Low-dose corticosteroids for adult patients with septic shock: A systematic review with meta-analysis and trial sequential analysis. *Intensive Care Med.* **2018**, *44*, 1003–1016. [CrossRef]
37. Torres, A.; Sibila, O.; Ferrer, M.; Polverino, E.; Mendendez, R.; Mensa, J.; Gabarrus, A.; Sellares, J.; Restrepo, M.; Anzueto, A.; et al. Effect of corticosteroids on treatment failure among hospitalized patients with severe community-acquired pneumonia and high inflammatory response: A randomized clinical trial. *Acute Critical Care* **2015**, *46*, 677–686. [CrossRef]
38. Recovery Collaborative Group; Horby, P.; Lim, W.S.; Emberson, J.; Mafham, M.; Bell, J.L.; Linsell, L.; Staplin, N.; Brightling, C.; Ustianowski, A.; et al. Dexamethasone in Hospitalized Patients with Covid-19—Preliminary Report. *N. Engl. J. Med.* **2021**, *384*, 693–704, (online ahead of print).
39. Metlay, J.P.; Waterer, G.W.; Long, A.C.; Anzueto, A.; Brozek, J.; Crothers, K.; Cooley, L.A.; Dean, N.C.; Fine, M.J.; Flanders, S.A.; et al. Diagnosis and treatment of adults with community-acquired pneumonia. An official clinical practice guideline of the american thoracic society and infectious diseases society of America. *Am. J. Respir. Crit. Care Med.* **2019**, *200*, e45–e67. [CrossRef]
40. Hayakawa, M.; Katabami, K.; Wada, T.; Sugano, M.; Hoshino, H.; Sawamura, A.; Gando, S. Sivelestat (Selective Neutrophil Elastase Inhibitor) improves the mortality rate of sepsis associated with both acute respiratory distress syndrome and disseminated intravascular coagulation patients. *Shock* **2010**, *33*, 14–18. [CrossRef]
41. Nakamori, Y.; Park, E.J.; Shimaoka, M. Immune Deregulation in Sepsis and Septic Shock: Reversing Immune Paralysis by Targeting PD-1/PD-L1 Pathway. *Front. Immunol.* **2021**, *11*, 624279. [CrossRef] [PubMed]
42. Ryter, S.W. Therapeutic Potential of Heme Oxygenase-1 and Carbon Monoxide in Acute Organ Injury, Critical Illness, and Inflammatory Disorders. *Antioxidants* **2020**, *9*, 1153. [CrossRef] [PubMed]
43. Bellomo, R.; Kellum, J.A.; Ronco, C.; Wald, R.; Martensson, J.; Maiden, M.; Bagshaw, S.M.; Glassford, N.J.; Lankadeva, Y.; Vaara, S.T.; et al. Acute kidney injury in sepsis. *Intensive Care Med.* **2017**, *43*, 816–828. [CrossRef]
44. Cutuli, S.; Grieco, D.; De Pascale, G.; Antonelli, M. Hemadsorption. *Curr. Opin. Anaesthesiol.* **2021**, *34*, 113–118, (online ahead of print). [CrossRef] [PubMed]
45. Douvris, A.; Malhi, G.; Hiremath, S.; McIntyre, L.; Silver, S.; Bagshaw, S.M.; Wald, R.; Ronco, C.; Sikora, L.; Weber, C.; et al. Interventions to prevent hemodynamic instability during renal replacement therapy in critically ill patients: A systematic review. *Crit. Care* **2018**, *22*, 41. [CrossRef]
46. Kushimoto, S.; Gando, S.; Saitoh, D.; Mayumi, T.; Ogura, H.; Fujishima, S.; Araki, T.; Ikeda, H.; Kotani, J.; Miki, Y.; et al. The impact of body temperature abnormalities on the disease severity and outcome in patients with severe sepsis: An analysis from a multicenter, prospective survey of severe sepsis. *Crit. Care* **2013**, *17*, R271. [CrossRef]
47. Malard, B.; Lambert, C.; Kellum, J. In vitro comparison of the adsorption of inflammatory mediators by blood purification devices. *Intensive Care Med. Exp.* **2018**, *6*, 12. [CrossRef]
48. Broman, M.E.; Hansson, F.; Vincent, J.-L.; Bodelsson, M. Endotoxin and cytokine reducing properties of the oXiris membrane in patients with septic shock: A randomized crossover double-blind study. *PLoS ONE* **2019**, *14*, e0220444. [CrossRef]
49. Villa, G.; Romagnoli, S.; De Rosa, S.; Greco, M.; Resta, M.; Montin, D.P.; Prato, F.; Patera, F.; Ferrari, F.; Rotondo, G.; et al. Blood purification therapy with a hemodiafilter featuring enhanced adsorptive properties for cytokine removal in patients presenting COVID-19: A pilot study. *Crit. Care* **2020**, *24*, 1–13. [CrossRef]
50. Cascarano, L.; Cutuli, S.L.; Pintaudi, G.; Tanzarella, E.S.; Carelli, S.; Anzellotti, G.; Grieco, D.L.; DE Pascale, G.; Antonelli, M. Extracorporeal immune modulation in COVID-19 induced immune dysfunction and secondary infections: The role of oXiris® membrane. *Minerva Anestesiol.* **2021**, *87*. (online ahead of print). [CrossRef]
51. Harm, S.; Schildböck, C.; Hartmann, J. Cytokine Removal in Extracorporeal Blood Purification: An in vitro Study. *Blood Purif.* **2020**, *49*, 33–43. [CrossRef] [PubMed]
52. Schädler, D.; Pausch, C.; Heise, D.; Meier-Hellmann, A.; Brederlau, J.; Weiler, N.; Marx, G.; Putensen, C.; Spies, C.; Jörres, A.; et al. The effect of a novel extracorporeal cytokine hemoadsorption device on IL-6 elimination in septic patients: A randomized controlled trial. *PLoS ONE* **2017**, *12*, e0187015. [CrossRef] [PubMed]
53. Seffer, M.-T.; Cottam, D.; Forni, L.G.; Kielstein, J.T. Heparin 2.0: A New Approach to the Infection Crisis. *Blood Purif.* **2021**, *50*, 28–34, (online ahead of print). [CrossRef] [PubMed]
54. Livigni, S.; Bertolini, G.; Rossi, C.; Ferrari, F.; Giardino, M.; Pozzato, M.; Remuzzi, G. Efficacy of coupled plasma filtration adsorption (CPFA) in patients with septic shock: A multicenter randomised controlled clinical trial. *BMJ Open* **2014**, *4*, e003536. [CrossRef] [PubMed]
55. Ankawi, G.; Neri, M.; Zhang, J.; Breglia, A.; Ricci, Z.; Ronco, C. Extracorporeal techniques for the treatment of critically ill patients with sepsis beyond conventional blood purification therapy: The promises and the pitfalls. *Crit. Care* **2018**, *22*, 262. [CrossRef] [PubMed]
56. Morgera, S.; Slowinski, T.; Melzer, C.; Sobottke, V.; Vargas-Hein, O.; Volk, T.; Zuckermann-Becker, H.; Wegner, B.; Müller, J.M.; Baumann, G.; et al. Renal replacement therapy with high-cutoff hemofilters: Impact of convection and diffusion on cytokine clearances and protein status. *Am. J. Kidney Dis.* **2004**, *43*, 444–453. [CrossRef]

57. Haase, M.; Bellomo, R.; Baldwin, I.; Haase-Fielitz, A.; Fealy, N.; Davenport, P.; Morgera, S.; Goehl, H.; Storr, M.; Boyce, N.; et al. Hemodialysis Membrane With a High-Molecular-Weight Cutoff and Cytokine Levels in Sepsis Complicated by Acute Renal Failure: A Phase 1 Randomized Trial. *Am. J. Kidney Dis.* **2007**, *50*, 296–304. [CrossRef]
58. Morgera, S.; Haase, M.; Kuss, T.; Vargas-Hein, O.; Zuckermann-Becker, H.; Melzer, C.; Krieg, H.; Wegner, B.; Bellomo, R.; Neumayer, H.-H. Pilot study on the effects of high cutoff hemofiltration on the need for norepinephrine in septic patients with acute renal failure. *Crit. Care Med.* **2006**, *34*, 2099–2104. [CrossRef]
59. Morgera, S.; Haase, M.; Rocktäschel, J.; Böhler, T.; Vargas-Hein, O.; Melzer, C.; Krausch, D.; Kox, W.J.; Baumann, G.; Beck, W.; et al. Intermittent High-Permeability Hemofiltration Modulates Inflammatory Response in Septic Patients with Multiorgan Failure. *Nephron Clin. Pract.* **2003**, *94*, c75–c80. [CrossRef]
60. Morgera, S.; Rocktäschel, J.; Haase, M.; Lehmann, C.; Von Heymann, C.; Ziemer, S.; Priem, F.; Hocher, B.; Göhl, H.; Kox, W.J.; et al. Intermittent high permeability hemofiltration in septic patients with acute renal failure. *Intensive Care Med.* **2003**, *29*, 1989–1995. [CrossRef]
61. Antonelli, M.; Bello, G.; Maviglia, R.; Cutuli, S.; Ronco, C.; Cruz, D.; Ranieri, V.M.; Martin, E.; Fumagalli, R.; Monti, G.; et al. Polymyxin B hemoperfusion in clinical practice: The picture from an unbound collaborative registry. *Blood Purif.* **2014**, *37*, 22–25.
62. Cutuli, S.L.; Artigas, A.; Fumagalli, R.; Monti, G.; Ranieri, V.M.; Ronco, C.; Antonelli, M. Polymyxin-B hemoperfusion in septic patients: Analysis of a multicenter registry. *Ann. Intensiv. Care* **2016**, *6*, 77. [CrossRef]
63. Fujii, T.; Ganeko, R.; Kataoka, Y.; Furukawa, T.; Featherstone, R.; Doi, K.; Vincent, J.; Pasero, D.; Robert, R.; Ronco, C.; et al. Polymyxin B-immobilized hemoperfusion and mortality in critically ill adult patients with sepsis/septic shock: A systematic review with meta-analysis and trial sequential analysis. *Intensive Care Med.* **2018**, *44*, 167–178. [CrossRef]
64. Chang, T.; Tu, Y.K.; Lee, C.T.; Chao, A.; Huang, C.H.; Wang, M.J.; Yeh, Y.C. Effects of Polymyxin B Hemoperfusion on Mortality in Patients with Severe Sepsis and Septic Shock: A Systemic Review, Meta-Analysis Update, and Disease Severity Subgroup Meta-Analysis. *Crit. Care Med.* **2017**, *45*, e858–e864. [CrossRef] [PubMed]
65. Romaschin, A.D.; Obiezu-Forster, C.V.; Shoji, H.; Klein, D.J. Novel Insights into the Direct Removal of Endotoxin by Polymyxin B Hemoperfusion. *Blood Purif.* **2017**, *44*, 193–197. [CrossRef] [PubMed]
66. Srisawat, N.; Tungsanga, S.; Lumlertgul, N.; Komaenthammasophon, C.; Peerapornratana, S.; Thamrongsat, N.; Tiranathanagul, K.; Praditpornsilpa, K.; Eiam-Ong, S.; Tungsanga, K.; et al. The effect of polymyxin B hemoperfusion on modulation of human leukocyte antigen DR in severe sepsis patients. *Crit. Care* **2018**, *22*, 1–10. [CrossRef] [PubMed]
67. De Rosa, S.; Cutuli, S.; Ferrer, R.; Antonelli, M.; Ronco, C.; the COVID-19 EUPHAS2 Collaborative Group. Polymyxin B hemoperfusion in COVID-19 Patients with endotoxic shock: Case Series from EUPHAS II registry. *Artif. Organs* **2020**. (online ahead of print). [CrossRef]
68. Scicluna, B.P.; Vught, L.A.; Zwinderman, A.H.; Wiewel, M.A.; Davenport, E.E.; Burnham, K.L.; Nürnberg, P.; Schultz, M.J.; Horn, J.; Cremer, O.L.; et al. Classification of patients with sepsis according to blood genomic endotype: A prospective cohort study. *Lancet Respir. Med.* **2017**, *5*, 816–826. [CrossRef]
69. Celi, L.; Mark, R.; Stone, D.; Montgomery, R. "Big data" in the intensive care unit. Closing the data loop. *Am. J. Respir. Crit. Care Med.* **2013**, *187*, 1157–1160. [CrossRef]
70. Mohammed, A.; Van Wyk, F.; Chinthala, L.K.; Khojandi, A.; Davis, R.L.; Coopersmith, C.M.; Kamaleswaran, R. Temporal Differential Expression of Physiomarkers Predicts Sepsis in Critically Ill Adults. *Shock* **2020**. (online ahead of print). [CrossRef]

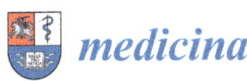

Review

Neutropenic Enterocolitis and Sepsis: Towards the Definition of a Pathologic Profile

Giuseppe Bertozzi [1], Aniello Maiese [2], Giovanna Passaro [3], Alberto Tosoni [4], Antonio Mirijello [5], Stefania De Simone [1], Benedetta Baldari [6], Luigi Cipolloni [1] and Raffaele La Russa [1,*]

1. Section of Legal Medicine, Department of Clinical and Experimental Medicine, University of Foggia, Ospedale Colonnello D'Avanzo, Viale Europa 12, 71100 Foggia, Italy; giuseppe.bertozzi@unifg.it (G.B.); stefania.desimone@unifg.it (S.D.S.); luigi.cipolloni@unifg.it (L.C.)
2. Department of Surgical Pathology, Medical, Molecular and Critical Area, Institute of Legal Medicine, University of Pisa, 56126 Pisa, Italy; aniellomaiese@msn.com
3. Fondazione Policlinico Universitario "A. Gemelli" IRCCS, 00168 Rome, Italy; passaro.giovanna@gmail.com
4. CEMAD Digestive Disease Center, Fondazione Policlinico Universitario "A. Gemelli" IRCCS, Università Cattolica del Sacro Cuore, 00168 Rome, Italy; alberto.tosoni@policlinicogemelli.it
5. Department of Medical Sciences, IRCCS Casa Sollievo della Sofferenza, 71013 San Giovanni Rotondo, Italy; a.mirijello@operapadrepio.it
6. Department of Anatomical, Histological, Forensic and Orthopedic Sciences, Sapienza University of Rome, 00186 Rome, Italy; benedetta.baldari@uniroma1.it
* Correspondence: raffaele.larussa@unifg.it

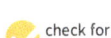

Citation: Bertozzi, G.; Maiese, A.; Passaro, G.; Tosoni, A.; Mirijello, A.; Simone, S.D.; Baldari, B.; Cipolloni, L.; La Russa, R. Neutropenic Enterocolitis and Sepsis: Towards the Definition of a Pathologic Profile. *Medicina* 2021, 57, 638. https://doi.org/10.3390/medicina57060638

Academic Editor: Salvatore Di Somma

Received: 6 May 2021
Accepted: 18 June 2021
Published: 20 June 2021

Publisher's Note: MDPI stays neutral with regard to jurisdictional claims in published maps and institutional affiliations.

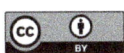

Copyright: © 2021 by the authors. Licensee MDPI, Basel, Switzerland. This article is an open access article distributed under the terms and conditions of the Creative Commons Attribution (CC BY) license (https://creativecommons.org/licenses/by/4.0/).

Abstract: *Background*: Neutropenic enterocolitis (NE), which in the past was also known as typhlitis or ileocecal syndrome for the segment of the gastrointestinal tract most affected, is a nosological entity that is difficult to diagnose and whose pathogenesis is not fully known to date. Initially described in pediatric patients with leukemic diseases, it has been gradually reported in adults with hematological malignancies and non-hematological conditions, such as leukemia, lymphoma, multiple myeloma, aplastic anemia, and also myelodysplastic syndromes, as well as being associated with other immunosuppressive causes such as AIDS treatment, therapy for solid tumors, and organ transplantation. Therefore, it is associated with high mortality due to the rapid evolution in worse clinical pictures: rapid progression to ischemia, necrosis, hemorrhage, perforation, multisystem organ failure, and sepsis. *Case report*: A case report is included to exemplify the clinical profile of patients with NE who develop sepsis. *Literature Review*: To identify a specific profile of subjects affected by neutropenic enterocolitis and the entity of the clinical condition most frequently associated with septic evolution, a systematic review of the literature was conducted. The inclusion criteria were as follows: English language, full-text availability, human subjects, and adult subjects. Finally, the papers were selected after the evaluation of the title and abstract to evaluate their congruity with the subject of this manuscript. Following these procedures, 19 eligible empirical studies were included in the present review. *Conclusions*: Despite the recent interest and the growing number of publications targeting sepsis and intending to identify biomarkers useful for its diagnosis, prognosis, and for the understanding of its pathogenesis, and especially for multi-organ dysfunction, and despite the extensive research period of the literature review, the number of publications on the topic "neutropenic enterocolitis and sepsis" appears to be very small. In any case, the extrapolated data allowed us to conclude that the integration of medical history, clinical and laboratory data, radiological imaging, and macroscopic and histological investigations can allow us to identify a specific pathological profile.

Keywords: neutropenic enterocolitis; sepsis; chemotherapy-induced damage

1. Introduction

Neutropenic enterocolitis (NE), as the phrase used to identify it suggests, is a severe inflammatory bowel disease that occurs in neutropenic patients. It is also known as ileocecal syndrome or "typhlitis", from the Greek word "typhon", used to indicate caecum or cecitis, since this is the site of the organism most frequently affected; it was a clinical entity initially described in pediatric leukemia patients. However, over the years, the diagnoses of adult subjects with neoplasms have increased (mainly hematological diagnoses, such as leukemia, lymphoma, multiple myeloma, aplastic anemia, and even myelodysplastic syndromes), as well as other immunosuppressive causes such as AIDS, therapy for solid tumors, and organ transplantation. However, since different tracts of the gastrointestinal (GI) system could be involved, it was considered more appropriate to use the definition of neutropenic enterocolitis [1–3].

The incidence of NE varies between studies. In a systemic review conducted by Gorschlüter et al., the incidence rate of 21 studies was 5.3% in patients hospitalized for hematologic malignancies, high-dose chemotherapy for solid tumors, or aplastic anemia, while another cohort study found it in 3.5% of 317 severely neutropenic patients [4,5].

The incidence of NE has increased with the increasing use of intensive chemotherapy [1]. Gastrointestinal toxicity, in fact, is a common complication of cytotoxic cancer chemotherapy. Currently available cytotoxic drugs do not discriminate between cancer cells and rapidly dividing normal cells. The toxicity of anticancer treatment will continue to be a significant problem until highly selective therapies for malignant cells are developed [6]. Combination regimens are often the standard treatment. The rapid extension of available antineoplastic drugs, however, has also underscored the urgent need for clinicians to better understand and detect the acute and late toxicity spectrum of these regimens.

In fact, exposure to cytotoxic drugs has been called into question as to the main mechanism in the pathogenesis of NE, although currently it is not yet fully understood. One of the mechanisms is the onset of mucositis with consequent interruption of the mucous barrier, which allows for bacterial translocation from the intestine. This mechanism is supported by histological findings of intestinal wall edema, swollen blood vessels, and mucosal surface rupture [7] with areas of ulceration and bleeding. Neutropenia further aggravates the risks, causing decreased immunity with the inability to control the transmural translocation of pathogens. There are also concerns that direct invasion of the interstitial wall by malignant cells may contribute to the disease. The cecum is more commonly involved in NE due to its distensibility and limited blood supply (elements which, by self-feeding, can in turn cause the clinical condition to worsen).

Therefore, it is associated with high mortality due to the rapid evolution in worse clinical pictures: rapid progression to ischemia, necrosis, hemorrhage, perforation, and multisystem organ failure and sepsis, which is defined as infection-induced organ dysfunction or hypoperfusion abnormalities that predispose to septic shock and increased mortality in neutropenic settings [8]. It is underrecognized clinically, with the diagnosis often being made on post-mortem examination.

This review of the literature, focusing on the relationship between NE and sepsis in comparison with a clinical case, thus aims to favor the gnoseological diffusion of this nosological entity, to support the etiopathological mechanism, as proposed above, and to define its main characteristics for its diagnostic framework.

2. Case Report

The case study involved a 56-year-old woman diagnosed with locally advanced infiltrating ductal carcinoma of the breast treated with chemotherapy according to the TAC scheme (Docetaxel, Doxorubicin, Cyclophosphamide). The blood tests at the beginning of chemotherapy were documented as follows: white blood cells $9630/mm^3$, of which $4860/mm^3$ were neutrophils. After 10 days from the start of chemotherapy, the woman in the case in question entered the local emergency department for abdominal pain refractory to medical pain-relieving therapy. Physical examination by the doctors documented the treatable abdomen on all quadrants with tenesmus, vomiting, and diarrhea, with the vital parameters of blood pressure at 110/70, 99% oxygen saturation, and body temperature at 38.0 °C. On laboratory tests, she had $560/mm^3$ of white blood cells, of which $290/mm^3$

were neutrophils. CT imaging showed the absence of pneumoperitoneum with a collapsed and thickened rectum, as well as fat stranding and intramural areas of low attenuation. A gastroenterological specialistic examination was also performed, which documented a smooth mucosa on rectal exploration, but with underlying layers there was increased consistency, circumferentially, and the presence of mucus bloody material into the lumen. During the diagnostic process, however, the patient's condition suddenly worsened, due to the onset of hyperlactacidemic metabolic acidosis, respiratory insufficiency, and a tendency to hypotension despite the massive volume filling and the aggressive life support, and she died. The autopsy examination allowed us to detect, upon isolation of the intestinal tract between the ileocecal valve and the anus, the presence of a focal pattern of circumferential thickening and edema of the rectum-sigma mucosa, in the context of which it was possible to observe the presence of small yellow membranes. Upon cutting of the bowel wall, diffuse submucosal hemorrhages were also noted. The histological investigations (Figure 1) conducted on the organ samples allowed us to confirm the presence of mucosal and submucosal edema, and well-defined agglomerations of inflammatory cells in the context of the bowel wall as well as Councilman bodies were observed in the study of the liver in association with biliary stasis. The histological study was completed with immunohistochemical staining with positive anti-TNF-alpha and anti-IL15 antibody reactions on the heart samples [9,10]. The cause of death was attributed to sepsis and multi-organ failure.

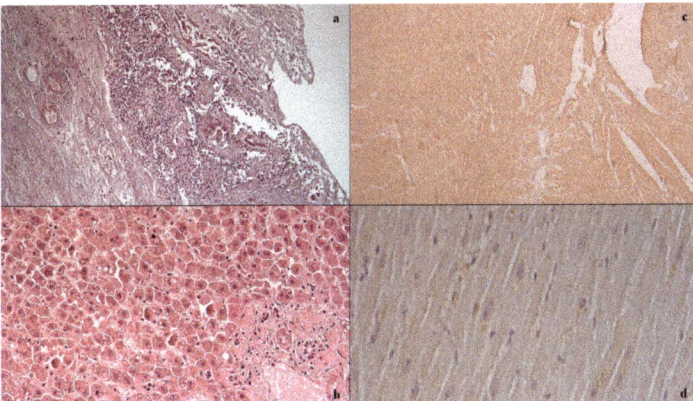

Figure 1. Histological investigation: mucosal and submucosal edema, and well-defined agglomerations of inflammatory cells in the context of the bowel wall (**a**); Councilman bodies of the liver (**b**); positive anti-IL15 (**c**) anti-TNF-alpha (**d**) antibody reactions on heart samples.

3. Side Effects of Chemotherapy

Chemotherapy drugs can cause damage to the wall of the various tracts of the gastrointestinal (GI) system, according to multiple mechanisms. On the one hand, in fact, the damage can be mediated by a direct effect on the mucosa that can lead to inflammation, edema, ulceration, and atrophy of the same. On the other hand, these alterations cause, consequently, increased permeability of the mucosa which, in association with the immunosuppressive effect of the drugs themselves, predispose to an increased risk of transparietal infections, resulting in septicemia and shock, with consequent mucosal ischemia. This would trigger a self-sufficient vicious circle [11,12].

Among the drugs most implicated in mucosal damage, taxanes, which act by stabilizing microtubules and inhibiting cellular mitosis [13], have been linked to a broad spectrum of colitis. Specifically, it was difficult to compare the effects induced by docetaxel and paclitaxel in terms of toxicity, although docetaxel appears to be associated with more side effects than paclitaxel. The most frequent type of illness induced is ischemic colitis, clinically characterized by acute abdominal pain and associated neutropenia, fever, and/or diarrhea, with or without blood. This condition can develop into serious complications such as intestinal necrosis, colonic perforation, or typhlitis. Septicemia occurs frequently and the most common etiopathology is aerobic Gram-negative bacteria infection. The mucosal histopathological analysis is compatible with a significant component of inflammatory changes such as mucosal and submucosal edema, hemorrhage, acute inflammatory infiltrates, and mucosal ulcerations [14].

Platinum compounds follow, the best known of which is cisplatin. It works by binding inside cells to nucleophiles, such as DNA, RNA, and bases, to form adducts, which induce apoptosis [15]. Vomiting is the earliest GI symptom and is usually associated with a peak in the urinary metabolites of serotonin, suggesting a strong correlation between the release of serotonin with this agent and vomiting [16]. Oxaliplatin, on the other hand, has a large number of GI side effects: diarrhea and nausea, vomiting, stomatitis, dry mouth, melaena, bleeding, proctitis, and tenesmus.

Furthermore, doxorubicin is a drug belonging to the category of DNA intercalators, and it acts mainly by inhibiting DNA topoisomerase II and DNA replication through epigenetic mechanisms of DNA methylation [17]. Stomatitis has been reported in up to 80% of patients, in other cases, ulceration of the esophagus and colon has been described following its use.

On the other hand, 5-fluorouracil (5-FU) and methotrexate belong to the category of antimetabolites, i.e., analogs of folic acid, pyrimidine, or purines that induce cell death during the phase following incorporation into RNA and in DNA, thus inhibiting the synthesis of nucleic acid [18,19]. 5-FU, in detail, causes gastrointestinal side effects that can be serious and life threatening. Stomatitis and esophagopharyngitis are commonly observed during therapy, with ulceration and necrosis of the visceral wall. In fact, subsequent diarrhea can be bloody. Methotrexate, on the other hand, has a severe toxicity profile manifesting in myelosuppression, oropharyngeal ulceration, and diarrhea. Other frequently reported gastrointestinal side effects include stomatitis, hematemesis, melaena, and other types of bleeding. Extremely rare cases of toxic megacolon have been associated with the use of methotrexate.

4. Literature Review

Information Sources and Search: For this literature review the PubMed database was questioned on 30 April 2021. A primary selection was conducted with this search strategy: (neutropenic enterocolitis) showing 491 results. In order to focus on the link between neutropenic enterocolitis and sepsis, this search was narrowed to [(neutropenic enterocolitis) AND (sepsis)], resulting in 72 manuscripts.

Study Selection: The inclusion criteria were being in the English language and being published in a scholarly peer-reviewed journal. Full-length articles were preferred; duplicate manuscript or only abstract-available texts were excluded. Studies involving human targets were further selected. Moreover, the references of the selected articles were also reviewed.

Synthesis: Following these procedures, 30 eligible studies were included in present review. Then potentially relevant studies were further assessed, excluding other-than-neutropenic-enterocolitis entities causing sepsis [20–26], pediatric subjects [27], and clinical trials [28–30]. After this literature review process, 19 papers were selected (Figure 2).

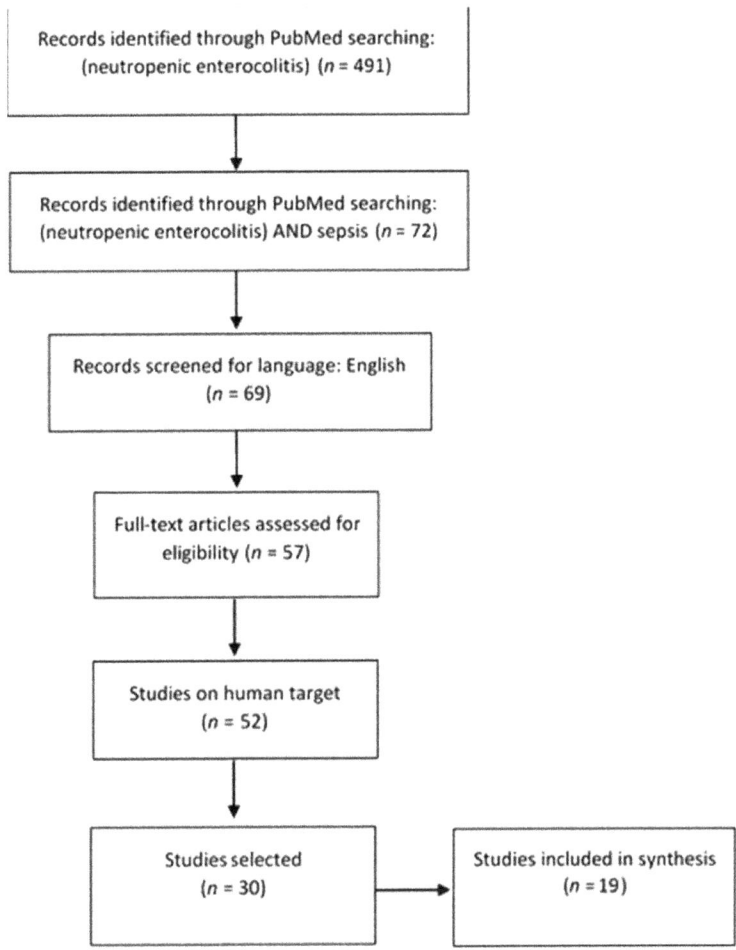

Figure 2. Review flow diagram, according to PRISMA guidelines.

5. Results

5.1. Etiology

From the literature review (Table 1), the most commonly isolated pathogens include *Pseudomonas aeruginosa*, *Escherichia coli*, *Bacillus cereus*, *Klebsiella* spp., *Enterococci*, *Clostridium* spp., and *Candida* spp. [31–35]. However, the organisms most frequently associated with sepsis or septic shock are Clostridium septicum, Citrobacter freundii, Stomatococcus mucilaginosus, and Stenotrophomonas maltophilia [36–40].

5.2. Kind of Neoplasia and Therapy

Regarding the history, all subjects identified from the reviewed literature were immunocompromised. In detail, the most frequently encountered pathologies were leukemia lymphoma [33,39,41–43]. Other pathological conditions associated with NE were found to be not only solid tumors, such as lung cancer and sarcoma [43], but also myelodysplasia or aplastic anemia [44].

Of those with a history of cancer and available clinical data, all had received chemotherapy in the previous month, particularly those agents that cause mucositis, such as taxanes [45].

Other documented chemotherapeutic agents included methotrexate, vincristine, cyclophosphamide, cytarabine, daunorubicin, cyclosporine, fludarabine, and/or doxorubicin or combinations, such as chemoradiotherapy (CRT) with 5-fluorouracil (5-FU) and mitomycin C [33,43,46].

5.3. Clinical and Imaging

Concerning the clinic complaints by the patient upon access to medical facilities, both general and specific GI involvement symptoms were reported for all confirmed NE patients when the next medical history was available. In particular, fever appeared in almost all patients, followed by pain or abdominal pain and diarrhea [47].

The reported laboratory tests identified as a common feature in all cases of major neutropenia with absolute neutrophil count <1500 mm^3 [33,43]. Besides, subjects with absolute neutrophil count <500/mm^3 more frequently had abdominal pain and higher fever as the main symptoms and more frequently encountered hemodynamic instability.

The diagnostic method most frequently used to reach the diagnosis was the CT scan of the abdomen, with signs of cecal inflammation and thickened edematous colon.

5.4. Macroscopic and Microscopic Features

Alterations were described in all segments of the GI including the ileus, left or right colon, or both, with involvement of different entities and considered mainly segmental or irregular (although diffuse or focal were also described) [33–47].

In order to macroscopically document these macroscopic alterations, endoscopic studies in NE cases have shown the following: mucosal ulceration, edema, erosions, pseudomembranes, nodularity, friability, or bleeding [33,43,48,49].

The histological features, on the other hand, of NE included the presence of intracellular organisms, necrosis, hemorrhage, ulceration, erosion, and pseudomembranes. However, a depleted inflammatory background was also described in some cases [33].

5.5. Treatment and Outcomes

In the study from Sachak et al. 79% of patients with histologically confirmed NE died after a median survival of 1 day [33].

Most of the symptomatic patients were treated with antibiotics or supportive perfusion therapy [42], and only a few benefited from granulocyte transfusion (GT) therapy or granulocyte colony-stimulating factor therapy [35]. This non-conservative approach demonstrated its efficacy in retrospective and prospective case series, but no studies have been successful in demonstrating its benefits from a statistically significant advantage in controlled clinical trials. It has also been associated with prophylactic bowel rest and total parenteral nutrition instituted at the beginning of further chemotherapy, with surgery delayed until complications appear [41].

NE-reported complications were as follows: sepsis, intra-abdominal abscesses, colon perforation, and pneumatosis intestinalis.

Patients with ongoing severe systemic sepsis and those with established complications (perforation, obstruction, hemorrhage, or abscess) require surgical intervention consisting of all necrotic material removal, usually performed with resective surgery of the affected segment [50,51]. According to Abu-Sbeih et al., all patients that required surgery had hematologic malignancies and absolute neutrophil counts <500/mm^3 [43].

Table 1. Summary of the literature review.

Etiology	Kind of Neoplasia	Chemotherapy	Neutrophils	Imaging-CT	Macroscopic Examination	Microscopic Investigation
Escherichia coli [31,35,43,44,51,52]; Clostridium difficile [33,36,46,50,51]; Bacillus cereus [34]; Enterococcus sbb [33,35,43]; Clostridium septicum [33,36,37]; Stenotrophomonas maltophilia [38]; Citrobacter freundii [39]; Stomatococcos mucilaginosus [40]; Mucormycosis [42]; Fungi [33–35,50]; Viruses [33,35]; Aeromonas hydrophila [46]; Enterobacter cloacae [46]; Klebsiella pneumoniae [33,46]; Morganella morganii [52]; Streptococcus oralis [52]	Leukemia/lymphoma [31,33–38,42,43,46,50–52]; Lung carcinoma [33]; Sarcoma [33]; Breast cancer [39,45]; Vulvar cancer [47]	Cyclophosphamide [31,33,38–40,45,51]; Vincristine [31,33,40,51]; Methotrexate [33,40,51]; Cytarabine [33,36,42,51,52]; Daunorubicin [33]; Fludarabine [33]; Doxorubicin [33,45]; Idarubicina [34,42]; 6 thioguanine [36,40]; Daunorubicina [36,40,51]; Deoxycoformycin [37]; 5-fluorouracil [39,46]; Epirubicin [39]; Idarubicin [42]; Docetaxel [45]; Mitomycin C [47]	ANC = 1.2×10^9/L [31]; ANC < 0.1×10^9/L [35,44]; ANC < 0.5×10^9/L [35,36]; ANC < 100×10 cells/mm^3 [40,43]; 14.2% [42]; ANC = $500/mm^3$ [45]; ANC < 1000 cells/microL [50]	Thickened colon [33,34,42,44,45]; Small bowel dilatation [42]	Ulcerations [31,43]; Thickening and hemorrhagic walls [36,39,43,45]; Perforation [42,43]; Abscess [43,44]	Mucosal ulceration [31,33,34,36,38,43,51,52]; Granulation tissue [31,45]; Necrosis [33,35,42,43]; Edema [33]; Hemorrhage [33,36,38,43]; Infiltrating organisms in an inflammatory depleted background [33,36,38,39,45,52]; Microabscess [34]; Thrombosis [36,52]; Pseudomembranes [43]

6. Conclusions

Despite the recent interest and the growing number of publications targeting sepsis, intending to identify biomarkers useful both for its diagnosis, prognosis, and for the understanding of its pathogenesis, and especially for the multi-organ dysfunction, and despite the extensive research period of the literature review, the number of publications on the topic "neutropenic enterocolitis and sepsis" appears to be very small. In any case, the extrapolated data allowed us to conclude that the integration of medical history, clinical and laboratory data, radiological imaging, and macroscopic and histological investigations allowed us to identify a specific pathological profile. As regards the medical history, particular attention must be paid to subjects with onco-hematological neoplasia (in particular leukemia or solid tumors), in treatment with chemotherapeutic agents (among which particular attention must be paid to therapeutic schemes involving taxanes) [13,14,45]. An important clinical element is the triad composed of fever, abdominal pain, and diarrhea, but certainly the alarm bell is represented by marked neutropenia. In the case described, in fact, the patient had a history of solid tumor in treatment with poli-chemotherapy, according to an administration regimen that included taxanes, and entered the local hospital for fever, abdominal pain, and diarrhea. The most significant finding was the very low neutrophil count, which, as per the literature review, is more frequently associated with a worse prognostic characterized by hemodynamic instability and sepsis, which subsequently occurred. In the present case as in similar ones, a rapid diagnostic classification is essential to implement the earliest support measures, although based on the available data, neutropenic enterocolitis is characterized by high mortality even at early stages.

In this context, the case under examination is perfectly in line with the data from the literature review and seems to be an overlap of what Cornely and Schirmacher have already reported [52]. Even in our case, the demonstration of an altered intestinal mucosal barrier would seem to support the hypothesis of translocation as a prerequisite for subsequent bacteremia, sepsis, and multi-organ failure. Further studies are needed to better understand these aspects and if there are risk factors more correlated to a bad outcome.

Author Contributions: Conceptualization, G.B. and S.D.S.; methodology, B.B.; validation, L.C., R.L.R., and A.M. (Aniello Maiese); formal analysis, L.C. and G.P.; investigation, G.B.; resources, R.L.R. and B.B.; data curation, A.M. (Antonio Mirijello); writing—original draft preparation, G.B.; writing—review and editing, R.L.R. and A.M. (Aniello Maiese); visualization, G.P.; supervision, G.P., A.T., and A.M. (Antonio Mirijello); project administration, R.L.R. All authors have read and agreed to the published version of the manuscript.

Funding: This research received no external funding.

Institutional Review Board Statement: The study did not require ethical approval. Data processing complies with the general authorization for scientific research purposes granted by the Italian Data Protection Authority (1 March 2012 as published in Italy's Official Journal no. 72 dated 26 March 2012) since the data do not entail any significant personalized impact on data subjects. Approval by an institutional and/or licensing committee is not required since experimental protocols are not applied in the study. The case is judicial and ordered by local prosecutors.

Informed Consent Statement: No informed consent is required to use information from persons where the same in-formation is strictly indispensable and relevant for scientific and research purposes.

Data Availability Statement: Data available on request due to restrictions e.g., privacy or ethical reason.

Conflicts of Interest: The authors declare no conflict of interest.

References

1. Snydman, D.R.; Nesher, L.; Rolston, K.V.I. Neutropenic enterocolitis, a growing concern in the era of widespread use of aggressive chemotherapy. *Clin. Infect. Dis.* **2013**, *56*, 711–717. [CrossRef]
2. Davila, M.L. Neutropenic enterocolitis. *Curr. Treat. Options Gastroenterol.* **2006**, *9*, 249–255. [CrossRef] [PubMed]
3. Moran, H.; Yaniv, I.; Ashkenazi, S.; Schwartz, M.; Fisher, S.; Levy, I. Risk factors for typhlitis in pediatric patients with cancer. *J. Pediatr. Hematol. Oncol.* **2009**, *31*, 630–634. [CrossRef] [PubMed]

4. Gorschlüter, M.; Mey, U.; Strehl, J.; Ziske, C.; Schepke, M.; Schmidt-Wolf, I.G.H.; Sauerbruch, T.; Glasmacher, A. Neutropenic enterocolitis in adults: Systematic analysis of evidence quality. *Eur. J. Haematol.* **2005**, *75*, 1–13. [CrossRef] [PubMed]
5. Aksoy, D.Y.; Tanriover, M.D.; Uzun, O.; Zarakolu, P.; Ercis, S.; Ergüven, S.; Oto, A.; Kerimoglu, U.; Hayran, M.; Abbasoglu, O. Diarrhea in neutropenic patients: A prospective cohort study with emphasis on neutropenic enterocolitis. *Ann. Oncol.* **2007**, *18*, 183–189. [CrossRef]
6. Andreyev, H.J.N.; Davidson, S.E.; Gillespie, C.; Allum, W.H.; Swarbrick, E. Practice guidance on the management of acute and chronic gastrointestinal problems arising as a result of treatment for cancer. *Gut* **2012**, *61*, 179–192. [CrossRef]
7. Katz, J.A.; Mahoney, D.H.; Fernbach, D.J.; Wagner, M.L.; Gresik, M.V. Typhlitis. An 18-year experience and postmortem review. *Cancer* **1990**, *65*, 1041–1047. [CrossRef]
8. Jeddi, R.; Achour, M.; Amor, R.B.; Aissaoui, L.; Bouterâa, W.; Kacem, K.; Lakhal, R.B.; Abid, H.B.; BelHadjAli, Z.; Turki, A.; et al. Factors associated with severe sepsis: Prospective study of 94 neutropenic febrile episodes. *Hematology* **2010**, *15*, 28–32. [CrossRef]
9. Pomara, C.; Riezzo, I.; Bello, S.; De Carlo, D.; Neri, M.; Turillazzi, E. A Pathophysiological Insight into Sepsis and Its Correlation with Postmortem Diagnosis. *Mediat. Inflamm.* **2016**, *2016*, 4062829. [CrossRef]
10. Chen, Y.; Pat, B.; Zheng, J.; Cain, L.; Powell, P.; Shi, K.; Sabri, A.; Husain, A.; Dell'italia, L.J. Tumor necrosis factor-α produced in cardiomyocytes mediates a predominant myocardial inflammatory response to stretch in early volume overload. *J. Mol. Cell Cardiol.* **2010**, *49*, 70–78. [CrossRef]
11. Stemmler, H.J.; Kenngott, S.; Diepolder, H.; Heinemann, V. Gastrointestinal toxicity associated with weekly docetaxel treatment. *Ann. Oncol.* **2002**, *13*, 978–981. [CrossRef] [PubMed]
12. Van Vuuren, R.J.; Visagie, M.H.; Theron, A.E.; Joubert, A.M. Antimitotic drugs in the treatment of cancer. *Cancer Chemother. Pharmacol.* **2015**, *76*, 1101–1112. [CrossRef]
13. Boussios, S.; Pentheroudakis, G.; Katsanos, K.; Pavlidis, N. Systemic treatment-induced gastrointestinal toxicity: Incidence, clinical presentation and management. *Ann. Gastroenterol.* **2012**, *25*, 106–118.
14. Chen, E.; Abu-Sbeih, H.; Thirumurthi, S.; Mallepally, N.; Khurana, S.; Wei, D.; Altan, M.; Morris, V.K.; Tan, D.; Barcenas, C.H.; et al. Clinical characteristics of colitis induced by taxane-based chemotherapy. *Ann. Gastroenterol.* **2020**, *33*, 59–67. [CrossRef]
15. Dasari, S.; Bernard Tchounwou, P. Cisplatin in cancer therapy: Molecular mechanisms of action. *Eur. J. Pharmacol.* **2014**, *740*, 364–378. [CrossRef]
16. Weber, G.F.; Weber, G.F. DNA Damaging Drugs. In *Molecular Therapies of Cancer*; Springer International Publishing: Cham, Switzerland, 2015; pp. 9–112. [CrossRef]
17. Yang, F.; Teves, S.S.; Kemp, C.J.; Henikoff, S. Doxorubicin, DNA torsion, and chromatin dynamics. *Biochim. Biophys. Acta Rev. Cancer* **2014**, *1845*, 84–89. [CrossRef] [PubMed]
18. Thymidylate Synthase Inhibitor—An Overview I ScienceDirect Topics n.d. Available online: https://www.sciencedirect.com/topics/chemistry/thymidylate-synthase-inhibitor (accessed on 17 April 2021).
19. Lee, C.S.; Ryan, E.J.; Doherty, G.A. Gastro-intestinal toxicity of chemotherapeutics in colorectal cancer: The role of inflammation. *World J. Gastroenterol.* **2014**, *20*, 3751–3761. [CrossRef] [PubMed]
20. Tascini, C.; Menichetti, F.; Stefanelli, A.; Loni, C.; Lambelet, P. Clinical efficacy of intravenous colistin therapy in combination with ceftazidime in severe MDR P. aeruginosa systemic infections in two haematological patients. *Le Infez. Med.* **2006**, *14*, 41–44.
21. Garrett, J.; Klimberg, V.S.; Anaissie, E.; Barlogie, B.; Turnage, R.; Badgwell, B.D. The surgical management of abdominal pain in the multiple myeloma patient. *Am. J. Surg.* **2012**, *203*, 127–131. [CrossRef] [PubMed]
22. Teichmann, D.; Cummins, M.; Keogh, S.J.; Rogers, T. The complication of gastro-enteric fistulisation in neutropenic enterocolitis secondary to aplastic anaemia. *Pediatr. Blood Cancer* **2014**, *61*, 358–359. [CrossRef] [PubMed]
23. Royo-Cebrecos, C.; Gudiol, C.; Ardanuy, C.; Pomares, H.; Calvo, M.; Carratalà, J. A fresh look at polymicrobial bloodstream infection in cancer patients. *PLoS ONE* **2017**, *12*. [CrossRef]
24. Slavin, M.A.; Grigg, A.P.; Schwarer, A.P. Fatal anaerobic bacteremia after hematopoietic stem cell transplant. *Leuk. Lymphoma* **2004**, *45*, 143–145. [CrossRef]
25. Roghmann, M.C.; McCarter, R.J.; Brewrink, J.; Cross, A.S.; Glenn Morris, J. Clostridium difficile infection is a risk factor for bacteremia due to vancomycin-resistant enterococci (VRE) in VRE-colonized patients with acute leukemia. *Clin. Infect. Dis.* **1997**, *25*, 1056–1059. [CrossRef] [PubMed]
26. Gorschlüter, M.; Glasmacher, A.; Hahn, C.; Leutner, C.; Marklein, G.; Remig, J.; Schmidt-Wolf, I.G.; Sauerbruch, T. Severe abdominal infections in neutropenic patients. *Cancer Investig.* **2001**, *19*, 669–677. [CrossRef] [PubMed]
27. Maiese, A.; Bolino, G.; Mastracchio, A.; Frati, P.; Fineschi, V. An immunohistochemical study of the diagnostic value of TREM-1 as marker for fatal sepsis cases. *Biotech. Histochem.* **2019**, *94*, 159–166. [CrossRef]
28. Heng, M.S.; Barbon Gauro, J.; Yaxley, A.; Thomas, J. Does a neutropenic diet reduce adverse outcomes in patients undergoing chemotherapy? *Eur. J. Cancer Care (Engl.)* **2020**, *29*, e13155. [CrossRef]
29. Polee, M.B.; Verweij, J.; Siersema, P.D.; Tilanus, H.W.; Splinter, T.A.W.; Stoter, G.; Van der Gaast, A. Phase I study of a weekly schedule of a fixed dose of cisplatin and escalating doses of paclitaxel in patients with advanced oesophageal cancer. *Eur. J. Cancer* **2002**, *38*, 1495–1500. [CrossRef]
30. Cioch, M.; Jawniak, D.; Kotwica, K.; Wach, M.; Mańko, J.; Goracy, A.; Klimek, P.; Mazurkiewicz, E.; Jarosz, P.; Hus, M. Biosimilar granulocyte colony-stimulating factor is effective in reducing the duration of neutropenia after autologous peripheral blood stem cell transplantation. *Transplant. Proc.* **2014**, *46*, 2882–2884. [CrossRef] [PubMed]

31. Sadullah, S.; Nagesh, K.; Johnston, D.; McCullough, J.B.; Murray, F.; Cachia, P.G. Recurrent septicaemia in a neutropenic patient with typhlitis. *Clin. Lab. Haematol.* **1996**, *18*, 215–217. [CrossRef] [PubMed]
32. Qasim, A.; Nahas, J. *Neutropenic Enterocolitis (Typhlitis)*; StatPearls Publishing: Treasure Island, FL, USA, 2021.
33. Sachak, T.; Arnold, M.A.; Naini, B.V.; Graham, R.P.; Shah, S.S.; Cruise, M.; Park, J.Y.; Clark, L.; Lamps, L.; Frankel, W.L.; et al. Neutropenic enterocolitis. *Am. J. Surg. Pathol.* **2015**, *39*, 1635–1642. [CrossRef]
34. Ginsburg, A.S.; Salazar, L.G.; True, L.D.; Disis, M.L. Fatal Bacillus cereus sepsis following resolving neutropenic enterocolitis during the treatment of acute leukemia. *Am. J. Hematol.* **2003**, *72*, 204–208. [CrossRef]
35. Cherif, H.; Axdorph, U.; Kalin, M.; Björkholm, M. Clinical experience of granulocyte transfusion in the management of neutropenic patients with haematological malignancies and severe infection. *Scand. J. Infect. Dis.* **2013**, *45*, 112–116. [CrossRef]
36. King, A.; Rampling, A.; Wight, D.G.D.; Warren, R.E. Neutropenic enterocolitis due to Clostridium septicum infection. *J. Clin. Pathol.* **1984**, *37*, 335–343. [CrossRef]
37. Litam, P.P.; Loughran, T.P. Clostridium septicum bacteremia in a patient with large granular lymphocyte leukemia. *Cancer Investig.* **1995**, *13*, 492–494. [CrossRef] [PubMed]
38. Kaito, S.; Sekiya, N.; Najima, Y.; Sano, N.; Horiguchi, S.; Kakihana, K.; Hishima, T.; Ohashi, K. Fatal neutropenic enterocolitis caused by stenotrophomonas maltophilia: A rare and underrecognized entity. *Intern. Med.* **2018**, *57*, 3667–3671. [CrossRef] [PubMed]
39. Clemons, M.J.; Valle, J.W.; Harris, M.; Ellenbogen, S.; Howell, A. Citrobacter freundii and fatal neutropenic enterocolitis following adjuvant chemotherapy for breast cancer. *Clin. Oncol.* **1997**, *9*, 172–175. [CrossRef]
40. Fanourgiakis, P.; Georgala, A.; Vekemans, M.; Daneau, D.; Heymans, C.; Aoun, M. Bacteremia due to Stomatococcos mucilaginosus in neutropenic patients in the setting of a cancer institute. *Clin. Microbiol. Infect.* **2003**, *9*, 1068–1072. [CrossRef]
41. Moir, C.R.; Scudamore, C.H.; Benny, W.B. Typhlitis: Selective surgical management. *Am. J. Surg.* **1986**, *151*, 563–566. [CrossRef]
42. Yi, H.S.; Sym, S.J.; Park, J.; Cho, E.K.; Shin, D.B.; Lee, J.H. Typhlitis due to mucormycosis after chemotherapy in a patient with acute myeloid leukemia. *Leuk. Res.* **2010**, *34*. [CrossRef] [PubMed]
43. Abu-Sbeih, H.; Ali, F.S.; Chen, E.; Mallepally, N.; Luo, W.; Lu, Y.; Foo, W.C.; Qiao, W.; Okhuysen, P.C.; Adachi, J.A.; et al. Neutropenic enterocolitis: Clinical features and outcomes. *Dis. Colon. Rectum.* **2020**, *63*, 381–388. [CrossRef]
44. Youngs, J.; Suarez, C.; Koh, M.B.C. An unusual presentation of neutropenic enterocolitis (typhlitis). *Lancet Infect. Dis.* **2016**, *16*, 618. [CrossRef]
45. Cherri, S.; Prochilo, T.; Rota, L.; Mutti, S.; Garatti, M.; Liserre, B.; Alberto, Z. Neutropenic Enterocolitis in the Treatment of Solid Tumors: A Case Report and Review of the Literature. *Case Rep. Oncol.* **2020**, *13*, 442–448. [CrossRef] [PubMed]
46. Hsu, T.F.; Huang, H.H.; Yen, D.H.T.; Kao, W.F.; Chen, J.D.; Wang, L.M.; Lee, C.H. ED presentation of neutropenic enterocolitis in adult patients with acute leukemia. *Am. J. Emerg. Med.* **2004**, *22*, 276–279. [CrossRef] [PubMed]
47. Mulayim, N.; Silver, D.F.; Schwartz, P.E.; Higgins, S. Chemoradiation with 5-fluorouracil and mitomycin C in the treatment of vulvar squamous cell carcinoma. *Gynecol. Oncol.* **2004**, *93*, 659–666. [CrossRef]
48. Van Eyken, P.; Fanni, D.; Gerosa, C. Ischemic colitis. In *Colitis a Pract. Approach to Colon Biopsy Interpret*; Springer International Publishing: Cham, Switzerland, 2014; pp. 139–145. [CrossRef]
49. Villanacci, V.; Salemme, M. Microscopic colitis. In *Colitis a Pract. Approach to Colon Biopsy Interpret*; Springer International Publishing: Cham, Switzerland, 2014; pp. 155–163. [CrossRef]
50. Badgwell, B.D.; Cormier, J.N.; Wray, C.J.; Borthakur, G.; Qiao, W.; Rolston, K.V.; Pollock, R.E. Challenges in surgical management of abdominal pain in the neutropenic cancer patient. *Ann. Surg.* **2008**, *248*, 104–109. [CrossRef]
51. Koea, J.B.; Shaw, J.H.F. Surgical management of neutropenic enterocolitis. *Br. J. Surg.* **1989**, *76*, 821–824. [CrossRef]
52. Cornely, O.A.; Schirmacher, P. Clinical picture: Bacterial translocation in neutropenic sepsis. *Lancet* **2001**, *358*, 1842. [CrossRef]

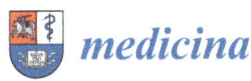

Case Report

Successful Treatment of *Klebsiella pneumoniae* NDM Sepsis and Intestinal Decolonization with Ceftazidime/Avibactam Plus Aztreonam Combination in a Patient with TTP Complicated by SARSCoV-2 Nosocomial Infection

Francesco Perrotta [1] and Marco Paolo Perrini [2,*]

1. Department of Anesthesia and Intensive Care Unit, IRCCS Casa Sollievo della Sofferenza, Viale Cappuccini, 1, 71013 San Giovanni Rotondo, FG, Italy; francperr72@yahoo.it
2. Department of Anesthesia and Intensive Care Unit, Università degli Studi di Foggia, Azienda Ospedaliero Universitaria Ospedali Riuniti di Foggia, 1, 71122 Viale Pinto, FG, Italy
* Correspondence: marco.perrini@unifg.it

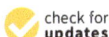

Citation: Perrotta, F.; Perrini, M.P. Successful Treatment of *Klebsiella pneumoniae* NDM Sepsis and Intestinal Decolonization with Ceftazidime/Avibactam Plus Aztreonam Combination in a Patient with TTP Complicated by SARSCoV-2 Nosocomial Infection. *Medicina* **2021**, *57*, 424. https://doi.org/10.3390/medicina57050424

Academic Editor: Antonio Mirijello

Received: 8 March 2021
Accepted: 23 April 2021
Published: 28 April 2021

Publisher's Note: MDPI stays neutral with regard to jurisdictional claims in published maps and institutional affiliations.

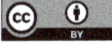

Copyright: © 2021 by the authors. Licensee MDPI, Basel, Switzerland. This article is an open access article distributed under the terms and conditions of the Creative Commons Attribution (CC BY) license (https://creativecommons.org/licenses/by/4.0/).

Abstract: Carbapenem-resistant *Enterobacteriaceae* (CRE) are a serious public health threat. Infections due to these organisms are associated with significant morbidity and mortality. Among them, metallo-β-lactamases (MBLs)-producing *Klebsiella pneumoniae* are of global concern today. The ceftazidime/avibactam combination and the ceftazidime/avibactam + aztreonam combination currently represent the most promising antibiotic strategies to stave off these kinds of infections. We describe the case of a patient affected by thrombotic thrombocytopenic purpura (TTP) admitted in our ICU after developing a hospital-acquired SarsCoV2 interstitial pneumonia during his stay in the hematology department. His medical conditions during his ICU stay were further complicated by a *K. Pneumoniae* NDM sepsis. To our knowledge, the patient had no risk factors for multidrug-resistant bacteria exposure or contamination during his stay in the hematology department. During his stay in the ICU, we treated the sepsis with a combination therapy of ceftazidime/avibactam + aztreonam. The therapy solved his septic state, allowing for a progressive improvement in his general condition. Moreover, we noticed that the negativization of the hemocultures was also associated to a decontamination of his known rectal colonization. The ceftazidime/avibactam + aztreonam treatment could not only be a valid therapeutic option for these kinds of infections, but it could also be considered as a useful tool in selected patients' intestinal decolonizations.

Keywords: multidrug-resistant bacteria; *Klebsiella* NDM; ceftazidime-avibactam

1. Introduction

The prevalence of multidrug-resistant organisms (MDROs), a major public health threat, continues to increase on a global level and is associated with significant morbidity and mortality.

Phenotypic resistance to carbapenems is typically caused by the β-lactamase activity combined with structural mutations and the production of carbapenemases, enzymes that hydrolyze carbapenem antibiotics.

Other mechanisms associated with carbapenem resistance in Gram-negative bacteria (GNB) include drug efflux pumps and alterations in penicillin-binding proteins.

These characteristics are generally located on mobile genetic elements (MGE) or linked to the hyperproduction of enzymes from inducible or derepressed chromosomal genes [1,2].

In a single-center longitudinal study in long-term acute care hospital, patients who were colonized with carbapenemase-producing *Klebsiella pneumoniae* (KPC-Kp) were studied by Shimasaki et al., who found that carbapenem use was associated with an increased hazard for high relative abundance of KPC-Kp in the gut microbiota. Additionally, high relative abundance of KPC-Kp was associated with KPC-Kp bacteremia [3].

As already known, bacteriemia can rapidly evolve into sepsis and septic shock, especially if it occurs in debilitated patients affected by systemic diseases and needing intensive care unit treatments.

In Italy, the national surveillance carried out in the period 2014–2017 reported 7632 carbapenemase-producing *Enterobacteriaceae* blood stream infections (CPE BSI) from all Italian regions and autonomous provinces.

Most of the cases (7490, 98.1%) were due to *K. pneumoniae*, while *E. coli* was reported in only 142 (1.9%) cases.

A carbapenemase enzyme identified in the CPE strains and isolated from BSI was reported in 60.4% (4612/7632) of cases.

In most cases, the enzyme reported was *Klebsiella pneumoniae* carbapenemase (in 95.2% of *K. pneumoniae* and 81.4% of *E. coli*). Metallo-beta-lactamases (MBL) were reported in 2.1% of cases, and carbapenem-hydrolyzing oxacillinase-48 (OXA-48) in 1.2%. Associations between MBL and KPC (0.9%) or MBL and OXA-48 (0.3%) were also identified in rare cases.

MBL-detected genes were mainly Verona integron-encoded metallo-beta-lactamase (VIM) (65/86, 75.6%) followed by New Delhi metallo-beta-lactamase (NDM) (21/86, 24.4%). NDM was reported only in the years 2016–2017, mainly in *K. pneumoniae* (20/21, 95.2%), and often in association with OXA-48 [4].

The high incidence of KPC-CPE in Italy favors the use of ceftazidime/avibactam (CAZ/AVI), a combination of a well-established β-lactam antibiotic, ceftazidime, with a novel β-lactamase inhibitor, avibactam, for treatment of serious infections caused by resistant Gram-negative pathogens. Ceftazidime/avibactam is active against OXA-48- and KPC-producing *Enterobacteriaceae*, but not NDM- or VIM-producing *Enterobacteriaceae*, and would offer a partial solution to treat infections due to XDR or PDR Gram-negative bacteria [5].

Metallo-β-lactamase (NDM) is the most recently discovered carbapenemase capable of hydrolyzing almost all β-lactams present in Gram-negative pathogens produced mainly by *K. pneumoniae* and *Escherichia coli*, and is responsible for hospital and acquired infections in community [6].

In vitro data support the use of aztreonam (ATM) with ceftazidime/avibactam (CAZ/AVI) combination, but clinical studies are lacking. In a recent study, the CAZ/AVI + ATM combination offered a therapeutic advantage over other antibiotics for patients with BSI due to MBL-producing *Enterobacterales* [7].

We describe the successful treatment of a patient with the ceftazidime/avibactam + aztreonam combination below. This was effective not only in the treatment of sepsis, but also in the intestinal decolonization.

To our knowledge, this is the first case report in literature on intestinal decontamination using the ceftazidime/avibactam + aztreonam combination as treatment for *Klebsiella pneumoniae* NDM sepsis.

2. Case Report

On 27 November 2020, during the main peak of the second wave of the Sars-CoV2 pandemic, a 57-year-old man was admitted to the hematology department of our hospital with a diagnosis of acute TTP.

On admission, the physical examination revealed jaundice and purpura throughout the body; the total Khellaf score was 9.

Laboratory evaluation revealed a total platelet count of $8 \times 10^3/\mu L$, increased levels of total bilirubine (6.2 mg/dL), and serum creatinine (2.2 mg/dL), LDH (1499 mU/mL), with an Adamts 13 value of <0.01. A peripheral blood smear showed numerous schistocytes. Direct and indirect Coombs tests came back negative.

On the basis of these findings, we started plasma exchange therapy (a total of six sessions) together with methylprednisolone at 40 mg twice daily, along with a treatment by the humanized anti-von Willebrand Factor (vWF) nanobody caplacizumab of 10 mg after each plasma exchange session.

Seven days after the beginning of the therapy we observed a complete remission of the TTP.

On day 10 of hospitalization, the patient suddenly developed a fever and dyspnea requiring continuous oxygen support; the chest X-ray showed an image of diffuse bilateral opacities suggestive of an extended interstitial evolving pneumonia, and a nasopharyngeal swab was therefore realized and tested positive for SARS-CoV 2.

The further necessity for non-invasive mechanical ventilation required an ICU hospitalization on 11 December 2021.

Because of the fast-increasing respiratory distress, at day 2 of ICU hospitalization, we proceeded with the sedation, curarization, orotracheal intubation, and connection to mechanical ventilatory support.

Upon admission, the patient's signs and symptoms and the biological response to TTP were in regression: the total platelets count was $240 \times 10^3/\mu L$, serum creatinine was 1.3 mg/dL, and the level of total bilirubine was 1.5 mg/dL.

A CPE surveillance rectal swab performed on admission in the ICU tested positive for *Klebsiella Pneumoniae* NDM.

The patient had no recent history of hospitalization and no other predisposing risk factors. Thus, a horizontal transfer during the stay in hematology or a rare community acquired colonization were conceivable.

Between day 2 and day 3 of hospitalization in the intensive care unit, the patient conditions worsened: the total platelets count dropped to $5 \times 10^3/\mu L$ together with an increase in the serum creatinine, increasing levels of total bilirubine associated to the hemolysis, and Pct levels up to 7.12 ng/mL and WBC up to $1.46 \times 10^3/\mu L$.

The patient had developed a severe septic condition (SOFA score 9) that was causing the exacerbation of the TTP, thus requiring further cycles of plasma exchange.

After performing blood and urine cultures, we started a therapy with CAZ/AVI 1.25 mg q8 h plus AZT 1 gr q8 h for up to 10 days; we decided not to use colistin because of the renal failure.

Both the blood and urine cultures tested positive for KPC NMD with the same antibiogram profile tested in the rectal swab (Table 1).

Table 1. Resistance profile of the *K. pneumoniae* NDM strain found in the blood samples.

Antibiotics		MIC	MIC Breakpoint MICS	MICR
Cefepime	R	≥ 32	1	4
Cefotaxime	R	≥ 64	1	2
Ceftazidime	R	≥ 64	1	4
Ceftazidime/Avibactam	R	≥ 16	8	8
Ceftolozane/Tazobactam	R	≥ 32	2	2
Ciprofloxacine	R	≥ 4	0.25	0.5
Colistin	S	≤ 0.5	2	2
Gentamicine	R	≥ 16	2	4
Imipenem	R	≥ 16	2	4
Meropenem	R	≥ 16	2	8
Piperacilline/Tazobactam	R	≥ 128	8	16
Tobramycin	R	≥ -16	2	2
Trimetoprim/Sulfam	R	≥ 320	40	80

The patient's clinical conditions improved soon after the therapy introduction and after 10 days of treatment, the blood culture and rectal swab both tested negative; the resolution of the sepsis and the clinical improvement of the patient's conditions allowed for a progressive weaning, and finally, extubation at day 28.

The patient was then transferred to the medical ward for post-ICU rehabilitation.

3. Discussion

New Delhi metallo-β-lactamase (NDM-1), is one of the most clinically significant carbapenemases. It was first reported in New Delhi, India [6], followed by several clinical cases in the UK, Pakistan, and now around the world [2].

A large outbreak sustained by New Delhi metallo-β-lactamase (NDM)-producing *Enterobacterales* was recently documented in Tuscany, Italy [8].

In 2020, NDM-9-producing *Klebsiella pneumoniae* were isolated in the same geographic area.

A genomic and phylogenetic study suggested the correlation of the 2018–2019 and 2020 strains, with a change from the NDM-1 to NDM-9 carbapenemase variant in the latter [9]. No apparent changes in beta-lactam susceptibility were detected, and in addiction, new mutations in chromosomally encoded genes showed an acquired resistance to tigecycline, fosfomycin, and colistin.

The plasmid-carried bla-NDM gene is a transferable gene and it is capable of extensive rearrangement. This strongly suggests a marked capability for horizontal transfer from a colonized patient and a greater likelihood of occurrence between different bacterial strains.

Aztreonam, a monobactam antibiotic, is active against MBL-producing bacteria, but it is hydrolyzed by Ambler class A beta-lactamases (e.g., ESBL and KPCs) and class C (e.g., AmpC) beta-lactamases [10].

Since many MBL-producing Gram-negative bacteria may simultaneously express beta-lactamases or carbapenemases that could hydrolyze aztreonam, the combination with avibactam is able to inhibit cell wall synthesis in MBL-producing strains despite the presence of other co-carried beta-lactamases.

Aztreonam–avibactam showed a potent in-vitro activity against ESBL, class C β-lactamase, MBL, and KPC-producing strains with an activity 10 times that of aztreonam alone.

However, limited activity has been shown against *A. baumannii* or *P. aeruginosa* compared with aztreonam alone [11].

The potential for the use of CZA in combination with MEM, AMK, AZT, COL, and FOS against MDR *P. aeruginosa* and carbapenemase-producing *K. pneumoniae* was investigated in a recent publication [12]. Unfortunately, this study was not focused on MBL-producing bacteria, and surely, further research is merited to clarify the mechanisms of enhanced activity between CZA with MEM and other antibiotics together with further tests in clinical settings.

A phase III clinical trial to compare aztreonam–avibactam (with or without metronidazole) with meropenem (with or without colistin) for the treatment of HAP, VAP, and cIAI due to Gram-negative bacteria, for which there are limited or no treatment options, started in March 2018 and will end in 2021 [NCT03329092].

In a 2017 publication, Marshal et al. showed the in vitro efficacy of a unique combination of CAZ/AVI and ATM against most of the 21 representative *Enterobacteriaceae* isolates, with a complex molecular background that included blaIMP, blaNDM, blaOXA-48, blaCTX-M, blaAmpC, and combinations thereof [13].

This opened the way for the most promising new combination, currently available for NDM- or VIM-producing KPC.

From another point of view, key synergies in treating MBL infections especially lie with the action of avibactam.

Avibactam, inhibiting class A, C, and D β-lactamases, is thus supposed to leave ceftazidime and aztreonam not hydrolyzed by MBL, allowing them to act [14].

Another propriety of non-β-lactam β-lactamase inhibitor avibactam, as reported by Asli et al., is the ability to covalently bind to some bacterial PBPs, such as *E. coli* and *H. influenzae* PBP2, PBPs 2 and 3 of *P. aeruginosa* and *S. aureus*, and PBP3 of *S. pneumoniae*.

This capacity may explain its moderate antibacterial activity against some bacterial strains and species [15].

Patients like the one reported in our case provide strong evidence that intestinal colonization with KPC-Kp is associated with an increased hazard for high relative abundance of KPC-Kp in the gut microbiota, and additionally, the increased risk of KPC-Kp bacteremia [3].

As is already known, bacteriemia can rapidly evolve into sepsis and septic shock, especially if it occurs in debilitated patients affected by systemic diseases and needing intensive care unit treatments.

The COVID-19 pandemic continues to challenge healthcare systems around the world, and is indeed adding further challenges that we still do not fully understand in the antibiotic-resistance field.

The dramatically increased number of ICU hospitalizations, the direct or indirect role of SarsCoV-2 in the individual augmented risk for developing superinfections, and the spreading of nosocomial infections requiring antibiotic treatments on such a large scale will be impactful, and precipitate further widespread adverse health outcomes that we should be prepared for.

Like what happened with our patient, a Sars-CoV2 infection could rapidly lead to the worsening of the previous clinical conditions and the need for ICU hospitalization.

There are many ways beyond interstitial pneumonia—linked to opportunistic infections—in which a COVID-19 infection could rapidly worsen already unstable conditions of a hospitalized patient.

SARS-CoV-2 has linked impaired antigen presentation or acquired immunosuppression with concomitant lymphopenia [16,17], and the macro- and microcirculation alterations associated to the SARSCoV-2 hypercoagulability [18] can likely increase the risk of bacterial translocation [19], the classic example being the intestinal tract.

Endothelial dysfunctions of the digestive tract were frequently observed in COVID-19 and were associated with different mesenteric infarctions [20] that could explain the gut flora alteration and increased risk of translocations.

These considerations have also been taken into account in a recent French case–cohort study from the multicentric OUTCOMEREA network that showed how the daily hazard rate of ICU BSI in critically ill COVID-19 patients increased, and that this was more frequent seven days after ICU admission [21].

The extended use of immune-modulatory treatments, such as IL-1 or IL-6 receptors or antagonists in critically ill patients affected by Sars-CoV2, could surely play a role in these findings, as suggested by the French study.

There is an open literature debate about this argument. On the one hand (like in work recently published by the RECOVERY collaborative group [NCT04381936]), some studies are showing the non-negligible benefits associated with dexamethasone without significant increased risk of developing secondary infections compared with standards of care. Similar findings about the risk of secondary infections were also shown in two other recent RCTs [22,23].

On the other hand, some randomized trials of tocilizumab in COVID-19 have so far shown mixed results for 28–83 day mortality, and in a recent randomized-controlled trial [24], there was an increased risk of superinfections, and a similar trend was shown in the BSI.

The last, and more particular point of view in our case, is how interestingly the ceftazidime/avibactam + aztreonam combination therapy used was able to succeed in eradicating the *Klebsiella* NDM strain from the patient's gut as confirmed by two molecular tests.

The eradication of carbapenemase-producing *Klebsiella* from the gut is still a challenge and a matter of discussion.

Although various efforts have been made with both oral drugs and combined oral and systemic drugs, only partial results have been obtained.

Ceftazidime/avibactam plus aztreonam therapy could be one of the more useful solutions to consider in this field for selected patients.

4. Conclusions

The ceftazidime/avibactam + aztreonam treatment could not only be a valid therapeutic option for MBL-producing *Enterobacterales* infections, but it could also be considered as a useful tool in selected patients' intestinal decolonization.

Author Contributions: Conceptualization, F.P. and M.P.P.; methodology, F.P.; validation, F.P., M.P.P.; resources, F.P.; data curation, M.P.P. and F.P.; writing—original draft preparation, F.P.; writing— review and editing, M.P.P. and F.P.; funding acquisition, F.P. All authors have read and agreed to the published version of the manuscript.

Funding: This research received no external funding.

Institutional Review Board Statement: Not applicable.

Informed Consent Statement: Written informed consent has been obtained from the patient(s) to publish this paper.

Acknowledgments: In this section, you can acknowledge any support given which is not covered by the author contribution or funding sections. This may include administrative and technical support, or donations in kind (e.g., materials used for experiments).

Conflicts of Interest: The authors declare no conflict of interest.

References

1. Logan, L.K.; Weinstein, R.A. The epidemiology of Carbapenem-resistant enterobacteriaceae: The impact and evolution of a global menace. *J. Infect. Dis.* **2017**, *215*, S28–S36. [CrossRef] [PubMed]
2. Nordmann, P.; Dortet, L.; Poirel, L. Carbapenem resistance in Enterobacteriaceae: Here is the storm! *Trends Mol. Med.* **2012**, *18*, 263–272. [CrossRef]
3. Shimasaki, T.; Seekatz, A.; Bassis, C.; Rhee, Y.; Yelin, R.D.; Fogg, L.; Dangana, T.; Cisneros, E.C.; Weinstein, R.A.; Okamoto, K.; et al. Increased Relative Abundance of Klebsiella pneumoniae Carbapenemase-producing Klebsiella pneumoniae within the Gut Microbiota Is Associated with Risk of Bloodstream Infection in Long-term Acute Care Hospital Patients. *Clin. Infect. Dis.* **2019**, *68*, 2053–2059. [CrossRef] [PubMed]
4. Iacchini, S.; Sabbatucci, M.; Gagliotti, C.; Rossolini, G.M.; Moro, M.L.; Iannazzo, S.; D'Ancona, F.; Pezzotti, P.; Pantosti, A. Bloodstream infections due to carbapenemaseproducing Enterobacteriaceae in Italy: Results from nationwide surveillance, 2014 to 2017. *Eurosurveillance* **2019**, *24*, 1800159. [CrossRef] [PubMed]
5. Albiger, B.; Glasner, C.; Struelens, M.J.; Grundmann, H.; Monnet, D.L. Carbapenemase-producing Enterobacteriaceae in Europe: Assessment by national experts from 38 countries, May 2015. *Eurosurveillance* **2015**, *20*, 30062. [CrossRef]
6. Yong, D.; Toleman, M.A.; Giske, C.G.; Cho, H.S.; Sundman, K.; Lee, K.; Walsh, T.R. Characterization of a new metallo-β-lactamase gene, bla NDM-1, and a novel erythromycin esterase gene carried on a unique genetic structure in Klebsiella pneumoniae sequence type 14 from India. *Antimicrob. Agents Chemother.* **2009**, *53*, 5046–5054. [CrossRef] [PubMed]
7. Falcone, M.; Daikos, G.L.; Tiseo, G.; Bassoulis, D.; Giordano, C.; Galfo, V.; Leonildi, A.; Tagliaferri, E.; Barnini, S.; Sani, S.; et al. Efficacy of Ceftazidime-avibactam Plus Aztreonam in Patients with Bloodstream Infections Caused by Metallo-β-lactamase– Producing Enterobacterales. *Clin. Infect. Dis.* **2020**. [CrossRef]
8. Tavoschi, L.; Forni, S.; Porretta, A.; Righi, L.; Pieralli, F.; Menichetti, F.; Falcone, M.; Gemignani, G.; Sani, S.; Vivani, P.; et al. Prolonged outbreak of New Delhi metallo-betalactamase-producing carbapenem-resistant Enterobacterales (NDM-CRE), Tuscany, Italy, 2018 to 2019. *Eurosurveillance* **2020**, *25*, 2000085. [CrossRef]
9. Falcone, M.; Giordano, C.; Barnini, S.; Tiseo, G.; Leonildi, A.; Malacarne, P.; Menichetti, F.; Carattoli, A. Extremely drug-resistant NDM-9-producing ST147 Klebsiella pneumoniae causing infections in Italy, May 2020. *Eurosurveillance* **2020**, *25*, 3–8.
10. Jean, S.-S.; Lee, W.-S.; Lam, C.; Hsu, C.-W.; Chen, R.-J.; Hsueh, P.-R. Carbapenemase-producing Gram-negative bacteria: Current epidemics, antimicrobial susceptibility and treatment options. *Future Microbiol.* **2015**, *10*, 407–425. [CrossRef]
11. Bassetti, M.; Vena, A.; Castaldo, N.; Righi, E.; Peghin, M. New antibiotics for ventilator-associated pneumonia. *Curr. Opin. Infect. Dis.* **2018**, *31*, 177–186. [CrossRef] [PubMed]
12. Mikhail, S.; Singh, N.B.; Kebriaei, R.; Rice, S.A.; Stamper, K.C.; Castanheira, M.; Rybak, M.J. Evaluation of the synergy of ceftazidime-avibactam in combination with meropenem, amikacin, aztreonam, colistin, or fosfomycin against well-characterized multidrug-resistant Klebsiella pneumoniae and Pseudomonas aeruginosa. *Antimicrob. Agents Chemother.* **2019**, *63*, e00779-19. [CrossRef] [PubMed]

13. Marshall, S.; Hujer, A.M.; Rojas, L.J.; Papp-Wallace, K.M.; Humphries, R.M.; Spellberg, B.; Hujer, K.M.; Marshall, E.K.; Rudin, S.D.; Perez, F.; et al. Can Ceftazidime-Avibactam and Aztreonam Overcome β-Lactam Resistance Conferred by Metallo-β-Lactamases in *Enterobacteriaceae*? *Antimicrob. Agents Chemother.* **2017**, *61*, 1–9. [CrossRef] [PubMed]
14. Drawz, S.M.; Papp-Wallace, K.M.; Bonomo, R.A. New β-lactamase inhibitors: A therapeutic renaissance in an MDR world. *Antimicrob. Agents Chemother.* **2014**, *58*, 1835–1846. [CrossRef]
15. Asli, A.; Brouillette, E.; Krause, K.M.; Nichols, W.W.; Malouin, F. Distinctive binding of avibactam to penicillin-binding proteins of gram-negative and gram-positive bacteria. *Antimicrob. Agents Chemother.* **2016**, *60*, 752–756. [CrossRef]
16. Giamarellos-Bourboulis, E.J.; Netea, M.G.; Rovina, N.; Akinosoglou, K.; Antoniadou, A.; Antonakos, N.; Damoraki, G.; Gkavogianni, T.; Adami, M.-E.; Katsaounou, P.; et al. Complex Immune Dysregulation in COVID-19 Patients with Severe Respiratory Failure. *Cell Host Microbe* **2020**, *27*, 992–1000.e3. [CrossRef] [PubMed]
17. Terpos, E.; Ntanasis-Stathopoulos, I.; Elalamy, I.; Kastritis, E.; Sergentanis, T.N.; Politou, M.; Psaltopoulou, T.; Gerotziafas, G.; Dimopoulos, M.A. Hematological findings and complications of COVID-19. *Am. J. Hematol.* **2020**, *95*, 834–847. [CrossRef]
18. Dobesh, P.P.; Trujillo, T.C. Coagulopathy, Venous Thromboembolism, and Anticoagulation in Patients with COVID-19. *Pharmacotherapy* **2020**, *40*, 1130–1151. [CrossRef] [PubMed]
19. Cardinale, V.; Capurso, G.; Ianiro, G.; Gasbarrini, A.; Arcidiacono, P.G.; Alvaro, D. Intestinal permeability changes with bacterial translocation as key events modulating systemic host immune response to SARS-CoV-2: A working hypothesis. *Dig. Liver Dis.* **2020**, *52*, 1383–1389. [CrossRef]
20. Cheung, K.S.; Hung, I.F.; Chan, P.P.; Lung, K.C.; Tso, E.; Liu, R.; Ng, Y.Y.; Chu, M.Y.; Chung, T.W.; Tam, A.R.; et al. Gastrointestinal Manifestations of SARS-CoV-2 Infection and Virus Load in Fecal Samples From a Hong Kong Cohort: Systematic Review and Meta-analysis. *Gastroenterology* **2020**, *159*, 81–95. [CrossRef]
21. Buetti, N.; Ruckly, S.; de Montmollin, E.; Reignier, J.; Terzi, N.; Cohen, Y.; Shiami, S.; Dupuis, C.; Timsit, J.-F. COVID-19 increased the risk of ICU-acquired bloodstream infections: A case–cohort study from the multicentric OUTCOMEREA network. *Intensive Care Med.* **2021**, *47*, 180–187. [CrossRef] [PubMed]
22. Salvarani, C.; Dolci, G.; Massari, M.; Merlo, D.F.; Cavuto, S.; Savoldi, L.; Bruzzi, P.; Boni, F.; Braglia, L.; Turrà, C.; et al. Effect of Tocilizumab vs. Standard Care on Clinical Worsening in Patients Hospitalized with COVID-19 Pneumonia: A Randomized Clinical Trial. *JAMA Intern. Med.* **2021**, *181*, 24–31. [CrossRef] [PubMed]
23. Hermine, O.; Mariette, X.; Tharaux, P.L.; Resche-Rigon, M.; Porcher, R.; Ravaud, P.; Bureau, S.; Dougados, M.; Tibi, A.; Azoulay, E.; et al. Effect of Tocilizumab vs. Usual Care in Adults Hospitalized with COVID-19 and Moderate or Severe Pneumonia: A Randomized Clinical Trial. *JAMA Intern. Med.* **2021**, *181*, 32–40. [CrossRef] [PubMed]
24. Aziz, M.; Haghbin, H.; Abu Sitta, E.; Nawras, Y.; Fatima, R.; Sharma, S.; Lee-Smith, W.; Duggan, J.; Kammeyer, J.A.; Hanrahan, J.; et al. Efficacy of tocilizumab in COVID-19: A systematic review and meta-analysis. *J. Med. Virol.* **2021**, *93*, 1620–1630. [CrossRef] [PubMed]

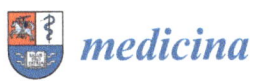

Article

Post-Prescription Audit Plus Beta-D-Glucan Assessment Decrease Echinocandin Use in People with Suspected Invasive Candidiasis

Rita Murri [1,2,*], Sara Lardo [3], Alessio De Luca [4], Brunella Posteraro [1,5], Riccardo Torelli [1,5], Giulia De Angelis [1,5], Francesca Giovannenze [1,2], Francesco Taccari [1], Lucia Pavan [4], Lucia Parroni [4], Maurizio Sanguinetti [1,5] and Massimo Fantoni [1,2]

1. Department of Laboratory and Infectious Diseases Sciences, A. Gemelli University Hospital Foundation IRCCS, 00168 Rome, Italy; brunella.posteraro@unicatt.it (B.P.); riccardo.torelli@policlinicogemelli.it (R.T.); giulia.deangelis@unicatt.it (G.D.A.); francesca.giovannenze@gmail.com (F.G.); francesco.taccari@policlinicogemelli.it (F.T.); maurizio.sanguinetti@unicatt.it (M.S.); massimo.fantoni@policlinicogemelli.it (M.F.)
2. Infectious Diseases Section, Department of Safety and Bioethics, Catholic University of the Sacred Heart, 00168 Rome, Italy
3. A. Gemelli University Hospital Foundation IRCCS, 00168 Rome, Italy; saralardo@gmail.com
4. Pharmacy Complex Operative Unit, A. Gemelli University Hospital Foundation IRCCS, 00168 Rome, Italy; alessio.deluca@policlinicogemelli.it (A.D.L.); lucia.pavan@policlinicogemelli.it (L.P.); lucia.parroni@policlinicogemelli.it (L.P.)
5. Department of Basic Biotechnology, Clinical Intensive Care and Perioperative Sciences, Catholic University of the Sacred Heart, 00168 Rome, Italy
* Correspondence: rita.murri@unicatt.it; Tel.: +39-333-456-2124

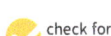

Abstract: *Background and Objectives:* Overtreatment with antifungal drugs is often observed. Antifungal stewardship (AFS) focuses on optimizing the treatment for invasive fungal diseases. The objective of the present study was to evaluate the utility of a post-prescription audit plus beta-D-glucan (BDG) assessment on reducing echinocandin use in persons with suspected invasive candidiasis. *Materials and Methods:* This is a prospective, pre-post quasi-experimental study of people starting echinocandins for suspected invasive candidiasis. The intervention of the study included review of each echinocandin prescription and discontinuation of treatment if a very low probability of fungal disease or a negative BDG value were found. Pre-intervention data were compared with the intervention phase. The primary outcome of the study was the duration of echinocandin therapy. Secondary outcomes were length of hospital stay and mortality. *Results:* Ninety-two echinocandin prescriptions were reviewed, 49 (53.3%) in the pre-intervention phase and 43 (46.7%) in the intervention phase. Discontinuation of antifungal therapy was possible in 21 of the 43 patients in the intervention phase (48.8%). The duration of echinocandin therapy was 7.4 (SD 4.7) in the pre-intervention phase, 4.1 days (SD 2.9) in persons undergoing the intervention, and 8.6 (SD 7.3) in persons in whom the intervention was not feasible (p at ANOVA = 0.016). Length of stay and mortality did not differ between pre-intervention and intervention phases. *Conclusions:* An intervention based on pre-prescription restriction and post-prescription audit when combined with BDG measurement is effective in optimizing antifungal therapy by significantly reducing excessive treatment duration.

Keywords: antifungal stewardship; *Candida* bloodstream infection; echinocandin

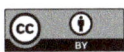

1. Introduction

Invasive candidiasis is becoming an emerging problem in hospital practice [1]. *Candida* is one of the leading causes of catheter-associated bloodstream infection (BSI) in the United States [2]. Mortality associated with invasive candidiasis is very high (51% in Internal Medicine in Italy) [3], and severely ill persons are more susceptible to *Candida* infections, leading to frequent antifungal drugs overtreatment. However, the diagnosis of invasive candidiasis and invasive fungal infection (IFI) is a complex task, because of the lack of standardized and widely accepted criteria. In addition, the large number of risk factors, limitations in diagnostic techniques, and lack of well-established criteria for initiating antifungal therapy are major problems in the approach to antifungal treatment. It follows that up to 42% of all antifungal therapies are empiric [4–7] and represent a huge field for potential optimization and antifungal stewardship (AFS) programs [8]. According to current definition, AFS refers to coordinated interventions to monitor and direct the appropriate use of antifungal agents in order to achieve the best clinical outcomes and minimize selective pressure and adverse events [9]. In some experiences, success in reducing overuse of antifungal therapies has been demonstrated, resulting in a containment of microbiological pressure on the ecosystem, which is recognized as the cause of resistance emergence [10]. In addition, the costs of antifungal therapies are often very high, and thus financial resource savings are an important driver of AFS. According to published guidelines [11,12], the optimal starting regimen for suspected invasive candidiasis are echinocandins, which mean high costs and potentially high selection pressure and induction of strains resistant to this crucial drug class. Thus, echinocandin discontinuation and de-escalation to azole-based therapies represents one of the cornerstones of any AFS programs.

Studies of beta-D-glucan (BDG) assessment have demonstrated its high negative predictive value [13,14]. Currently, BDG assessment has been widely introduced into clinical practice to discriminate people without candidemia and, when negative, offers valuable decision support for discontinuation of empiric antifungal therapy [13,15].

The objective of the present study was to evaluate the utility of a post-prescription audit plus BDG assessment on reducing echinocandin use in persons with suspected invasive candidiasis.

2. Materials and Methods

This is a prospective, pre-post quasi-experimental study of people starting echinocandins for suspected invasive candidiasis. The study was conducted at a 1100-bed university hospital in Italy (Fondazione Policlinico A. Gemelli IRCCS, Università Cattolica S. Cuore). An antimicrobial stewardship program has been active in the hospital since 2013; it is not active in hematological units and intensive care units (ICUs), and therefore patients in these units were not included in the study.

In our hospital, for an echinocandin treatment to be prescribed, a form is required from the hospital pharmacy. However, no restrictions were in place before the present intervention study, and every request was fulfilled. For fluconazole, the order is cumulative for the entire department, and the prescription is recorded on a nonelectronic form, and thus it was impossible to verify the prescription on a patient-by-patient basis. Therefore, patients who were prescribed fluconazole were excluded from the Intervention.

In the pre-intervention phase (Period 1), from January to May 2017, we reviewed all the echinocandins' prescription forms sent to the hospital pharmacy service and we collected patients' data. In the pre-intervention phase, we did not make any clinical suggestion, except when attending physicians actively requested an infectious diseases specialist advice. In the intervention phase (Period 2), from September 2017 to February 2018, we prospectively collected data of patients who were prescribed with echinocandins. Each echinocandin prescription was reviewed, IFI diagnosis was verified on both medical records and at the bedside, and inappropriate prescriptions were actively discussed with attending physicians who remained the final prescribers and could decide not to discontinue echinocandins. The intervention included discontinuation of treatment in patients with a very low probability of having IFI and with a negative BDG value, when available.

Risk factors for invasive candidiasis were considered according to a previous published article [16]: having a central venous catheter, total parenteral nutrition, recent surgery, previous admission to an ICU, previous antibiotic therapy, hemodialysis, solid organ transplantation, or multiple underlying medical conditions.

The primary outcome of the study was the duration of echinocandin therapy. Secondary outcomes were length of hospital stay (LOS) and mortality.

2.1. Microbiology

The Fungitell assay (Associates of Cape Cod, East Falmouth, MA, USA) was used to measure BDG. BDG results were evaluated using different cutoff values: 80, 200, 300, 400, and >500 pg/mL. For clinical use, the BDG test was considered positive if BDG had a result above the manufacturer's recommended cut-off (80 pg/mL). Only BDG available within +48 h after initiation of antifungal therapy was considered for analysis. Informed consent was not required because the activity does not alter routine clinical practice, and only cumulative and anonymized data were analyzed.

2.2. Statistical Analysis

Descriptive data are presented. Normally distributed values are expressed as mean (± standard deviation (SD)) and non-normally distributed values as median (interquartile range (IQR)). Chi-squared test or Fisher's exact test were used to compare the distribution of categorical variables, and Student's t or Mann–Whitney U test was used to compare quantitative variables. A two-sided p value < 0.05 was considered statistically significant. The Kaplan–Meier method was used to estimate the correlation between intervention and 30-day mortality. All statistical analyses were performed using SPSS 17.0 (IBM SPSS Statistics for Windows, SPSS Inc., Chicago, IL, USA).

3. Results

Since January 2017, all the echinocandin prescriptions (n = 92) were reviewed, 49 (53.3%) in the pre-intervention phase and 43 (46.7%) in the intervention phase. If a patient had more than one echinocandin prescription, only the first one was considered for the present study. The mean age of those enrolled was 67 years (SD 13.8), 31 (33.7%) were female, and 68 patients (73.9%) were admitted to a medical ward. None of the included patients were neutropenic (Table 1). Thirty-nine (42.4%) died within 30 days of starting antifungal therapy.

Table 1. Characteristics of the 92 patients for whom an echinocandin was prescribed.

Age, Mean (SD), Years.	67.0 (13.8)
Female (%)	31 (33.7)
Medical ward (%)	68 (73.9)
Surgical ward (%)	24 (26.1)
Anidulafungin	41 (44.6)
Caspofungin	51 (55.4)
Beta-D-glucan value	
<80 pg/mL	52 (56.5)
>80 pg/mL	27 (29.3)
>500 pg/mL	10 (10.9)
Not done	13 (14.1)

All the patients who began empirical antifungal therapy had clinical signs consistent with invasive candidiasis and at least one risk factor for invasive candidiasis.

None of the patients who received an empiric antifungal regimen were subsequently found to have culture-proved evidence of invasive candidiasis. No treatment was prescribed for prophylactic purposes.

Discontinuation of antifungal therapy was possible in 21 of the 43 patients in the intervention phase (48.8%). Of these 21 patients, BDG was available in 19 (in 14 cases, BDG was <80 pg/mL). In five cases, BDG >80 pg/mL was considered a false positive. In all patients who discontinued antifungal therapy, blood cultures (and peritoneal fluid cultures when indicated) were negative. Discontinuation of therapy was not possible in 22 cases: 17 patients were too sick, and in five cases, BDG was very high (>500 pg/mL) (Figure 1). The very high levels of BDG in these patients confirmed the suspicion of invasive candidiasis, contraindicating discontinuation of antifungal therapy, but it was not sufficient in the absence of positive cultures to establish a definite diagnosis of invasive candidiasis.

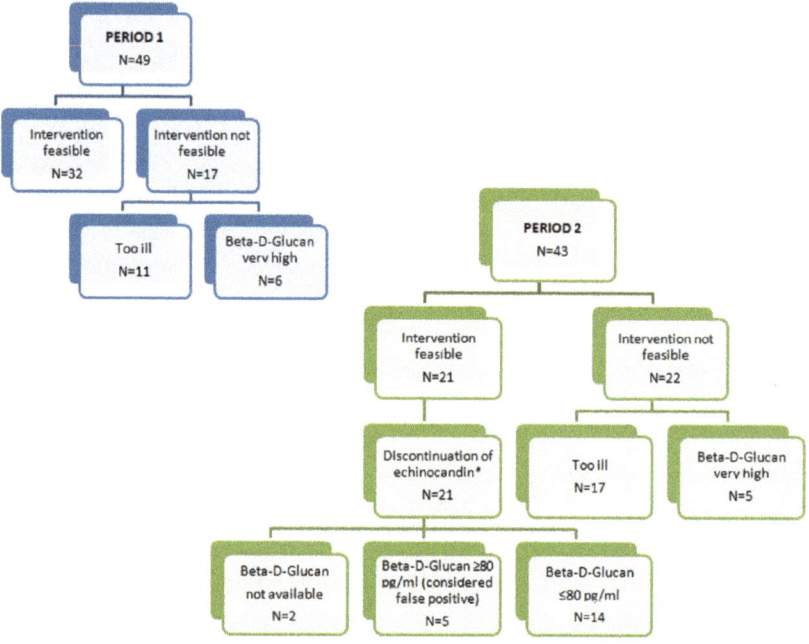

Figure 1. Flowchart of the study. * All patients who discontinued echinocandin had negative blood cultures for *Candida* spp.

Individuals with BDG < 80 pg/mL or not done, when compared with patients with BDG > 80 pg/mL, had shorter duration of therapy (6.1 days (SD 5.0) versus 9.8 (SD 7.5); $p = 0.007$) and shorter length of stay (23.7 days (SD 31.4) versus 19.8 (SD 21.2); $p = 0.06$). The correlation between BDG outcome and duration of therapy was significant only in the intervention phase (Table 2).

Table 2. Correlation between beta-D-glucan results with duration of therapy and length of stay.

Duration of Antifungal Therapy, Days, Mean (SD)	Beta-D-Glucan < 80 pg/mL or not Done	Beta-D-Glucan > 80 pg/mL	p
Total	6.1 (5.0)	9.8 (7.5)	0.007
Pre-intervention period	6.4 (4.9)	8.4 (5.9)	0.29
Intervention period	5.5 (5.2)	10.8 (7.9)	0.026
Length of stay, days, mean (SD)	Beta-D-glucan <80 pg/mL or not done	Beta-D-glucan >80 pg/mL	p
Total	23.7 (31.4)	19.8 (21.2)	0.06

Acceptance of the intervention from the treating physician, who remained the final prescriber and who could decide not to discontinue echinocandins, was very high, although this was not formally recorded. The requested time in terms of human resources was estimated at 1–1.5 days per week.

The duration of echinocandin therapy was 4.1 days (SD 2.9) in persons undergoing the intervention, 8.6 (SD 7.3) in persons in whom the intervention was not feasible, and 7.4 (SD 4.7) in persons in the pre-intervention period (p at ANOVA = 0.016). The mean duration of therapy in persons who did not receive an intervention was 8.1 days (SD 6.3). Duration of therapy was shorter in the intervention group than in people who did not receive an intervention ($p < 0.001$). Length of stay was 19.1 days (SD 25.3) in persons who received the intervention, 21.2 days (SD 33.8) in persons in whom the intervention was not feasible, and 26.6 (SD 23.9) in persons in the pre-intervention phase (p at ANOVA 0.61) (Table 3).

Table 3. Outcomes of the study.

Outcomes	Intervention not Done N = 71	Intervention Done N = 21	p
Antifungal therapy duration, days, mean (SD)	8.1 (6.3)	4.1 (2.9)	<0.001
Length of hospitalization, days, mean (SD)	23.6 (29.8)	19.1 (25.3)	0.54
Death (%)	30 (42.3)	9 (42.8)	0.96

Outcomes	Period 1 N = 49	Period 2, not feasible N = 22	Period 2, feasible N = 21	p at ANOVA
Antifungal therapy duration, days, mean (SD)	7.4 (4.7)	8.6 (7.3)	4.1 (2.9)	0.016
Length of hospitalization, days, mean (SD)	26.6 (23.9)	21.2 (33.8)	19.1 (25.3)	0.61
Death (%)	17 (34.7)	13 (59.1)	9 (42.8)	0.57

Nine persons died in the intervention group (42.8%), 17 (34.7%) in persons in whom the intervention was not done, and 13 (59.1%) in persons for whom an intervention was not feasible (log-rank at Kaplan–Meier estimate = 0.64).

4. Discussion

In the present study, we demonstrated that an intervention based on pre-prescription restriction and post-prescription audit when combined with BDG measurement is effective in optimizing antifungal therapy by significantly reducing excessive treatment duration.

Several predictive scores of invasive fungal infections are available [17–19] and include variables that are largely present in most hospitalized patients or are very impractical to obtain in non-intensive care units, such as the number of *Candida* colonization sites. The predictive power of these variables is therefore poor. This uncertainty about the likelihood of diagnosis as well as awareness of the high mortality of invasive fungal infections likely underlies widely recognized overtreatment. In one study, more than half of antifungal prescriptions were described as suboptimal, with 16% considered unnecessary [6]. Overtreatment may be associated with several disadvantages. First, unnecessary pressure on the local ecology may contribute to increased antifungal resistance [10]. An increased incidence of *Candida* infections caused by strains resistant to fluconazole or to echinocandin has been reported [20–22]. In addition, many antifungals have complex pharmacokinetics and require careful consideration of drug–drug interactions [23]. Moreover, adverse events should be considered in the cost-effectiveness of any antifungal treatment [24]. Finally, antifungal treatments are often associated with high costs.

AFS programs are designed to reduce the overuse of empiric antifungal therapies and to optimize individualized regimens. The cornerstones of these programs are post-prescription audits, formulary restrictions (preauthorization strategies), discontinuation of therapies when they are not needed, and de-escalation from echinocandin to oral fluconazole when appropriate [8]. To date, published studies on the effectiveness of AFS programs are not numerous, and the most effective type of intervention remains unclear. Post-prescription audits, often associated with pre-prescription restrictions, have demonstrated a significant reduction in antifungal consumption [8,25–28]. In a Spanish study of 100 patients admitted to different hospital wards, a non-mandatory bedside intervention significantly reduced consumption and cost of antifungal treatments [29]. Whitney et al. published the results on a 6-year AFS program on more than 400 patients with a comprehensive approach that included stewardship rounds. The authors found a significant decrease in overall antifungal consumption and financial costs [29]. A few other studies have shown significant decrease in costs [26,30] and adverse events [31], without a different impact on survival. However, some of them identified a very small sample size [30,32], and most of them focused on optimizing only high-cost antifungal treatment [26]. Few studies incorporated therapeutic drug monitoring (TDM) measurement into AFS programs.

Several papers have previously demonstrated a very high negative predictive value of BDG, and clinicians can use a negative result to discontinue empiric antifungal therapy. However, only one published study has shown results on the implementation of BDG within AFS programs [32]. In the present study, negative BDG results were used to discontinue antifungals in 14 of 43 patients in the intervention phase (32.5%). Considering only patients for whom an intervention was feasible, BDG was used to discontinue unnecessary antifungal treatments in 14 of 21 cases (66.7%). Because spending on antifungals in our hospital was approximately EUR 1,200,000, a 32.5% savings would allow us to reduce costs by 390,000 per year. The cost of the BDG test was less than savings. Moreover, it should be taken into account that the time needed to get BDG results is shorter (few hours, depending on laboratory's capacity) than classic culture methods, thus representing a fundamental tool for early unnecessary antifungal discontinuation in AFS programs.

In the present study, the duration of empiric therapy was longer for patients without an intervention. Possibly, without the intervention of the AFS team, noninfectious disease physicians are more reluctant to de-escalate or discontinue antimicrobial treatments.

The overall 30-day mortality in the present study was 42.4%, similar to previously published studies [1,8], demonstrating that antifungal discontinuation was safe and did not result in unintended increased mortality.

Previously published studies included mainly patients with hematological diseases, and the most represented disease was aspergillosis. Hematological patients have peculiar characteristics such as the use of a high rate of antifungal prophylaxis, specific guidelines for antifungal treatment management, and noninfectious disease specialists as primary prescribers (so-called champions). In our study, hematologic patients were excluded, and results included, through a bedside approach, a hospital-level approach in a nonspecific setting.

It may be argued that fluconazole-treated patients should be included in AFS programs and that excluding them from this intervention may have reduced study size and statistical significance. However, after IDSA guidelines published in 2016 [12], echinocandins are considered the agent of choice in the suspicion of invasive candidiasis, even in non-neutropenic patients, and the use of fluconazole is restricted as an alternative agent in patients not critically ill and in those who have a low risk of fluconazole-resistant organisms. It follows that the use of fluconazole as empiric starting therapy in patients with suspected IFI has markedly decreased in clinical practice. For example, the use of echinocandins as initial antifungal therapy in *Candida* bloodstream infections at our institution has increased from 60.7% in 2013 to 88% in 2019 (unpublished data). Thus, despite its potential role in widening the pool of suitable patients for AFS, adding fluconazole-treated patients to this study population would not have had a great statistical impact.

Nevertheless, it is reasonable that our intervention will be effective, even in patients receiving fluconazole as empiric antifungal therapy. Actually, in previous studies on AFS programs including fluconazole-treated patients, the majority of those who received empiric antifungal therapy had no diagnostic criteria for invasive fungal infection, and stopping antifungal therapy was one of the most commonly applied interventions [29].

Lack of staff time is one of the most frequent factors considered as a barrier to AFS, according to a UK survey [26]. However, time spent on the intervention in our experience has been limited and low-cost infrastructure is needed for the program. This suggests easy reproducibility of the intervention in other clinical centers.

Our study has several limitations. First, the single-center design limits the generalizability of the results to hospitals with different patient populations. Second, because hematologic patients are not included, neutropenic patients are very rare, and no conclusions can be drawn for this population. Third, adverse effects of antifungals and readmission rates were not evaluated.

5. Conclusions

In conclusions, we demonstrated significant resource savings through reduction in the duration of antifungal therapy by means of an easily reproducible intervention. AFS programs are feasible and cost-effective, especially when combined with the use of well-validated biomarkers such as BDG. AFS could be a standard of care in hospitals with specialized units as well as a reference point for noninfectious disease specialists.

Author Contributions: Conceptualization, R.M., M.S., and M.F.; data curation, R.M., S.L., F.G., and F.T.; formal analysis, R.M. and B.P.; investigation, M.F.; methodology, A.D.L., B.P., R.T., G.D.A., F.G., F.T., L.P. (Laura Pavan), and L.P. (Lucia Parroni); project administration, R.M.; resources, S.L. and M.S.; supervision, M.F.; writing—original draft, R.M.; writing—review and editing, B.P., G.D.A., M.S., and M.F. All authors have read and agreed to the published version of the manuscript.

Funding: This research received no external funding.

Institutional Review Board Statement: Not applicable.

Informed Consent Statement: Not applicable.

Data Availability Statement: Data are available from the corresponding author upon request.

Conflicts of Interest: The authors declare no conflict of interest.

References

1. Pappas, P.G.; Lionakis, M.S.; Arendrup, M.C.; Ostrosky-Zeichner, L.; Kullberg, B.J. Invasive candidiasis. *Nat. Rev. Dis. Primers* **2018**, *4*, 18026. [CrossRef]
2. Pfaller, M.A.; Castanheira, M. Nosocomial Candidiasis: Antifungal Stewardship and the Importance of Rapid Diagnosis. *Med. Mycol.* **2016**, *54*, 1–22. [CrossRef] [PubMed]
3. Bassetti, M.; Merelli, M.; Righi, E.; Diaz-Martin, A.; Rosello, E.M.; Luzzati, R.; Parra, A.; Trecarichi, E.M.; Sanguinetti, M.; Posteraro, B.; et al. Epidemiology, species distribution, antifungal susceptibility, and outcome of candidemia across five sites in Italy and Spain. *J. Clin. Microbiol.* **2013**, *51*, 4167–4172. [CrossRef]
4. Martínez-Jiménez, M.C.; Muñoz, P.; Valerio, M.; Vena, A.; Guinea, J.; Bouza, E. Combination of *Candida* biomarkers in patients receiving empirical antifungal therapy in a Spanish tertiary hospital: A potential role in reducing the duration of treatment. *J. Antimicrob. Chemother.* **2015**, *70*, 3107–3115. [CrossRef] [PubMed]
5. Leon, C.; Ostrosky-Zeichner, L.; Schuster, M. What it's new in the clinical and diagnostic management of invasive candidiasis in critically ill patients. *Intensive Care Med.* **2014**, *40*, 808–819. [CrossRef]
6. Valerio, M.; Rodriguez-Gonzalez, C.G.; Muñoz, P.; Caliz, B.; Sanjurjo, M.; Bouza, E.; COMIC Study Group (Collaborative Group on Mycoses). Evaluation of antifungal use in a tertiary care institution: Antifungal stewardship urgently needed. *J. Antimicrob. Chemother.* **2014**, *69*, 1993–1999. [CrossRef] [PubMed]
7. Ruhnke, M. Antifungal stewardship in invasive *Candida* infections. *Clin. Microbiol. Infect.* **2014**, *20* (Suppl. 6), 11–18. [CrossRef]
8. Ananda-Rajah, M.R.; Slavin, M.A.; Thursky, K.T. The case for an-tifungal stewardship. *Curr. Opin. Infect. Dis.* **2012**, *25*, 107–115. [CrossRef]
9. Hamdy, R.F.; Zaoutis, T.E.; Seo, S.K. Antifungal stewardship considerations for adults and pediatrics. *Virulence* **2017**, *8*, 658–672. [CrossRef]

10. Perlin, D.S.; Rautemaa-Richardson, R.; Alastruey-Izquierdo, A. The global problem of antifungal resistance: Prevalence, mechanisms, and management. *Lancet Infect. Dis.* **2017**, *17*, e383–e392. [CrossRef]
11. Cornely, O.A.; Bassetti, M.; Calandra, T.; Garbino, J.; Kullberg, B.J.; Lortholary, O.; Meersseman, W.; Akova, M.; Arendrup, M.C.; Arikan-Akdagli, S.; et al. ESCMID* guideline for the diagnosis and management of Candida diseases 2012: Non-neutropenic adult patients. *Clin. Microbiol. Infect.* **2012**, *18* (Suppl. 7), 19–37. [CrossRef] [PubMed]
12. Pappas, P.G.; Kauffman, C.A.; Andes, D.R.; Clancy, C.J.; Marr, K.A.; Ostrosky-Zeichner, L.; Reboli, A.C.; Schuster, M.G.; Vazquez, J.A.; Walsh, T.J.; et al. Clinical Practice Guideline for the Management of Candidiasis: 2016 Update by the Infectious Diseases Society of America. *Clin. Infect. Dis.* **2016**, *62*, e1–e50. [CrossRef]
13. Murri, R.; Camici, M.; Posteraro, B.; Giovannenze, F.; Taccari, F.; Ventura, G.; Scoppettuolo, G.; Sanguinetti, M.; Cauda, R.; Fantoni, M. Performance evaluation of the (1,3)-β-D-glucan detection assay in non-intensive care unit adult patients. *Infect. Drug Resist.* **2018**, *12*, 19–24. [CrossRef] [PubMed]
14. Posteraro, B.; De Pascale, G.; Tumbarello, M.; Torelli, R.; Pennisi, M.A.; Bello, G.; Maviglia, R.; Fadda, G.; Sanguinetti, M.; Antonelli, M. Early diagnosis of candidemia in intensive care unit patients with sepsis: A prospective comparison of (1→3)-β-D-glucan assay, Candida score, and colonization index. *Crit. Care* **2011**, *15*, R249. [CrossRef] [PubMed]
15. Posteraro, B.; Tumbarello, M.; De Pascale, G.; Liberto, E.; Vallecoccia, M.S.; De Carolisn, E.; Di Gravio, V.; Trecarichi, E.M.; Sanguinetti, M.; Antonelli, M. (1,3)-β-d-Glucan-based antifungal treatment in critically ill adults at high risk of candidaemia: An observational study. *J. Antimicrob. Chemother.* **2016**, *71*, 2262–2269. [CrossRef]
16. Scudeller, L.; Viscoli, C.; Menichetti, F.; del Bono, V.; Cristini, F.; Tascini, C.; Bassetti, M.; Viale, P.; ITALIC Group. An Italian consensus for invasive candidiasis management (ITALIC). *Infection* **2014**, *42*, 263–279. [CrossRef]
17. León, C.; Ruiz-Santana, S.; Saavedra, P.; Almirante, B.; Nolla-Salas, J.; Alvarez-Lerma, F.; Garnacho-Montero, J.; León, M.A.; EPCAN Study Group. A bedside scoring system ("Candida score") for early antifungal treatment in nonneutropenic critically ill patients with Candida colonization. *Crit. Care Med.* **2006**, *34*, 730–737. [CrossRef]
18. Ostrosky-Zeichner, L.; Sable, C.; Sobel, J.; Alexander, B.D.; Donowitz, G.; Kan, V.; Kauffman, C.A.; Kett, D.; Larsen, R.A.; Morrison, V.; et al. Multicenter retrospective development and validation of a clinical prediction rule for nosocomial invasive candidiasis in the intensive care setting. *Eur. J. Clin. Microbiol. Infect. Dis.* **2007**, *26*, 271–276. [CrossRef]
19. Sozio, E.; Pieralli, F.; Azzini, A.M.; Tintori, G.; Demma, F.; Furneri, G.; Sbrana, F.; Bertolino, G.; Fortunato, S.; Meini, S.; et al. A prediction rule for early recognition of patients with candidemia in Internal Medicine: Results from an Italian, multicentric, case-control study. *Infection* **2018**, *46*, 625–633. [CrossRef]
20. Beyda, N.D.; John, J.; Kilic, A.; Alam, M.J.; Lasco, T.M.; Garey, K.W. FKS mutant *Candida* glabrata: Risk factors and outcomes in patients with candidemia. *Clin. Infect. Dis.* **2014**, *59*, 819–825. [CrossRef]
21. Slavin, M.A.; Sorrell, T.C.; Marriott, D.; Thursky, K.A.; Nguyen, Q.; Ellis, D.H.; Morrissey, C.O.; Chen, S.C.; Australian Candidemia Study, Australasian Society for Infectious Diseases. Candidaemia in adult cancer patients: Risks for fluconazole-resistant isolates and death. *J. Antimicrob. Chemother.* **2010**, *65*, 1042–1051. [CrossRef]
22. Lortholary, O.; Desnos-Ollivier, M.; Sitbon, K.; Fontanet, A.; Bretagne, S.; Dromer, F.; French Mycosis Study Group. Recent exposure to caspofungin or fluconazole influences the epidemiology of candidemia: A prospective multicenter study involving 2441 patients. *Antimicrob. Agents Chemother.* **2011**, *55*, 532–538. [CrossRef]
23. Andes, D.; Azie, N.; Yang, H.; Harrington, R.; Kelley, C.; Tan, R.D.; Wu, E.Q.; Franks, B.; Kristy, R.; Lee, E.; et al. Drug-Drug Interaction Associated with Mold-Active Triazoles among Hospitalized Patients. *Antimicrob. Agents Chemother.* **2016**, *60*, 3398–3406. [CrossRef]
24. Mourad, A.; Perfect, J.R. Tolerability profile of the current antifungal armoury. *J. Antimicrob. Chemother.* **2018**, *73* (Suppl. 1), i26–i32. [CrossRef]
25. Bienvenu, A.L.; Argaud, L.; Aubrun, F.; Fellahi, J.L.; Guerin, C.; Javouhey, E.; Piriou, V.; Rimmele, T.; Chidiac, C.; Leboucher, G. A systematic review of interventions and performance measures for antifungal stewardship programmes. *J. Antimicrob. Chemother.* **2018**, *73*, 297–305. [CrossRef]
26. Micallef, C.; Ashiru-Oredope, D.; Hansraj, S.; Denning, D.W.; Agrawal, S.G.; Manuel, R.J.; Schelenz, S.; Guy, R.; Muller-Pebody, B.; Patel, R.; et al. An investigation of antifungal stewardship programmes in England. *J. Med. Microbiol.* **2017**, *66*, 1581–1589. [CrossRef] [PubMed]
27. Lachenmayr, S.J.; Berking, S.; Horns, H.; Strobach, D.; Ostermann, H.; Berger, K. Antifungal treatment in haematological and oncological patients: Need for quality assessment in routine care. *Mycoses* **2018**, *61*, 464–471. [CrossRef]
28. Standiford, H.C.; Chan, S.; Tripoli, M.; Weekes, E.; Forrest, G.N. Antimicrobial stewardship at a large tertiary care academic medical center: Cost analysis before, during, and after a 7-year program. *Infect. Control Hosp. Epidemiol.* **2012**, *33*, 338–345. [CrossRef] [PubMed]
29. Whitney, L.; Al-Ghusein, H.; Glass, S.; Koh, M.; Klammer, M.; Ball, J.; Youngs, J.; Wake, R.; Houston, A.; Bicanic, T. Effectiveness of an antifungal stewardship programme at a London teaching hospital 2010-16. *J. Antimicrob. Chemother.* **2019**, *74*, 234–241. [CrossRef] [PubMed]
30. Benoist, H.; Rodier, S.; de La Blanchardière, A.; Bonhomme, J.; Cormier, H.; Thibon, P.; Saint-Lorant, G. Appropriate use of antifungals: Impact of an antifungal stewardship program on the clinical outcome of candidaemia in a French University Hospital. *Infection* **2019**, *47*, 435–440. [CrossRef]

31. Valerio, M.; Muñoz, P.; Rodríguez, C.G.; Caliz, B.; Padilla, B.; Fernández-Cruz, A.; Sánchez-Somolinos, M.; Gijón, P.; Peral, J.; Gayoso, J.; et al. Antifungal stewardship in a tertiary-care institution: A bedside intervention. *Clin. Microbiol. Infect.* **2015**, *21*, e1–e9. [CrossRef] [PubMed]
32. Ito-Takeichi, S.; Niwa, T.; Fujibayashi, A.; Suzuki, K.; Ohta, H.; Niwa, A.; Tsuchiya, M.; Yamamoto, M.; Hatakeyama, D.; Suzuki, A.; et al. The impact of implementing an antifungal stewardship with monitoring of 1-3, β-D-glucan values on antifungal consumption and clinical outcomes. *J. Clin. Pharm. Ther.* **2019**, *44*, 454–462. [CrossRef] [PubMed]

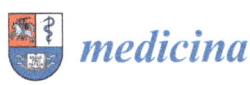

Article

The Role of Early Procalcitonin Determination in the Emergency Department in Adults Hospitalized with Fever

Marcello Covino [1,2,*], Antonella Gallo [3], Massimo Montalto [2,3], Giuseppe De Matteis [3], Maria Livia Burzo [4], Benedetta Simeoni [1], Rita Murri [2,5], Marcello Candelli [1], Veronica Ojetti [1,2] and Francesco Franceschi [1,2]

1. Emergency Medicine, Fondazione Policlinico Universitario A. Gemelli, IRCSS, 00168 Rome, Italy; bsimeoni@gmail.com (B.S.); marcello.candelli@policlinicogemelli.it (M.C.); vojetty@gmail.com (V.O.); francesco.franceschi@unicatt.it (F.F.)
2. Faculty of Medicine and Surgery, Università Cattolica del Sacro Cuore, 00168 Rome, Italy; massimo.montalto@unicatt.it (M.M.); rita.murri@unicatt.it (R.M.)
3. Department of Internal Medicine, Fondazione Policlinico Universitario A. Gemelli, IRCSS, 00168 Rome, Italy; antonella.gallo@policlinicogemelli.it (A.G.); dr.giuseppedematteis@gmail.com (G.D.M.)
4. Emergency Department, Ospedale Generale M.G. Vannini, Istituto Figlie di San Camillo, 00177 Rome, Italy; maliburzo@gmail.com
5. Department of Infectious Diseases, Fondazione Policlinico Universitario A. Gemelli IRCCS, 00168 Rome, Italy
* Correspondence: Marcello.covino@policlinicogemelli.it

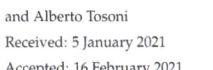

Citation: Covino, M.; Gallo, A.; Montalto, M.; De Matteis, G.; Burzo, M.L.; Simeoni, B.; Murri, R.; Candelli, M.; Ojetti, V.; Franceschi, F. The Role of Early Procalcitonin Determination in the Emergency Department in Adults Hospitalized with Fever. *Medicina* **2021**, *57*, 179. https://doi.org/10.3390/medicina57020179

Academic Editors: Antonio Mirijello and Alberto Tosoni

Received: 5 January 2021
Accepted: 16 February 2021
Published: 19 February 2021

Publisher's Note: MDPI stays neutral with regard to jurisdictional claims in published maps and institutional affiliations.

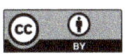

Copyright: © 2021 by the authors. Licensee MDPI, Basel, Switzerland. This article is an open access article distributed under the terms and conditions of the Creative Commons Attribution (CC BY) license (https://creativecommons.org/licenses/by/4.0/).

Abstract: *Background and Objectives:* Fever is one of the most common presenting complaints in the Emergency Department (ED). The role of serum procalcitonin (PCT) determination in the ED evaluation of adults presenting with fever is still debated. The aim of this study was to evaluate if, in adults presenting to the ED with fever and then hospitalized, the early PCT determination could improve prognosis. *Materials and Methods.* This is a retrospective, mono-centric study, conducted over a 10-year period (2009–2018). We analyzed consecutive patients ≥18 years admitted to ED with fever and then hospitalized. According to quick sequential organ failure assessment (qSOFA) at admission, we compared patients that had a PCT determination vs. controls. Primary endpoint was overall in-hospital mortality; secondary endpoints were in-hospital length of stay, and mortality in patients with bloodstream infection and acute respiratory infections. *Results.* The sample included 12,062 patients, median age was 71 years and 55.1% were men. In patients with qSOFA ≥ 2 overall mortality was significantly lower if they had a PCT-guided management in ED, (20.5% vs. 26.5%; $p = 0.046$). In the qSOFA < 2 group the mortality was not significantly different in PCT patients, except for those with a final diagnosis of bloodstream infection. *Conclusions.* Among adults hospitalized with fever, the PCT evaluation at ED admission was not associated with better outcomes, with the possible exception of patients affected by bloodstream infections. However, in febrile patients presenting to the ED with qSOFA ≥ 2, the early PCT evaluation could improve the overall in-hospital survival.

Keywords: procalcitonin; emergency department; qSOFA; sepsis; fever

1. Introduction

Fever is one of the most common cause of Emergency Department (ED) access, accounting for 5% up to 15% of adult visits [1]. It represents an early warning sign of most infections, but could also be present in several non-infectious diseases, such as autoimmune diseases, and neoplasms [1].

An early antimicrobial administration demonstrated to be associated with reduced mortality in patients with bacterial infection and sepsis [1], thus the identification of fever of bacterial origin is essential for clinicians. Several clinical and laboratory tests were evaluated for this purpose, but none of them demonstrated an adequate sensitivity and specificity to definitively rule in a bacterial cause of fever [1].

Procalcitonin (PCT) is a precursor protein of calcitonin, expressed by human cells [2]. Its production is upregulated by pro-inflammatory cytokines like interleukin (IL)-1, IL-2,

IL-6 and tumor necrosis factor alpha, and by bacterial endotoxins and lipopolysaccharide, while it is downregulated during viral infections [2,3]. Moreover, patients with autoimmune diseases or malignancies usually have low levels of PCT [4].

Several trials have reliably demonstrated the good performance of PCT in supporting the decision to start or stop antibiotic therapy in patients with suspected bacterial infections, leading to potential benefit in term of reduced length of in-hospital stays (LOS) and survival [5–7]. On these bases, in 2017 the United States Food and Drug Administration approved the use of PCT for guiding antibiotic therapy in acute respiratory infections and sepsis [8]. However, although PCT-guided management showed a good performance in selected populations, its role in patients with undifferentiated fever in ED is still unclear [9–12].

The aim of this study is to evaluate, in adults hospitalized with fever, if an early PCT determination at ED admission was associated to an improvement of the patient's level outcomes, defined as the reduction of overall in-hospital mortality and LOS.

2. Materials and Methods

This is a retrospective study conducted in an academic medical center with an average attendance at the ED of about 75,000 patients annually (more than 87% adults). Based on electronic health records, we identified all consecutive patients admitted in ED for fever and then hospitalized during a 10-year period, between 1st January 2009 and 31 December 2018. We included in the analysis all patients with fever at presentation to ED or which reported fever within 24 h before ED access.

We excluded from our cohort patients with age <18 years, known HIV infection, acute leukemia or lymphoma, and patients in immunosuppressive treatment due to transplant.

2.1. Patients Characteristics and Clinical History

All the demographic and clinical variables were collected from hospital-based electronic health records. For each patient included in the analysis, we evaluated vital signs (systolic and diastolic blood pressure, heart rate, respiratory rate, peripheral oxygen saturation, body temperature) and clinical symptoms (including neurological impairment and acute respiratory failure) to assess the quick Sepsis Related Organ Failure Assessment (qSOFA) score [13] at ED admission.

Computerized clinical records were reviewed to acquire information about patient's comorbidities, based on prior medical history and on the listing in the hospital discharge diagnosis. The comorbidities were used to assess the Charlson's comorbidity score [14].

Chart review protocol is described in Supplementary Materials.

2.2. Procalcitonin Sampling and Group Definition

The PCT was obtained in ED based on the clinical judgment of emergency physician at admission visit. Cutoff value of PCT serum level predictive of sepsis was set at 1 ng/mL, and a PCT interval between 0.5 and 1 ng/mL was considered as uncertain area. Procalcitonin determination was available 24 h a day.

All patients were categorized according to PCT determination. If PCT was assessed at ED presentation, patients were defined as "early PCT"; if PCT was not assessed at ED presentation, patients had a standard clinical-guided management and were defined as "controls".

All patients with suspect infection and high PCT received empirical antibiotic therapy according to current guidelines. For patients in the "uncertain area" the antibiotic therapy was evaluated case by case. Local protocols for empirical therapy were stable during the study period.

2.3. Outcome Measures

The primary endpoint of the study was the all-cause in-hospital mortality.

As secondary endpoints, we evaluated the in-hospital mortality in the subgroups of patients with a discharge diagnosis of bloodstream infections, acute respiratory infections, and other site infections (cumulative).

Finally, we evaluated the overall length of hospital stay (LOS), calculated from the time of ED admission to the hospital discharge or death in PCT groups vs. controls.

Discharge diagnosis were ascertained by ICD code at hospital discharge.

2.4. Statistical Analysis and Chart Review Methodology

Six board certified emergency physicians reviewed the clinical records and inserted study variable in a digital database. Variables were determined according to a pre-definite patient's form, based on the study protocol. To assess the intra-operator agreement of data extraction, 60 clinical records were randomly selected, and evaluated by all the six chart reviewers. We assessed the intra-operator reproducibility by Cohen's kappa measured on categorical variables in the forms.

Categorical variables are presented as absolute numbers and percentages; continuous variables are presented as median [interquartile range]. Categorical variables were statistically compared by Chi-square test or Fisher exact test as appropriate. Continuous variables were compared by Mann Whitney U test.

We analyzed mortality rates and LOS in patients that had an early PCT in ED, compared to controls. Study endpoints were assessed separately in patients with qSOFA $\geq$ 2 and qSOFA < 2. p values were 2-sided, with a significance threshold of 0.05, and corrected in case of multiple groups comparison. Study analysis was conducted by SPSS version 25 (IBM, Armonk, NY, USA)

3. Results

3.1. Study Cohort

During the study period, 14,697 adult patients were hospitalized with a diagnosis of fever. Among these, 2635 patients were excluded, because not meeting inclusion criteria or for incomplete or inconsistent clinical records, yielding to a final study cohort of 12,062 patients. Chart review process demonstrated a good reproducibility in the randomly selected records, with a Cohen's k 0.98 (95% CI 0.97–0.99). Enrollment details are reported in Supplementary Materials. Baseline characteristics are shown in Table 1.

Table 1. Demographic and clinical characteristics of the 12,062 patients included in the study.

Variable	Total Patients 12,062 pts	qSOFA < 2 11,136 pts	qSOFA $\geq$ 2 826 pts
Sex (Male)	6644 (55.1%)	6206 (55.2%)	438 (53.0)
Age (years)	71 (55–81)	70 (54–81)	78 (67–85)
Temperature °C	37.9 (37.0–38.8)	37.8 (36.9–38.7)	38.2 (37.5–39.1)
Heart Rate (b/min)	95 (80–110)	95 (80–110)	99 (83–114)
Systolic Blood Pressure (mmHg)	127 (110–145)	130 (114–145)	100 (90–110)
Diastolic Blood Pressure (mmHg)	70 (60–80)	71 (61–81)	60 (50–76)
Peripheral SaO$_2$	95 (92–97)	95 (92–97)	94 (89–96)
Procalcitonin in Emergency Department	3402 (28.2%)	3022 (26.9%)	380 (46.0%)
Blood Culture in Emergency Department	2261 (18.7%)	1991 (17.7%)	270 (32.7%)
Charlson score $\geq$ 2	3244 (26.9%)	3010 (26.8%)	234 (28.3%)
Outcomes			
Infectious diagnosis (any) ‡	7437 (61.7)	6844 (60.9%)	593 (71.8%)

Table 1. Cont.

Variable	Total Patients 12,062 pts	qSOFA < 2 11,136 pts	qSOFA ≥ 2 826 pts
• Acute respiratory inf. ‡	4525 (37.5)	4177 (37.2%)	348 (42.1%)
• Bloodstream inf. ‡	919 (7.6%)	778 (6.9%)	141 (17.1%)
• Other site infection ‡	3066 (25.4%)	2844 (25.3%)	222 (26.9%)
LOS # (days)	10 (6–17)	10 (6–17)	11 (7–18)
Deceased	1533 (12.7%)	1337 (11.9%)	196 (23.7%)

‡ Acute respiratory infections, Bloodstream infections, and other site infections were defined at hospital discharge; # Lenght of Hospital Stay; qSOFA: quick sequential organ failure assessment.

The serum PCT at ED access was determined in 3402 patients (28%), that represents the early PCT group. The remaining 8660 patients were used as control group.

A qSOFA < 2 was attributed to 11,136 (92.3%) patients; among them 3022 (27.1%) had a PCT determination in ED. A total of 826 patients (7.7%) had a qSOFA ≥ 2; 380 (46.0%) of them had a PCT determination in ED.

3.2. Early PCT Determination and In-Hospital Death

Overall, 1533 patients died (12.7%), and no differences were observed in death rates between patients in the early PCT group, compared to controls (Table 2).

Table 2. In-hospital mortality rate in patients that an early procalcitonin (PCT) determination in emergency department (ED) vs. controls. Data are shown for all population and according to qSOFA at ED admission.

	Controls n 8860	Ealry PCT n 3402	p Value
All patients	1070/8660 (12.4%)	463/3402 (13.6%)	0.063
qSOFA < 2	Controls n 8214	Early PCT n 3022	p Value
All patients	952/8214 (11.6%)	385/3022 (12.7%)	0.095
Infectious diagnosis (any)	568/4831 (11.7%)	251/2013 (12.5%)	0.381
• Acute respiratory inf.	459/3073 (14.9%)	174/1104 (15.8%)	0.512
• Bloodstream infection	142/464 (30.6%)	66/248 (21.0%)	0.003
• Other site infection	136/1974 (6.9%)	77/870 (8.9%)	0.067
qSOFA ≥ 2	Controls n 446	Early PCT n 380	p Value
All patients	118/446 (26.5%)	78/380 (20.5%)	0.046
Infectious diagnosis (any)	80/322 (24.8%)	55/271 (20.3%)	0.188
• Acute respiratory inf.	66/218 (30.3%)	44/130 (33.8%)	0.488
• Bloodstream infection	25/62 (40.3%)	25/79 (31.6%)	0.285
• Other site infection	13/100 (13.0%)	10/122 (8.2%)	0.243

In patients with qSOFA < 2, the early PCT determination in ED was not associated to a different mortality rate in the overall population. However, when considering the subgroup of patients with a final diagnosis of bloodstream infection the early PCT was associated to a significant better survival when compared to controls (21.0% vs. 30.6%; $p = 0.003$) (Table 2).

In patients with qSOFA $\geq$ 2, overall mortality was lower in patients which received a PCT assessment ED, being respectively 20.5% for early PCT group and 26.5% for controls ($p = 0.046$). When considering specific subgroups of infective diagnosis, the early PCT was generally associated to better survival rates, although not reaching statistical significance.

3.3. LOS and Early PCT Determination

Cumulative LOS of our patients was 10 (6–17) days. The early PCT patients had a significantly higher LOS compared to controls. This result was confirmed for both patients with qSOFA $\geq$ 2 and qSOFA < 2 (Table 3).

Table 3. Length of hospital stay (LOS) rate in patients that an early procalcitonin (PCT) determination in emergency department (ED) vs. controls. Data are shown for all population and according to qSOFA at ED admission.

	Controls n 8860	Early PCT n 3402	p Value
All Population	10 (6–17)	11 (7–18)	<0.001
qSOFA < 2	Controls n 8214	Early PCT n 3022	p Value
All patients	10 (6–17)	11 (7–18)	<0.001
Infectious disease diagnosis (any)	10 (6–17)	11 (7–18)	<0.001
qSOFA $\geq$ 2	Controls n 446	Ealry PCT n 380	p Value
All patients	10 (7–17)	11 (7–19)	0.044
Infectious disease diagnosis (any)	11 (7–17)	11 (7–19)	0.136

4. Discussion

The main finding of this study was that among adults admitted to ED with fever and subsequently hospitalized, an early PCT determination could improve prognosis in the group at higher risk of sepsis (qSOFA $\geq$ 2). Conversely, in patients with a low qSOFA score (<2), the early PCT determination was not associated to different outcomes, with the possible exception of patients affected by bloodstream infections.

The clinical management of patients with fever often represents a challenge for physicians, and determine whether fever is the expression of a harmful bacterial infection could be a challenging task in the ED setting. The available clinical and laboratory diagnostic tools could not be sufficient for an early diagnosis, and this particularly happens when the patient lacks the cognitive or physical ability to relay symptoms [15,16].

Direct identification of bacteria from blood culture and non-culture-based methodologies is expensive and time-consuming, and patients admitted to ED with fever are often exposed to an excess of broad-spectrum antibiotic therapy [17–20]. As a result, the interest on PCT to reduce both unnecessary and prolonged antibiotic therapy in these patients has grown in recent years.

In intensive care unit (ICU), the PCT-guided management of antibiotic therapy was associated to a mortality reduction [21]. At the same time, patients receiving PCT guided management had a shorter duration of antibiotic treatments [6–11]. This was confirmed by a meta-analysis on ICU patients with acute respiratory infections [8].

In study conducted in the ED setting, the early PCT was associated to a better discrimination of acute respiratory tract infections [16], and to a better prognosis in elderly patients with community-acquired pneumonia [22]. However, a multicenter randomized trial in patients admitted to ED with un-discriminate fever, showed that PCT testing did not reduce antibiotic prescription and 30-day mortality [12]. Similarly, patient benefit in term of mortality was not confirmed in the ED setting both for lower respiratory tract infections [23,24], and urinary tract infections [19,25].

As a whole, the PCT-guided management seems to have the most clinical benefit in high-risk populations while its utility in low-risk patients remains unclear [11]. Thus, conclusive evidence on the utility of early PCT determination in the ED is still lacking.

In our retrospective study, conducted in a large and heterogeneous population admitted to ED with fever, the early PCT showed a potential association to better survival in patients with qSOFA ≥ 2. This could likely be ascribed to an early start of antibiotic therapy or to a more aggressive clinical approach. These findings are in line with a recent meta-analysis confirming that in patients meeting sepsis-3 criteria, the PCT-guided management could be associated to an overall better survival [26]. However, analyzing the subgroups of patients with acute respiratory infections and bloodstream infections, our data demonstrate a slight reduction in overall mortality just in the latter ones, although not reaching the statistical significance. We can speculate that, in a population at high risk for sepsis (qSOFA ≥ 2), the overall effect of an early PCT management, although present, could be too low to be evidenced in a reduced sample size.

In patients with fever but at low risk of sepsis (qSOFA < 2), our data suggest that an extensive PCT determination in ED could have a limited influence on overall mortality. This is in line with a recent meta-analysis conducted on studies including septic and nonseptic patients, in which the PCT-guided management did not show a significant benefit compared to standard clinical management [27].

Interestingly, our data demonstrated a significant reduction of mortality rate in the subgroup of patients accessing with qSOFA < 2 and having a discharge diagnosis of bloodstream infection. Several studies showed that PCT has a high diagnostic accuracy for bloodstream infection [28,29], although the false negative ratio is too high to use PCT alone to address this diagnosis [30]. Nevertheless, the association between PCT sampling and better survival in these patients could be due to an increased awareness for potential bacterial infection in these otherwise low-risk patients. Indeed, apart from the qSOFA score assessment, the clinical judgment of ED physicians should always play a key role in recognizing the most complex patients (i.e., patients with central venous catheter or other risk factors for bloodstream infection) [31]. In this setting, the role of PCT could be enhanced, increasing the confidence of ED physician for the need of an aggressive antibiotic therapy [31].

Study Limitations

Although conducted on a large cohort of patients, some limitations are worth considering. First, this is a single center observational study, thus our result could not be generalizable to all EDs. Second, no established rule was defined to determine PCT assessment in ED, nor a specific PCT result management was operated. However, this latter limitation is diminished by the presence in our institution of an antibiotic stewardship team, which coordinate antibiotic prescriptions for every admitted patient. Finally, our observational study spans a decade, and the PCT sampling in ED considerably raised over the years (Figure S1).

5. Conclusions

Among adults admitted to ED with fever and hospitalized, those at high risk for sepsis (qSOFA ≥ 2) could have a better in-hospital survival if an early PCT determination is obtained in ED.

Conversely, in febrile patients with qSOFA < 2 at ED access, the early determination of PCT have a limited influence on overall prognosis, although in patients with high clinical suspicion of bloodstream infection it could be associated to improved outcomes if compared to standard clinical management.

As a result, a case-by-case analysis, and antibiotic stewardship are always recommended to maximize the clinical usefulness of the early PCT sampling for febrile adults in ED.

Supplementary Materials: The following are available online at https://www.mdpi.com/1010-660X/57/2/179/s1, Figure S1: Distribution of PCT determinations and controls during the study period.

Author Contributions: Conceptualization, methodology, original manuscript preparation. M.C. (Marcello Covino), A.G., and M.M.; Formal analysis: M.C. (Marcello Covino) and G.D.M.; data curation and retrieval: M.L.B., B.S., M.C. (Marcello Candelli); writing—review and editing: R.M., V.O., M.C. (Marcello Covino); Supervision and funding acquisition, F.F. All authors have read and agreed to the published version of the manuscript.

Funding: This research received no external fundings.

Institutional Review Board Statement: The study was conducted according to the principles expressed in the Declaration of Helsinki and its later amendments, and approved by local Institutional Review Board (0051814/19 released 04 December 2019).

Informed Consent Statement: Being a retrospective study performed on a database of anonymized patients, patient's informed consent was waived.

Data Availability Statement: The data presented in this study are available on reasonably request from the corresponding author.

Conflicts of Interest: The authors declare no conflict of interest.

References

1. DeWitt, S.; Chavez, S.A.; Perkins, J.; Long, B.; Koyfman, A. Evaluation of fever in the emergency department. *Am. J. Emerg. Med.* **2017**, *35*, 1755–1758. [CrossRef]
2. Becker, K.L.; Nylén, E.S.; White, J.C.; Müller, B.; Snider, R.H., Jr. Procalcitonin and the calcitonin gene family of peptides in inflammation, infection, and sepsis: A journey from calcitonin back to its precursors. *J. Clin. Endocrinol. Metab.* **2004**, *89*, 1512–1525. [CrossRef]
3. Simon, L.; Gauvin, F.; Amre, D.K.; Saint-Louis, P.; Lacroix, J. Serum procalcitonin and C-reactive protein levels as markers of bacterial infection: A systematic review and meta-analysis. *Clin. Infect. Dis.* **2004**, *39*, 206–217. [CrossRef]
4. Limper, M.; de Kruif, M.D.; Duits, A.J.; Brandjes, D.P.; van Gorp, E.C. The diagnostic role of procalcitonin and other biomarkers in discriminating infectious from noninfectious fever. *J. Infect.* **2010**, *60*, 409–416. [CrossRef]
5. Christ-Crain, M.; Stolz, D.; Bingisser, R.; Müller, C.; Miedinger, D.; Huber, P.R.; Zimmerli, W.; Harbarth, S.; Tamm, M.; Müller, B. Procalcitonin guidance of antibiotic therapy in community-acquired pneumonia: A randomized trial. *Am. J. Respir. Crit. Care Med.* **2006**, *174*, 84–93. [CrossRef]
6. Burkhardt, O.; Ewig, S.; Haagen, U.; Giersdorf, S.; Hartmann, O.; Wegscheider, K.; Hummers-Pradier, E.; Welte, T. Procalcitonin guidance and reduction of antibiotic use in acute respiratory tract infection. *Eur. Respir. J.* **2010**, *36*, 601–607. [CrossRef]
7. Schuetz, P.; Wirz, Y.; Sager, R.; Christ-Crain, M.; Stolz, D.; Tamm, M.; Bouadma, L.; Luyt, C.E.; Wolff, M.; Chastre, J.; et al. Effect of procalcitonin-guided antibiotic treatment on mortality in acute respiratory infections: A patient level meta-analysis. *Lancet Infect. Dis.* **2018**, *18*, 95–107. [CrossRef]
8. US Food and Drug Administration. FDA Press Release. FDA Clears Test to Help Manage Antibiotic Treatment for Lower Respiratory Tract Infections and Sepsis. 23 February 2017. Available online: https://www.fda.gov/NewsEvents/Newsroom/PressAnnouncements/ucm543160.htm (accessed on 2 October 2017).
9. De Kruif, M.D.; Limper, M.; Gerritsen, H.; Spek, C.A.; Brandjes, D.P.; ten Cate, H.; Bossuyt, P.M.; Reitsma, P.H.; van Gorp, E.C.M. Additional value of procalcitonin for diagnosis of infection in patients with fever at the emergency department. *Crit. Care Med.* **2010**, *38*, 457–463. [CrossRef] [PubMed]
10. Van der Does, Y.; Rood, P.P.; Haagsma, J.A.; Patka, P.; van Gorp, E.C.; Limper, M. Procalcitonin-guided therapy for the initiation of antibiotics in the ED: A systematic review. *Am. J. Emerg. Med.* **2016**, *34*, 1286–1293. [CrossRef] [PubMed]
11. Schuetz, P.; Falsey, A.R. Procalcitonin in patients with fever: One approach does not fit all. *Clin. Microbiol. Infect.* **2018**, *24*, 1229–1230. [CrossRef] [PubMed]
12. Van der Does, Y.; Limper, M.; Jie, K.E.; Schuit, S.C.E.; Jansen, H.; Pernot, N.; van Rosmalen, J.; Poley, M.J.; Ramakers, C.; Patka, P.; et al. Procalcitonin-guided antibiotic therapy in patients with fever in a general emergency department population: A multicentre non-inferiority randomized clinical trial (HiTEMP study). *Clin. Microbiol. Infect.* **2018**, *24*, 1282–1289. [CrossRef] [PubMed]
13. Singer, M.; Deutschman, C.S.; Seymour, C.W.; Shankar-Hari, M.; Annane, D.; Bauer, M.; Bellomo, R.; Bernard, G.R.; Chiche, J.D.; Coopersmith, C.M.; et al. The Third International Consensus Definitions for Sepsis and Septic Shock (Sepsis-3). *JAMA* **2016**, *315*, 801–810. [CrossRef]
14. Charlson, M.E.; Pompei, P.; Ales, K.L.; MacKenzie, C.R. A new method of classifying prognostic comorbidity in longitudinal studies: Development and validation. *J. Chronic Dis.* **1987**, *40*, 373–383. [CrossRef]
15. Myint, P.K.; Kamath, A.V.; Vowler, S.L.; Maisey, D.N.; Harrison, B.D. The CURB (confusion, urea, respiratory rate and blood pressure) criteria in community-acquired pneumonia (CAP) in hospitalized elderly patients aged 65 years and over: A prospective observational cohort study. *Age Ageing* **2005**, *34*, 75–77. [CrossRef]

16. Covino, M.; Petruzziello, C.; Onder, G.; Migneco, A.; Simeoni, B.; Franceschi, F.; Ojetti, V. A 12-year retrospective analysis of differences between elderly and oldest old patients referred to the emergency department of a large tertiary hospital. *Maturitas* **2019**, *120*, 7–11. [CrossRef] [PubMed]
17. British Thoracic Society Standards of Care Committee. BTS Guidelines for the Management of Community Acquired Pneumonia in Adults. *Thorax* **2001**, *56* (Suppl. 4), IV1–IV64. [CrossRef]
18. Aujesky, D.; Auble, T.E.; Yealy, D.M.; Stone, R.A.; Obrosky, D.S.; Meehan, T.P.; Graff, L.G.; Fine, J.M.; Fine, M.J. Fine, Prospective comparison of three validated prediction rules for prognosis in community-acquired pneumonia. *Am. J. Med.* **2005**, *118*, 384–392. [CrossRef] [PubMed]
19. Makam, A.N.; Auerbach, A.D.; Steinman, M.A. Blood culture use in the emergency department in patients hospitalized for community-acquired pneumonia. *JAMA Intern. Med.* **2014**, *174*, 803–806. [CrossRef]
20. Castellanos-Ortega, A.; Suberviola, B.; García-Astudillo, L.A.; Holanda, M.S.; Ortiz, F.; Llorca, J.; Delgado-Rodríguez, M. Impact of the Surviving Sepsis Campaign protocols on hospital length of stay and mortality in septic shock patients: Results of a three-year follow-up quasi-experimental study. *Crit. Care Med.* **2010**, *38*, 1036–1043. [CrossRef] [PubMed]
21. De Jong, E.; van Oers, J.A.; Beishuizen, A.; Vos, P.; Vermeijden, W.J.; Haas, L.E.; Loef, B.G.; Dormans, T.; Melsen, G.C.; Kluiters, Y.C.; et al. Efficacy and safety of procalcitonin guidance in reducing the duration of antibiotic treatment in critically ill patients: A randomised, controlled, open-label trial. *Lancet Infect. Dis.* **2016**, *16*, 819–827. [CrossRef]
22. Covino, M.; Piccioni, A.; Bonadia, N.; Onder, G.; Sabia, L.; Carbone, L.; Candelli, M.; Ojetti, V.; Murri, R.; Franceschi, F. Early procalcitonin determination in the emergency department and clinical outcome of community-acquired pneumonia in old and oldest old patients. *Eur. J. Intern. Med.* **2020**, *79*, 51–57. [CrossRef] [PubMed]
23. Alba, G.A.; Truong, Q.A.; Gaggin, H.K.; Gandhi, P.U.; De Berardinis, B.; Magrini, L. Global Research on Acute Conditions Team (GREAT) Network. Diagnostic and Prognostic Utility of Procalcitonin in Patients Presenting to the Emergency Department with Dyspnea. *Am. J. Med.* **2016**, *129*, 96–104.e7. [CrossRef]
24. Huang, D.T.; Yealy, D.M.; Filbin, M.R.; Brown, A.M.; Chang, C.H.; Doi, Y.; Donnino, M.W.; Fine, J.; Fine, M.J.; Fischer, M.A.; et al. ProACT Investigators. Procalcitonin-Guided Use of Antibiotics for Lower Respiratory Tract Infection. *N. Engl. J. Med.* **2018**, *379*, 236–249. [CrossRef]
25. Covino, M.; Manno, A.; Merra, G.; Simeoni, B.; Piccioni, A.; Carbone, L.; Forte, E.; Ojetti, V.; Franceschi, F.; Murri, R.; et al. Reduced utility of early procalcitonin and blood culture determination in patients with febrile urinary tract infections in the emergency department. *Intern. Emerg. Med.* **2019**. [CrossRef] [PubMed]
26. Wirz, Y.; Meier, M.A.; Bouadma, L.; Luyt, C.E.; Wolff, M.; Chastre, J. Effect of procalcitonin-guided antibiotic treatment on clinical outcomes in intensive care unit patients with infection and sepsis patients: A patient-level meta-analysis of randomized trials. *Crit. Care* **2018**, *15*, 191. [CrossRef]
27. Peng, F.; Chang, W.; Xie, J.F.; Sun, Q.; Qiu, H.B.; Yang, Y. Ineffectiveness of procalcitonin-guided antibiotic therapy in severely critically ill patients: A meta-analysis. *Int. J. Infect. Dis.* **2019**, *85*, 158–166. [CrossRef]
28. Wacker, C.; Prkno, A.; Brunkhorst, F.M.; Schlattmann, P. Procalcitonin as a diagnostic marker for sepsis: A systematic review and meta-analysis. *Lancet Infect. Dis.* **2013**, *13*, 426–435. [CrossRef]
29. Hoenigl, M.; Raggam, R.B.; Wagner, J.; Prueller, F.; Grisold, A.J.; Leitner, E.; Seeber, K.; Prattes, J.; Valentin, T.; Zollner-Schwetz, I.; et al. Procalcitonin fails to predict bacteremia in SIRS patients: A cohort study. *Int. J. Clin. Pract.* **2014**, *68*, 1278–1281. [CrossRef] [PubMed]
30. Long, B.; Koyfman, A. Best Clinical Practice: Blood Culture Utility in the Emergency Department. *J. Emerg. Med.* **2016**, *51*, 529–539. [CrossRef]
31. Sager, R.; Kutz, A.; Mueller, B.; Schuetz, P. Procalcitonin-guided diagnosis and antibiotic stewardship revisited. *BMC Med.* **2017**, *15*, 15. [CrossRef]

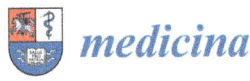

Article

Recognition in Emergency Department of Septic Patients at Higher Risk of Death: Beware of Patients without Fever

Emanuela Sozio [1,2], Alessio Bertini [3], Giacomo Bertolino [4], Francesco Sbrana [5,*], Andrea Ripoli [6], Fabio Carfagna [7], Alessandro Giacinta [1,2], Bruno Viaggi [8], Simone Meini [9], Lorenzo Ghiadoni [10,11] and Carlo Tascini [1,2]

1. Infectious Disease Unit, Azienda Sanitaria Universitaria Integrata di Udine (ASU FC), 33100 Udine, Italy; emanuela.sozio@gmail.com (E.S.); alessandro.giacinta@gmail.com (A.G.); c.tascini@gmail.com (C.T.)
2. Department of Medicine (DAME), University of Udine, 33100 Udine, Italy
3. Emergency Department, North-West District, Tuscany Health Care, Spedali Riuniti Livorno, 57124 Livorno, Italy; alessio.bertini@uslnordovest.toscana.it
4. Department of Public Health, Clinical and Molecular Medicine, Università degli Studi di Cagliari, 09124 Cagliari, Italy; giacomo.bertolino1985@gmail.com
5. U.O. Lipoaferesi, Fondazione Toscana "Gabriele Monasterio", Via Moruzzi,1, 1, 56124 Pisa, Italy
6. Deep Health Unit, Fondazione Toscana "Gabriele Monasterio", Via Moruzzi, 1, 56124 Pisa, Italy; ripoli@ftgm.it
7. SIMNOVA-Interdepartment Centre for Innovative Teaching and Simulation in Medicine and the Health Professions (Centro Interdipartimentale di Didattica Innovativa e di Simulazione in Medicina e Professioni Sanitarie), University of Eastern Piedmont, 28100 Novara, Italy; carfagna.fabio@gmail.com
8. Neuro Intensive Care Unit, Department of Anesthesia, Careggi Universital Hospital, 50139 Florence, Italy; bruno.viaggi@gmail.com
9. Internal Medicine Unit, Felice Lotti Hospital, Pontedera, Azienda USL Toscana Nord-Ovest, 1, 56124 Pisa, Italy; simonemeini2@gmail.com
10. Emergency Medicine, University Hospital of Pisa, 56124 Pisa, Italy; lorenzo.ghiadoni@unipi.it
11. Department of Clinical and Experimental Medicine, University of Pisa, 56124 Pisa, Italy
* Correspondence: francesco.sbrana@ftgm.it

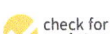

Citation: Sozio, E.; Bertini, A.; Bertolino, G.; Sbrana, F.; Ripoli, A.; Carfagna, F.; Giacinta, A.; Viaggi, B.; Meini, S.; Ghiadoni, L.; et al. Recognition in Emergency Department of Septic Patients at Higher Risk of Death: Beware of Patients without Fever. *Medicina* **2021**, *57*, 612. https://doi.org/10.3390/medicina57060612

Academic Editors: Antonio Mirijello and Alberto Tosoni

Received: 29 April 2021
Accepted: 10 June 2021
Published: 12 June 2021

Publisher's Note: MDPI stays neutral with regard to jurisdictional claims in published maps and institutional affiliations.

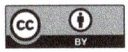

Copyright: © 2021 by the authors. Licensee MDPI, Basel, Switzerland. This article is an open access article distributed under the terms and conditions of the Creative Commons Attribution (CC BY) license (https://creativecommons.org/licenses/by/4.0/).

Abstract: *Background and Objectives*: Chances of surviving sepsis increase markedly upon prompt diagnosis and treatment. As most sepsis cases initially show-up in the Emergency Department (ED), early recognition of a septic patient has a pivotal role in sepsis management, despite the lack of precise guidelines. The aim of this study was to identify the most accurate predictors of in-hospital mortality outcome in septic patients admitted to the ED. *Materials and Methods*: We compared 651 patients admitted to ED for sepsis (cases) with 363 controls (non-septic patients). A Bayesian mean multivariate logistic regression model was performed in order to identify the most accurate predictors of in-hospital mortality outcomes in septic patients. *Results*: Septic shock and positive qSOFA were identified as risk factors for in-hospital mortality among septic patients admitted to the ED. Hyperthermia was a protective factor for in-hospital mortality. *Conclusions*: Physicians should bear in mind that fever is not a criterium for defining sepsis; according to our results, absence of fever upon presentation might be indicative of greater severity and diagnosis of sepsis should not be delayed.

Keywords: afebrile patients; emergency department; sepsis; septic shock; qSOFA

1. Introduction

Sepsis is a life-threatening condition whereby the risk of mortality exceeds that associated with acute coronary syndrome [1,2]. Its definition has been widely debated for several years [3,4], until in 2016 it was defined as "a life-threatening organ dysfunction caused by a dysregulated host response to infection" [5–7]. The Sequential Organ Failure Assessment (SOFA) score was proposed as a proxy for evaluating the organ dysfunction occurring during sepsis: an increase by two or more points was established as a necessary diagnostic criterium [5,8].

Notably, the concept of systemic inflammatory response syndrome (SIRS) and its determinants, such as body temperature, are no longer considered.

Sepsis is a time-dependent condition. Hence, early identification and treatment increase chances of survival [9]. As a result, the 2016 Task Force recommended the use of the quick SOFA (qSOFA) score as an early screening tool for discriminating patients with likelihood of sepsis: as qSOFA does not require diagnostic blood testing, it provides an advantage as its timely use may be implemented in every setting [5,10].

The qSOFA score has shown to be a good predictor of mortality, length of hospitalization and requirement of admission in Intensive Care Units (ICU) [11–13]. It also proved to be better than the SIRS criteria in identifying septic patients at higher risk of admission in the ICU or death [14,15]. In 2018, a meta-analysis concluded that SIRS criteria are more adequate than qSOFA for the diagnosis of sepsis, while qSOFA is a better predictor of in-hospital mortality [16].

On the other hand, both qSOFA and SIRS criteria are suboptimal predictors of outcome [2], whereas the Early Warning Score (EWS) has demonstrated superiority in selecting the most critically ill among septic patients [17,18].

The incidence of sepsis is increasing worldwide, with an estimated 270 cases per 100,000 inhabitants/year [9,19]. Indeed, most cases initially refer to the Emergency Department (ED) [20]; thus, proper assignment of the priority code at triage could lead to shorter lag time before clinical evaluation and to the administration of the most appropriate treatment [21]. Unfortunately, early recognition of sepsis is still challenging since validated systems and tools for prompt identification are found lacking.

The aim of this study was to define the most accurate mortality outcome predictors for identifying patients with sepsis referring to the ED.

2. Materials and Methods

2.1. Study Sample and Data Collection

A total of 1014 patients admitted to the ED of Pisa and Leghorn Hospitals, Italy, between March 2017 and December 2019 were included in this retrospective cohort study.

During their stay in the ED, 651 patients had a confirmed diagnosis of sepsis or septic shock (cases) in accordance with the new definitions of sepsis and septic shock (Sepsis-3) [5]. On the other hand, the 363 controls included patients admitted to ED on the same days of the cases, with similar triage diagnosis, which was subsequently corrected with a different condition other than sepsis or septic shock (e.g., consciousness disorders, dyspnea, hypotension, etc.).

Patients meeting sepsis criteria in the ED were identified among patients with infection and a SOFA score of two or more.

Patients who developed septic shock in the ED were identified according to a clinical scheme of sepsis with persisting hypotension requiring vasopressors to maintain MAP $\geq$65 mmHg and serum lactate levels >2 mmol/L (18 mg/dL) despite adequate volume resuscitation, according to Sepsis-3 definitions [5].

We excluded 114 septic patients whose blood test results or clinical data were not available.

Data were collected from the patients' records and included the following information: demographic features; risk factors for infection (prosthetic devices, immunosuppression, steroid therapy in the previous 30 days, trauma in the previous 30 days, surgery in the previous 30 days and presence of CVCs and/or bladder catheters); comorbidities (Charlson Comorbidity Index, Cardiovascular disease, Renal insufficiency, Diabetes, COPD, Chronic hepatopathy and Cancer); vital parameters (Body temperature and Mean Arterial Pressure-MAP); clinical parameters for assessing degree of illness (Sequential Organ Failure Assessment-SOFA- Score, quick SOFA-qSOFA, Glasgow Coma Scale-GCS and Shock index), laboratory investigations available in the ED (white blood cells count-WBC-platelet count; bilirubin, creatinine and procalcitonin (PCT) levels; lactate levels in arterial blood); details regarding hospitalization (length of stay and subsequent admission in the ICU); and in-hospital mortality or early death occurring in the ED.

This study did not require an institutional review board oversight due to its retrospective nature and the anonymity of pooled data.

2.2. Statistical Analysis

This study aimed primarily at uncovering factors related to in-hospital mortality among the overall septic population of patients referring to the ED. All variables were expressed as mean +/− standard deviation, median and interquartile range or percentage where appropriate. Normality of quantitative variables was assessed with the Shapiro–Wilk test and Q–Q plots. Depending on the distribution of variables, comparisons between groups were performed with unpaired two-tailed t-test, Mann–Whitney test or chi-squared test with continuity correction. A p value below 0.05 was considered statistically significant. Univariable logistic regression was performed to evaluate the association of each covariate with in-hospital mortality; covariates with a p value less than 0.10 were considered for multivariable analysis. A Bayesian averaging of logistic regression multivariable models (BMA) [22] was computed to address model uncertainty, which produces a posterior probability for each possible model and covariate. As a result of BMA, in addition to OR, the probability that the single covariate has a non-zero effect in the final averaged model (posterior probability, $p\,(b \neq 0)$) was reported. Covariates with $p\,(b \neq 0) > 0.80$ were considered as independently associated to the outcome. Analyses were performed using the R open-source statistical software.

3. Results

A total of 1014 patients admitted to the ED were enrolled. Among these, 651 patients received a diagnosis of sepsis or septic shock (cases) while the remaining 363 patients were diagnosed with a different condition other than sepsis or septic shock (controls).

The clinical characteristics of patients are reported in Table 1. The overall median age was 77.7 ± 13.5 years. Most patients were hospitalized (91.3%). Overall, in-hospital mortality was 15.9%.

There were no differences among age and gender between the two patient groups. On the other hand, patients with sepsis required hospitalization more frequently than those within the control group (94.5% vs. 85.7%, <0.0001) and showed higher mortality both early in ED (3.2 vs. 0.56, p = 0.0001) and during hospitalization (20.1% vs. 9.7%). Septic shock occurred in 14.8% of sepsis cases admitted to ED but no differences in ICU admissions were observed between the two groups (7.5% vs. 5.2%, p = 0.2047).

As opposed to controls, patients with sepsis displayed the following risk factors more frequently: history of trauma within the previous 30 days (6.1% vs. 3.0%, p = 0.0428), history of surgery within the previous 30 days (5.2% vs. 0.8%, p = 0.0007), presence of central venous catheters—CVCs (8.5% vs. 1.9%, p = 0.0001)—and presence of urinary catheters (15.7% vs. 3.3%, <0.0001).

In addition, septic patients were characterized by the following features as opposed to controls: higher body temperature (37.8 ± 1.2 °C vs. 36.9 ± 1.0 °C, p < 0.0001); lower MAP (101.0 ± 33.7 vs. 152.8 ± 33.8, p < 0.0001), platelet count (/mmc) (200 (142–293) vs. 226.5 (178–291), p < 0.0001) and GCS; higher SOFA Score (4 (3–6) vs. 2 (2–4), p < 0.00010), shock index (0.9 ± 0.3 vs. 0.7 ± 0.2, p = < 0.0001), lactate value (mmol/L) (2.1 (1.2–3.8) vs. 1.2 (0.8–1.9), p < 0.0001), white blood cells count (/mmc) (13.4 (9.3–19.6) vs. 10.0 (7.3–13.3), p < 0.0001), PCT (ng/mL) (2.9 (0.9–13.1) vs. 0.1 (0.1–0.2), p < 0.0001), creatinine (mg/dl) (1.3 (0.9–2.1) vs. 1.0 (0.8–1.4), p < 0.0001) and bilirubin (mg/dl) (0.9 (0.6–1.3) vs. 1.0 (0.8–1.4), p < 0.0001).

A positive qSOFA was reported in 38.9% of septic patients vs. 8.1% of non-septic controls, p < 0.0001.

Table 1. Comparison between septic patients (n 651) and controls (n 363).

	Over All (n 1014)	Controls (n 363)	Sepsis (n 651)	p
Gender (male)	537 (53.0%)	180 (49.6%)	357 (54.8%)	0.123
Age (years)	77.7 ± 13.5	77.6 ± 13.4	77.8 ± 13.5	0.857
Hospital admission	926 (91.3%)	311 (85.7%)	615 (94.5%)	<0.001
ICU admission	68 (6.7%)	19 (5.2%)	49 (7.5%)	0.205
ED discharge	65 (6.4%)	50 (13.8%)	15 (2.3%)	<0.001
Death in ED	23 (2.3%)	2 (0.56%)	21 (3.2%)	0.012
Death during hospitalization	161 (15.9%)	30 (9.7%)	131 (20.1%)	0.001
Charlson Comorbidity Index	2 (1.0–4.0)	2 (1–4)	2 (1–4)	0.239
Cardiovascular disease	550 (54.2%)	208 (57.3%)	342 (52.5%)	0.163
Renal insufficiency	23 (2.3%)	9 (2.5%)	14 (2.2%)	0.907
Diabetes	250 (24.7%)	105 (28.9%)	145 (22.3%)	0.023
COPD	176 (17.4%)	104 (28.7%)	72 (11.1%)	<0.001
Prosthetic device	157 (15.5%)	73 (20.1%)	84 (12.9%)	0.003
Chronic hepatopathy	46 (4.5%)	18 (5.0%)	28 (4.3%)	0.745
Immunosuppression	88 (8.7%)	33 (9.1%)	55 (8.5%)	0.817
Cancer	145 (14.3%)	66 (18.2%)	79 (12.1%)	0.011
Steroid therapy (in 30 days)	154 (15.2%)	77 (21.2%)	77 (11.8%)	<0.001
Trauma (in 30 days)	51 (5.0%)	11 (3.0%)	40 (6.1%)	0.043
Surgery (in 30 days)	37 (3.7%)	3 (0.8%)	34 (5.2%)	0.001
Presence of CVC	62 (6.1%)	7 (1.9%)	55 (8.5%)	<0.001
Presence of urinary catheter	112 (11.1%)	12 (3.3%)	100 (15.7%)	<0.001
Body temperature (°C)	37.6 ± 1.2	36.9 ± 1.0	37.8 ± 1.2	<0.001
MAP	119.2 ± 41.8	152.8 ± 33.8	101.0 ± 33.7	<0.001
GCS	13.7 ± 3.0	14.2 ± 2.5	13.3 ± 3.2	<0.001
Septic shock	96 (9.5%)	0 (0.0%)	96 (14.8%)	<0.001
Shock index	0.8 ± 0.3	0.7 ± 0.2	0.9 ± 0.3	<0.001
Positive qSOFA	277 (27.3%)	24 (8.1%)	253 (38.9%)	<0.001
SOFA score	3 (2.0–5.0)	2 (2–4)	4 (3–6)	<0.001
Lactate (mmol/L)	1.6 (1.0–2.9)	1.2 (0.8–1.9)	2.1 (1.2–3.8)	<0.001
WBC (/mmc)	11.9 (8.4–16.9)	10.0 (7.3–13.3)	13.4 (9.3–19.6)	<0.001
PCT (ng/mL)	1.4 (0.3–7.8)	0.1 (0.1–0.2)	2.9 (0.9–13.1)	<0.001
Creatinine (mg/dl)	1.2 (0.8–1.8)	1.0 (0.8–1.4)	1.3 (0.9–2.1)	<0.001
Bilirubin (mg/dl)	0.8 (0.5–1.2)	0.5 (0.3–0.9)	0.9 (0.6–1.3)	<0.001
Platelet count (/mmc)	213 (153–293)	226.5 (178–291)	200 (142–293)	<0.001

Figure 1 shows the result of the Bayesian model averaging in septic cases. The 50 distinct selected models are indicated on the x-axis. In correspondence with each model, the selected variable is marked with a blue rectangle if it is deemed as "protective" (the probability of the event decreases upon its increase). Variables are depicted as red rectangles if selected and deemed as "non-protective" (the probability of the event increases upon its increase). The spacing of the 50 models on the x-axis is representative of the posterior probability (of the goodness) of the individual model.

For septic patients admitted to the ED, the Bayesian mean of multivariate logistic regression models (Table 2) identified both septic shock and positive qSOFA as risk factors for in-hospital mortality outcome, while higher temperatures appeared as a protective factor vs. in-hospital mortality outcome.

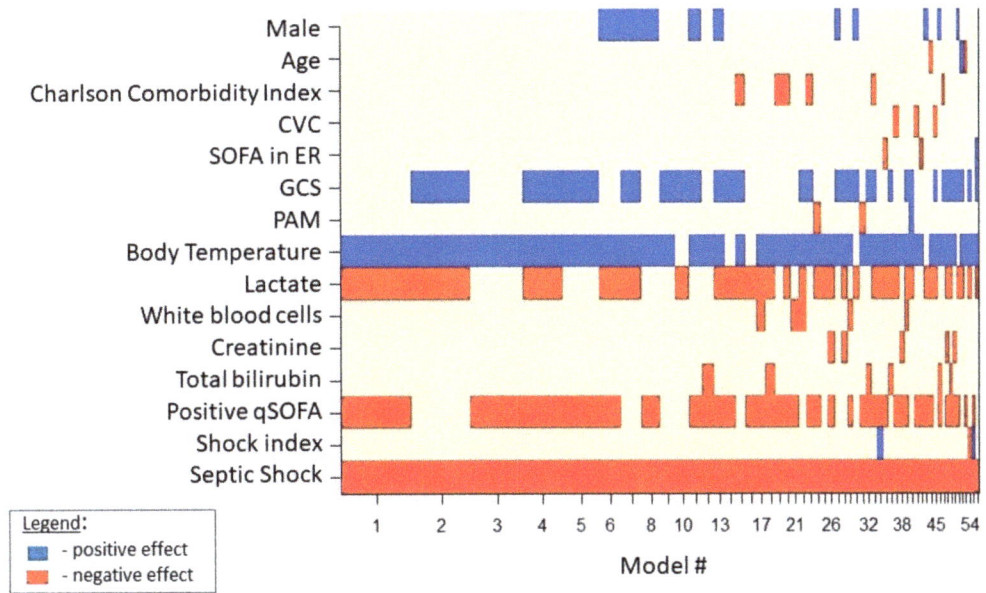

Figure 1. Model selected by BMA for in-hospital mortality in septic cases.

Table 2. Bayesian mean of multivariate logistic regression performed to investigate the association with the in-hospital mortality outcome in septic cases.

Variable	OR	95% CI OR	p (B! = 0)
Male	0.902	0.874–0.931	17
Age	1.000	0.999–1.001	1.8
Charlson Comorbidity Index	1.008	1.004–1.013	6.9
CVC	1.009	0.997–1.021	2.3
SOFA score	1.001	0.999–1.002	2.2
GCS	0.936	0.928–0.944	51.6
PAM	1.000	0.999–1.000	2.8
Body Temperature	0.687	0.673–0.701	92.5
Lactate	1.107	1.095–1.120	63.7
White blood cells	1.001	1.000–1.002	5.7
Creatinine	1.004	1.001–1.007	4.1
Total bilirubin	1.011	1.004–1.017	6.4
Positive qSOFA	2.144	2.002–2.297	71.7
Shock index	0.995	0.985–1.005	2
Septic Shock	6.582	6.289–6.88	100

Legend: the variables in italics are those that possess independent effect on mortality. Septic shock and positive qSOFA are risk factors for in-hospital mortality, while higher temperature is a protective factor.

4. Discussion

Sepsis is a time-dependent disease, as reported by a consistent body of evidence [8,23,24]. This implies that early identification and prompt administration of therapy are crucial in order to increase chances of survival. Early recognition of the affected patients is not always easy; indeed, symptoms may be atypical or appear evident only when the condition is very severe [25]. In 2016, along with the new definitions of sepsis and septic shock, both the qSOFA and SOFA scores were proposed as clinical tools for early recognition and definite diagnosis of infections complicated by sepsis, respectively [26].

Despite the uncertainty related to the choice of the best systems of early recognition and hemodynamic management, crucial actions currently recognized for decreasing sepsis related mortality include early recognition and management protocols in the ED [27,28]. When sepsis is readily identified in the ED and severe forms are treated aggressively with sepsis specific care bundles, mortality improvements are significant [8,23,24].

Regarding in-hospital mortality outcomes in septic patients admitted to the ED, our analysis confirmed the presence of septic shock and positive qSOFA as risk factors, while higher body temperature appeared as a protective factor.

Singer et al. demonstrated that qSOFA is a good predictor of mortality, length of hospitalization and ICU admission requirement [11–13]. Freund et al. added that qSOFA and SOFA scores are both better than the SIRS criteria at identifying septic patients at risk of death or transfer to the ICU [14,15]. In 2018, a meta-analysis concluded that SIRS criteria are more adequate than qSOFA for diagnosing sepsis, while qSOFA is a better predictor of in-hospital mortality [16].

Our data hereby confirms that qSOFA is a good predictor of mortality in septic patients admitted to ED.

Septic shock is well known to correlate with high mortality rates. Indeed, its definition comprises underlying circulatory and cellular/metabolic abnormalities associated to increased mortality in a subset of patients with sepsis.

The protective role of hyperthermia could have two alternative (but not necessarily mutually exclusive) explanations. Firstly, fever is one of the most prominent symptoms of infection as part of the host acute-phase response to pathogens: It is believed to reduce bacterial growth and promote cytokines synthesis and antibody production, thereby activating immune cell response [29,30]. Secondly, it represents a wake up call that immediately alerts doctors, thus speeding up the diagnostic process [31].

On the other hand, other reports confirm that the presence of hypothermia in patients with severe sepsis was an independent predictor of 28 day mortality and is associated with organ failure [31,32].

A recent study assessed 378 patients admitted to the ED with septic shock. Fever was reported in only 55% of them and afebrile patients had lower rates of antibiotic administration and intravenous fluids. Moreover, the afebrile status was shown to be a significant predictor of in-hospital mortality [33]. Afebrile patients, in our experience, were older and showed higher rates of organ dysfunction.

In recent observations, the absence of fever was associated with suppressed HLA-DR expression over time and findings suggested monocyte dysfunction in sepsis. Afebrile patients had higher rates of 28 day mortality and increased acquisition of secondary infections [34].

Unfortunately, these valuable clinical factors of immune dysfunction have not been taken into account in the present study since they are not commonly used in clinical practice in the ED.

This study has strengths and limitations. Among the study's strengths, we highlight the use of real-world data, the evaluation of a large number of predictive factors and the availability of the information at admission time in the ED. However, the study has some limitations as well. Firstly, due to the retrospective nature of the study, prospective validations in larger patient cohorts are needed to confirm these preliminary findings. Secondly, retrieving all requested information was at times challenging, as expected in settings burdened by overcrowding such as the ED.

Larger prospective and controlled studies are needed to confirm these findings.

5. Conclusions

Early recognition is crucial when managing sepsis. Identifying sepsis is often quite challenging and no single test offers diagnostic certainty in the early stages.

Our data showing hyperthermia as a protective factor for in-hospital mortality suggests the underlying importance of host immune response to sepsis. Furthermore, clinicians should bear in mind that fever is not a criterium for the definition of sepsis. Hence, early diagnosis of sepsis among afebrile patients should not be delayed.

Author Contributions: Conceptualization and writing—original draft preparation, E.S.; formal analysis, G.B. and A.R.; investigation F.C., B.V., A.B. and L.G.; data curation, F.S., S.M. and A.G.; writing—review and editing, C.T. All authors have read and agreed to the published version of the manuscript.

Funding: This research received no external funding.

Institutional Review Board Statement: Ethical review and approval were waived for this study, due to its retrospective nature and the anonymity of pooled data.

Informed Consent Statement: Informed consent was obtained from all subjects involved in the study.

Data Availability Statement: Data are available upon contacting the corresponding author.

Conflicts of Interest: C.T. has received funds for speaking at a symposium organized on behalf of Pfizer, Novartis, Merck, Angelini, Zambon, Thermofischer, Biotest, Gilead, Hikma, Biomerieux and Astellas. All other authors: none.

References

1. Fleischmann, M.C.; Scherag, A.; Adhikari, N.K.J.; Hartog, C.S.; Tsaganos, T.; Schlattmann, P.; Angus, D.C.; Reinhart, K. Assessment of Global Incidence and Mortality of Hospital-treated Sepsis. Current Estimates and Limitations. *Am. J. Respir. Crit. Care Med.* **2016**, *193*, 259–272. [CrossRef]
2. Tusgul, S.; Carron, P.-N.; Yersin, B.; Calandra, T.; Dami, F. Low sensitivity of qSOFA, SIRS criteria and sepsis definition to identify infected patients at risk of complication in the prehospital setting and at the emergency department triage. *Scand. J. Trauma Resusc. Emerg. Med.* **2017**, *25*, 108. [CrossRef] [PubMed]
3. Bone, R.; Balk, R.; Cerra, F.; Dellinger, R.; Fein, A.; Knaus, W.; Schein, R.; Sibbald, W. Definitions for sepsis and organ failure and guidelines for the use of innovative therapies in sepsis. The accp/sccm consensus conference committee. american college of chest physicians/society of crit care med. *Chest* **1992**, *101* (Suppl. S5), 1644–1655. [CrossRef] [PubMed]
4. Levy, M.M.; Fink, M.P.; Marshall, J.C.; Abraham, E.; Angus, D.; Cook, D.; Cohen, J.; Opal, S.M.; Vincent, J.L.; Ramsay, G.; et al. 2001 SCCM/ESICM/ACCP/ATS/SIS International Sepsis Definitions Conference. *Intensive Care Med.* **2003**, *29*, 530–538. [CrossRef] [PubMed]
5. Singer, M.; Deutschman, C.S.; Seymour, C.W.; Shankar-Hari, M.; Annane, D.; Bauer, M.; Bellomo, R.; Bernard, G.R.; Chiche, J.-D.; Coopersmith, C.M.; et al. The Third International Consensus Definitions for Sepsis and Septic Shock (Sepsis-3). *JAMA* **2016**, *315*, 801–810. [CrossRef] [PubMed]
6. Shankar-Hari, M.; Phillips, G.S.; Levy, M.L.; Seymour, C.W.; Liu, V.X.; Deutschman, C.S.; Angus, D.C.; Rubenfeld, G.D.; Singer, M. Developing a new definition and assessing new clinical criteria for septic shock: For the third international consensus Definitions for sepsis and septic shock (sepsis-3). *JAMA* **2016**, *315*, 775–787. [CrossRef]
7. Jacob, J.A. New sepsis diagnostic guidelines shift focus to organ dysfunction. *JAMA* **2016**, *315*, 739–740. [CrossRef]
8. Dellinger, R.P.; The Surviving Sepsis Campaign Guidelines Committee including The Pediatric Subgroup*; Levy, M.M.; Rhodes, A.; Annane, D.; Gerlach, H.; Opal, S.M.; Sevransky, J.E.; Sprung, C.L.; Douglas, I.; et al. Surviving Sepsis Campaign: International Guidelines for Management of Severe Sepsis and Septic Shock, 2012. *Intensive Care Med.* **2013**, *39*, 165–228. [CrossRef]
9. Hayden, G.E.; Tuuri, R.E.; Scott, R.; Losek, J.D.; Blackshaw, A.M.; Schoenling, A.J.; Nietert, P.J.; Hall, G.A. Triage sepsis alert and sepsis protocol lower times to fluids and antibiotics in the ed. *Am. J. Emerg. Med.* **2016**, *34*, 1–9. [CrossRef]
10. Giorgi-Pierfranceschi, M. Sepsis and septic shock: A practical management according to Sepsis-3 diagnostic criteria. *Ital. J. Med.* **2016**, *10*, 376. [CrossRef]
11. Singer, A.J.; Ng, J.; Thode, H.C., Jr.; Spiegel, R.; Weingart, S. Quick sofa scores predict mortality in adult emergency department patients with and without suspected infection. *Ann. Emerg. Med.* **2017**, *69*, 475–479. [CrossRef] [PubMed]
12. Khwannimit, B.; Bhurayanontachai, R.; Vattanavanit, V. Comparison of the performance of SOFA, qSOFA and SIRS for predicting mortality and organ failure among sepsis patients admitted to the intensive care unit in a middle-income country. *J. Crit. Care* **2018**, *44*, 156–160. [CrossRef] [PubMed]
13. Finkelsztein, E.J.; Jones, D.S.; Ma, K.C.; Pabón, M.A.; Delgado, T.; Nakahira, K.; Arbo, J.E.; Berlin, D.A.; Schenck, E.J.; Choi, A.M.K.; et al. Comparison of qSOFA and SIRS for predicting adverse outcomes of patients with suspicion of sepsis outside the intensive care unit. *Crit. Care* **2017**, *21*, 1–10. [CrossRef] [PubMed]
14. Freund, Y.; Lemachatti, N.; Krastinova, E.; Van Laer, M.; Claessens, Y.-E.; Avondo, A.; Occelli, C.; Feral-Pierssens, A.-L.; Truchot, J.; Ortega, M.; et al. Prognostic Accuracy of Sepsis-3 Criteria for In-Hospital Mortality Among Patients With Suspected Infection Presenting to the Emergency Department. *JAMA* **2017**, *317*, 301–308. [CrossRef]
15. Raith, E.; Udy, A.; Bailey, M.; McGloughlin, S.; MacIsaac, C.; Bellomo, R.; Pilcher, D.V.; Australian and New Zealand Intensive Care Society (ANZICS) Centre for Outcomes and Resource Evaluation (CORE). Prognostic Accuracy of the SOFA Score, SIRS Criteria, and qSOFA Score for In-Hospital Mortality Among Adults With Suspected Infection Admitted to the Intensive Care Unit. *JAMA* **2017**, *317*, 290–300. [CrossRef] [PubMed]

16. Churpek, M.M.; Snyder, A.; Han, X.; Sokol, S.; Pettit, N.; Howell, M.D.; Edelson, D.P. Quick Sepsis-related Organ Failure Assessment, Systemic Inflammatory Response Syndrome, and Early Warning Scores for Detecting Clinical Deterioration in Infected Patients outside the Intensive Care Unit. *Am. J. Respir. Crit. Care Med.* **2017**, *195*, 906–911. [CrossRef] [PubMed]
17. Siddiqui, S.; Chua, M.; Kumaresh, V.; Choo, R. A comparison of pre icu admission sirs, ews and q sofa scores for predicting mortality and length of stay in icu. *J. Crit. Care* **2017**, *41*, 191–193. [CrossRef]
18. Serafim, R.; Gomes, J.A.; Salluh, J.; Povoa, P. A comparison of the quick-sofa and systemic inflammatory response syndrome criteria for the diagnosis of sepsis and prediction of mortality: A systematic review and meta-analysis. *Chest* **2018**, *153*, 646–655. [CrossRef]
19. Gaieski, D.F.; Edwards, J.M.; Kallan, M.J.; Carr, B.G. Benchmarking the Incidence and Mortality of Severe Sepsis in the United States*. *Crit. Care Med.* **2013**, *41*, 1167–1174. [CrossRef]
20. Angus, D.C.; Linde-Zwirble, W.T.; Lidicker, J.; Clermont, G.; Carcillo, J.; Pinsky, M.R. Epidemiology of severe sepsis in the United States: Analysis of incidence, outcome, and associated costs of care. *Crit. Care Med.* **2001**, *29*, 1303–1310. [CrossRef]
21. Rhodes, A.A.; Evans, L.E.; Alhazzani, W.; Levy, M.M.; Antonelli, M.; Ferrer, R.; Kumar, A.; Sevransky, J.E.; Sprung, C.L.; Nunnally, M.E.; et al. Surviving Sepsis Campaign: International Guidelines for Management of Sepsis and Septic Shock: 2016. *Crit. Care Med.* **2017**, *45*, 486–552. [CrossRef] [PubMed]
22. Wang, D.; Zhang, W.; Bakhai, A. Comparison of Bayesian model averaging and stepwise methods for model selection in logistic regression. *Stat. Med.* **2004**, *23*, 3451–3467. [CrossRef] [PubMed]
23. Rivers, E.; Nguyen, B.; Havstad, S.; Ressler, J.; Muzzin, A.; Knoblich, B.; Peterson, E.; Tomlanovich, M. Early Goal-Directed Therapy in the Treatment of Severe Sepsis and Septic Shock. *New Engl. J. Med.* **2001**, *345*, 1368–1377. [CrossRef]
24. Osborn, T.M.; Nguyen, H.B.; Rivers, E.P. Emergency Medicine and the Surviving Sepsis Campaign: An International Approach to Managing Severe Sepsis and Septic Shock. *Ann. Emerg. Med.* **2005**, *46*, 228–231. [CrossRef] [PubMed]
25. Prescott, H.C.; Langa, K.M.; Iwashyna, T. Readmission Diagnoses After Hospitalization for Severe Sepsis and Other Acute Medical Conditions. *JAMA* **2015**, *313*, 1055–1057. [CrossRef] [PubMed]
26. Seymour, C.W.; Liu, V.X.; Iwashyna, T.J.; Brunkhorst, F.M.; Rea, T.D.; Scherag, A.; Rubenfeld, G.; Kahn, J.M.; Shankar-Hari, M.; Singer, M.; et al. Assessment of clinical criteria for sepsis: For the third international consensus Definitions for sepsis and septic shock (sepsis-3). *JAMA* **2016**, *315*, 762–774. [CrossRef]
27. Daniels, R.; Nutbeam, T.; McNamara, G.; Galvin, C. The sepsis six and the severe sepsis resuscitation bundle: A prospective observational cohort study. *Emerg. Med. J.* **2010**, *28*, 507–512. [CrossRef] [PubMed]
28. Ferrer, R.; Martin-Loeches, I.; Phillips, G.; Osborn, T.M.; Townsend, S.; Dellinger, R.P.; Artigas, A.; Schorr, C.; Levy, M.M. Empiric antibiotic treatment reduces mortality in severe sepsis and septic shock from the first hour: Results from a guideline-based performance improvement program. *Crit. Care Med.* **2014**, *42*, 1749–1755. [CrossRef]
29. Kluger, M.J.; Kozak, W.; Conn, C.A.; Leon, L.R.; Soszynski, D. THE ADAPTIVE VALUE OF FEVER. *Infect. Dis. Clin. North Am.* **1996**, *10*, 1–20. [CrossRef]
30. Mackowiak, P.A. Fever: Blessing or curse? a unify-ing hypothesis. *Ann. Intern. Med.* **1994**, *120*, 1037–1040. [CrossRef] [PubMed]
31. Rumbus, Z.; Matics, R.; Hegyi, P.; Zsiboras, C.; Szabo, I.; Illes, A.; Petervari, E.; Balasko, M.; Marta, K.; Miko, A.; et al. Fever Is Associated with Reduced, Hypothermia with Increased Mortality in Septic Patients: A Meta-Analysis of Clinical Trials. *PLoS ONE* **2017**, *12*, e0170152. [CrossRef]
32. Kushimoto, S.; Gando, S.; Saitoh, D.; Mayumi, T.; Ogura, H.; Fujishima, S.; Araki, T.; Ikeda, H.; Kotani, J.; Miki, Y.; et al. The impact of body temperature abnormalities on the disease severity and outcome in patients with severe sepsis: An analysis from a multicenter, prospective survey of severe sepsis. *Crit. Care* **2013**, *17*, R271. [CrossRef]
33. Henning, D.J.; Carey, J.R.; Oedorf, K.; Day, D.E.; Redfield, C.S.; Huguenel, C.J.; Roberts, J.C.; Sanchez, L.D.; Wolfe, R.E.; Shapiro, N.I. The absence of fever is associated with higher mortality and decreased antibiotic and iv fluid administration in emergency department patients with suspected septic shock. *Crit. Care Med.* **2017**, *45*, e575–e582. [CrossRef]
34. Drewry, A.; Ablordeppey, E.; Murray, E.; Fuller, B.; Kollef, M.; Hotchkiss, R. 1483: Monocyte function and clinical outcomes in febrile and afebrile patients with severe sepsis. *Crit. Care Med.* **2018**, *46*, 725. [CrossRef]

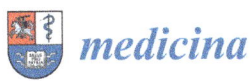

Article

Delta-Procalcitonin and Vitamin D Can Predict Mortality of Internal Medicine Patients with Microbiological Identified Sepsis

Alberto Tosoni [1,*], Anthony Cossari [2], Mattia Paratore [1], Michele Impagnatiello [1], Giovanna Passaro [3], Carla Vincenza Vallone [4], Vincenzo Zaccone [5], Antonio Gasbarrini [1], Giovanni Addolorato [1], Salvatore De Cosmo [6], Antonio Mirijello [6,*] and on behalf of the Internal Medicine Sepsis Study Group [†]

1 CEMAD Digestive Disease Center, Fondazione Policlinico Universitario "A. Gemelli" IRCCS, Università Cattolica del Sacro Cuore, 00168 Rome, Italy; mattia_paratore@virgilio.it (M.P.); mikimpa@libero.it (M.I.); antonio.gasbarrini@unicatt.it (A.G.); giovanni.addolorato@unicatt.it (G.A.)
2 Department of Economics, Statistics and Finance "Giovanni Anania", University of Calabria, 87036 Rende, Italy; anthony.cossari@unical.it
3 Department of Geriatrics, Fondazione Policlinico Universitario "A. Gemelli" IRCCS, 00168 Rome, Italy; passaro.giovanna@gmail.com
4 Department of Emergency and Critical Care, Azienda Ospedaliera Universitaria San Giovanni di Dio e Ruggi D'Aragona, 84125 Salerno, Italy; carlavallone@hotmail.it
5 Department of Internal and Subintensive Medicine, Azienda Ospedaliero-Universitaria "Ospedali Riuniti", 60126 Ancona, Italy; vincenzozaccone@libero.it
6 Department of Medical Sciences, IRCCS Casa Sollievo della Sofferenza, 71013 San Giovanni Rotondo, Italy; s.decosmo@operapadrepio.it
* Correspondence: alberto.tosoni@policlinicogemelli.it (A.T.); a.mirijello@operapadrepio.it (A.M.)
† The Internal Medicine Sepsis Study Group (alphabetic order): Stefano Carughi, Maria Maddalena D'Errico, Angela de Matthaeis, Antonio Pio Greco, Pamela Piscitelli, Leonardo Sacco (IRCCS Casa Sollievo della Sofferenza, 71013 San Giovanni Rotondo, Italy), Tommaso Dionisi (CEMAD Digestive Disease Center, Fondazione Policlinico Universitario "A. Gemelli" IRCCS, 00168 Rome, Italy).

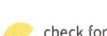

Citation: Tosoni, A.; Cossari, A.; Paratore, M.; Impagnatiello, M.; Passaro, G.; Vallone, C.V.; Zaccone, V.; Gasbarrini, A.; Addolorato, G.; De Cosmo, S.; et al. Delta-Procalcitonin and Vitamin D Can Predict Mortality of Internal Medicine Patients with Microbiological Identified Sepsis. *Medicina* 2021, 57, 331. https://doi.org/10.3390/medicina57040331

Academic Editor: Salvatore Di Somma

Received: 5 February 2021
Accepted: 25 March 2021
Published: 1 April 2021

Publisher's Note: MDPI stays neutral with regard to jurisdictional claims in published maps and institutional affiliations.

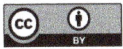

Copyright: © 2021 by the authors. Licensee MDPI, Basel, Switzerland. This article is an open access article distributed under the terms and conditions of the Creative Commons Attribution (CC BY) license (https://creativecommons.org/licenses/by/4.0/).

Abstract: *Background*: The management of septic patients hospitalized in Internal Medicine wards represents a challenge due to their complexity and heterogeneity, and a high mortality rate. Among the available prognostic tools, procalcitonin (PCT) is considered a marker of bacterial infection. Furthermore, an association between vitamin D deficiency and poor sepsis-related outcomes has been described. *Objectives:* To evaluate the prognostic accuracy of two consecutive PCT determinations (Delta-PCT) and of vitamin D levels in predicting mortality in a population of patients with microbiological identified sepsis admitted to Internal Medicine wards. *Methods*: This is a sub-analysis of a previous prospective study. A total of 80 patients had at least two available consecutive PCT determinations, while 63 had also vitamin D. Delta-PCT was defined as a reduction of PCT > 50% after 48 h, >75% after 72 h, and >85% after 96 h. Mortality rate at 28- and 90-days were considered as main outcome. *Results:* Mortality rate was 18.7% at 28-days and 30.0% at 90-days. Baseline PCT levels did not differ between survived and deceased patients (28-days: $p = 0.525$; 90-days: $p = 0.088$). A significantly higher proportion of survived patients showed Delta-PCT (28-days: $p = 0.002$; 90-days: $p < 0.001$). Delta-PCT was associated with a lower 28-days ($p = 0.007$; OR = 0.12, 95%CI 0.02–0.46) and 90-days mortality ($p = 0.001$; OR = 0.17, 95%CI 0.06–0.48). A significantly higher proportion of deceased patients showed severe vitamin D deficiency (28-days: $p = 0.047$; 90-days: $p = 0.049$). Severe vitamin D deficiency was associated with a higher 28-days ($p = 0.058$; OR = 3.95, 95%CI 1.04–19.43) and 90-days mortality ($p = 0.054$; OR = 2.94, 95%CI 1.00–9.23). *Conclusions*: Delta-PCT and vitamin D represent two useful tests for predicting prognosis of septic patients admitted to Internal Medicine wards.

Keywords: procalcitonin kinetics; prognostication; sepsis biomarkers

1. Introduction

Sepsis is a leading cause of death and health care systems major burden worldwide [1]. Sepsis has been estimated to cause about half of all deaths occurring in hospitals [2]. The prevention, diagnosis, and treatment of sepsis should be considered a global health priority according to the World Health Assembly.

Medical tools available for the management of septic patients, and used in daily clinical practice, have been mainly developed in Intensive Care Units (ICUs) and have not been extensively validated in Internal Medicine (IM) wards [3]. Among the evaluated scores, only a few showed good reliability in predicting mortality [4]. In particular, the accuracy of these scores could be low or inadequate for IM patients; this population is characterized by high heterogeneity, advanced age, and multiple comorbidities impacting on prognosis [5]. At present, there is uncertainty about the optimal clinical score to be used for septic IM patients.

Procalcitonin (PCT) is a polypeptide released after the interaction between cytokine-activated macrophages and endothelial cells in response to bacterial components, particularly lipopolysaccharide [6]. Circulating PCT levels rapidly raise during the early phase of sepsis, reaching a peak value proportionally correlated with the severity of bacterial infection and rapidly decrease, due to its short half-life, after the resolution of disease [7]. Thanks to these characteristics, PCT can be considered a fundamental marker for the recognition of bacterial infection and sepsis. Moreover, PCT could play a role as prognostic marker for predicting outcomes [8], and it can be used as a guide to antibiotic therapy, although not as a stand-alone test [9]. In fact, it must be considered that there are differences in the observed levels of PCT in relation to several variables (e.g., type and site of infection, host's comorbidities, etc.) [10]. Most of the evidence in the literature suggests that baseline PCT levels are helpful in identifying the sickest patients, but not in predicting outcome. Multiple PCT determinations (PCT kinetics) appear to be more adequate for this purpose [11].

Vitamin D is a hormone playing its primary role in the bone homeostasis, but it is also involved in regulating immunity, both innate and adaptive [12]. The prevalence of vitamin D deficiency is particularly high among institutionalized subjects or those with other concomitant diseases [13]. As described in a previous study, the prevalence of vitamin D insufficiency was high in patients with bloodstream infection and sepsis admitted to Internal Medicine wards [4]. Low vitamin D levels can also be associated with a worse prognosis in patients with sepsis, but the results of studies performed in ICUs are heterogeneous [14–16].

The aim of the present study was to evaluate the accuracy of two consecutive PCT determinations (Delta-PCT) and vitamin D levels in predicting mortality, among a population of IM inpatients with microbiological identified sepsis.

2. Patients and Methods

2.1. Patients

The Internal Medicine Sepsis Study Group has promoted a 12-months sepsis surveillance program in two Internal Medicine Units of the "Agostino Gemelli" University Hospital, Catholic University of Rome, Rome, Italy [4]. Sepsis was defined according Sepsis-2 definition [17], while Quick SOFA (qSOFA) score was calculated according to Sepsis-3 definition [18]. During a screening phase, clinical information, laboratory data (including PCT and vitamin D), and clinical scores of 226 consecutive patients were recorded. Successively, after excluding patients with negative blood cultures, absence of SIRS criteria or non-clinically significant pathogens isolated on blood cultures, a total of 88 microbiologically-identified septic patients were included in the main study [4]. A total of 80 patients had at least two consecutive PCT determinations, thus they represent the sample evaluated in the present paper for statistical purposes.

2.2. Methods

This is a sub-analysis of a database including prospectively collected data of a cohort of consecutive patients with microbiological-identified sepsis admitted to an IM Unit [4]. The study was conducted according to local Ethical Committee guidelines. Anonymized clinical data were extracted from clinical records and recorded; thus informed consent was waived due to the observational, non-interventional design of the study.

Data regarding 28- and 90-days mortality were retained from the initial study [4].

PCT was assessed at the time of collection of blood cultures (T0, baseline) and during antimicrobial treatment (T1, 48–96 h from baseline). As previously reported, a PCT level > 2 ng/mL was considered a significant cut-off for sepsis. Delta-PCT was calculated as the percentual variation of PCT at T1 compared to T0. We defined Delta-PCT as a reduction of PCT levels > 50% after 48 h or >75% after 72 h or >85% after 96 h from T0. Thus, a reduction of PCT levels lower than these cut-offs or a baseline PCT < 2 ng/mL was considered as "absence of Delta-PCT."

Vitamin D assay was available in 63 out 80 (78.7%) patients. Although the Endocrine Society suggests specific categories for different vitamin D levels (e.g., vitamin D deficiency: 25(OH)D $\leq$ 19.9 ng/mL; vitamin D insufficiency: 20–29.9 ng/mL; vitamin D normal group: $\geq$30 ng/mL) [19], we adopted a dichotomous classification based on the presence of severe vitamin D deficiency (<7 ng/mL). This choice was done on the basis of literature data showing an association between severe vitamin D deficiency and mortality, in both critically ill and non-critically ill patients [15,20,21].

2.3. Statistical Analysis

A number of statistical procedures were applied for analysis of data, both descriptive and inferential, including numerical summaries (reported throughout the paper), Wilcoxon tests, Chi-square tests of independence, and logistic regression. The ultimate goal of the analysis was to primarily study the effect of Delta-PCT on 28-days and, respectively, 90-days mortality in a logistic regression framework. Moreover, vitamin D deficiency was studied in a similar way. First, a two-sample Wilcoxon test was run for assessing location differences of PCT levels at T0 between the group of deceased versus that of non-deceased patients. Then, a standard chi-squared test of independence in a two-way contingency table was used for tentatively testing the influence of both Delta-PCT and vitamin D deficiency on mortality. Afterwards, logistic regression was performed for an in-depth study of the effect of Delta-PCT as well as vitamin D deficiency on mortality. Obviously, all these analyses were repeated for both 28- and 90-days mortality. For the correct application of logistic regression, standard model checking techniques were run to assess model adequacy and thus validate the analysis method. All the computations were carried out by using the free software R [22].

3. Results

Main characteristics of the studied population have already been described [4] and are summarized in Table 1. Median age of patients was 75 years old. A significant proportion of them had a history of immunosuppression (40.9%), neoplasm (39.3%), diabetes (35.9%), or end-stage illness (23.9%). The majority of patients had received an antibiotic treatment in the previous 6 months (70.4%).

Table 1. Clinical characteristics of the 80 evaluated patients expressed as median (IQR; range); median values of survived or deceased patients at 28- and 90-days and statistical comparison.

	Study Patients (n = 80)	Survived 28-Days (n = 65)	Deceased 28-Days (n = 15)	p-Value	Survived 90-Days (n = 53)	Deceased 90-Days (n = 27)	p-Value
Male sex	46 (57.5%)	–	–	–	–	–	–
Age (years)	75 (64–83; 39–90)	72	83	0.068	73	81	0.032
BMI	24.7 (22.1–27.6; 19–44)	25	23	0.087	24.9	24.3	0.440
Procalcitonin (ng/mL)	2.91 (0.6–17.9; 0.1–100)	4.03	2.26	0.525	5.54	1.83	0.088
Vitamin D (ng/mL)	<7 (<7–9.9; <7–55.7)	7.7	<7	0.044	8.5	<7	0.032

A total of 15 out 80 patients (18.7%) died at 28-days and 27 out 80 (30.0%) died at 90-days. Baseline PCT levels did not differ between survived and deceased patients. A total of 39 patients (48.7%) showed Delta-PCT. A total of 31 out 63 patients (49.2%) patients showed severe vitamin D deficiency. Vitamin D levels were significantly lower in deceased than survived patients.

3.1. PCT and Mortality

The two-sample Wilcoxon tests showed that location values (specifically medians) of PCT levels at T0 did not differ between survived and deceased patients at 28-days (4.03 vs. 2.26; $p = 0.525$) nor at 90-days (5.54 vs. 1.83; $p = 0.088$). The Chi-square tests of independence showed a significantly higher proportion of patients with Delta-PCT among survivors at 28-days ($p = 0.002$) (Table 2) and at 90-days ($p < 0.001$) (Table 2). The accuracy of Delta-PCT (sensitivity, specificity, positive, and negative predictive values) in predicting 28- and 90-days patient's mortality are reported in Table 2. The logistic regression showed that the presence of Delta-PCT was associated with a lower 28-days ($p = 0.007$; OR = 0.12, 95%CI 0.02–0.46) and 90-days mortality ($p = 0.001$; OR = 0.17, 95%CI 0.06–0.48).

Table 2. Number and percentage of patients survived or deceased at 28-days and at 90-days according to the presence of Delta-procalcitonin (DELTA-PCT) and statistical significance at chi-square tests of independence. (Sens = sensitivity; Spec = specificity; PPV = positive predictive value, NPV = negative predictive value).

Table 2—28-days	Survived	Deceased	Total	
Delta-PCT = 1, n (%)	37 (94.9)	2 (5.1)	39	PPV 0.95 (0.87–0.98)
Delta-PCT = 0, n (%)	28 (68.3)	13 (31.7)	41	NPV 0.32 (0.22–0.43)
Total	65	15	80	
	Sens. 0.57 (0.45–0.68)	Spec. 0.87 (0.62–0.96)		$p = 0.002$
Table 2—90 days	Survived	Deceased	Total	
Delta-PCT = 1, n (%)	33 (84.6)	6 (15.4)	39	PPV 0.85 (0.74–0.91)
Delta-PCT = 0, n (%)	20 (48.8)	21 (51.2)	41	NPV 0.51 (0.40–0.62)
Total	53	27	80	
	Sens. 0.62 (0.49–0.74)	Spec. 0.78 (0.59–0.89)		$p < 0.0001$

3.2. Vitamin D and Mortality

The Chi-squared tests of independence showed a higher proportion of patients with severe vitamin D deficiency among deceased patients at 28-days ($p = 0.047$) (Table 3) and at 90-days ($p = 0.049$) (Table 3). The accuracy of vitamin D (sensitivity, specificity, positive, and negative predictive values) in predicting 28- and 90-days patient's mortality is reported in Table 3. The logistic regression showed that severe vitamin D deficiency was associated with a higher 28-days ($p = 0.058$; OR = 3.95, 95%CI 1.04–19.43) and 90-days mortality ($p = 0.054$; OR = 2.94, 95%CI 1.00–9.23), even if the level of significance was borderline.

Table 3. Number and percentage of patients survived or deceased at 28-days and at 90-days according to the presence of vitamin D deficiency (>/<7 ng/mL) and statistical significance at chi-square tests of independence. (Sens = sensitivity; Spec = specificity; PPV = positive predictive value, NPV = negative predictive value).

Table 3—28-days	Survived	Deceased	Total	
Vitamin D > 7 ng/mL, n (%)	29 (90.6)	3 (9.4)	32	PPV 0.91 (0.80–0.96)
Vitamin D < 7 ng/mL, n (%)	22 (71.0)	9 (29.0)	31	NPV 0.29 (0.19–0.42)
Total	51	12	63	
	Sens. 0.57 (0.43–0.69)	Spec. 0.75 (0.47–0.91)		$p = 0.046$
Table 3—90-days	Survived	Deceased	Total	
Vitamin D > 7 ng/mL, n (%)	25 (78.1)	7 (21.9)	32	PPV 0.78 (0.66–0.87)
Vitamin D < 7 ng/mL, n (%)	17 (54.8)	14 (45.2)	31	NPV 0.45 (0.33–0.58)
Total	42	21	63	
	Sens. 0.60 (0.44–0.73)	Spec. 0.67 (0.45–0.83)		$p = 0.049$

3.3. Two-Factors Logistic Regression Analysis

Finally, a two factors logistic regression confirmed previous results in terms of a negative effect of Delta-PCT on mortality both at 28-days ($p = 0.012$, OR = 0.06, 95%CI 0.003–0.38) and 90-days ($p = 0.003$, OR = 0.13, 95%CI 0.03–0.46) and a positive effect of severe vitamin D deficiency on mortality both at 28-days ($p = 0.056$; OR = 4.43, 95%CI 1.05–23.82) and 90-days ($p = 0.053$; OR = 3.31, 95%CI 1.02–11.83).

4. Discussion

The present study shows that Delta-PCT represents an independent predictor of outcome in a cohort of IM patients affected by bloodstream infection and sepsis. Literature data on prognostic performances of PCT in the IM setting are few and controversial.

We previously showed in the main cohort of this study that baseline PCT did not predict mortality [4]. In line with our results, Papadimitriou-Olivgeris and colleagues showed that baseline PCT levels did not differ between survivors and non-survivors and PCT was not an independent predictor of mortality in a cohort of patients with similar characteristics [23]. However, although similar, IM patients are likely to show a high heterogeneity limiting the generalizability of results derived by single cohorts [5].

The prognostic performances of Delta-PCT (PCT kinetics) in the IM setting have been evaluated by a few studies. To the best of our knowledge, the study by Pieralli and colleagues is the only one conducted in a non-ICU setting, aiming to evaluate the role of PCT kinetics in predicting 30-days mortality in a sample of 144 patients with severe sepsis and/or septic shock admitted to Emergency Departments (EDs) or general wards [24]. As main result, Delta-PCT independently predicted 30-day mortality. The present study confirms that repeated PCT determinations with Delta-PCT assessment could be a useful tool to assess both 28- and 90-days risk of mortality in IM septic patients.

The ability of Delta-PCT to be a better prognostic marker than single PCT measurement has several explanations. First, the value of a single PCT measurement as a predictor of outcome is poor given the large overlap between false negative and false positive values, different normal ranges and high interindividual variability due to acute comorbid states [5,25]. Moreover, in patients with BSIs, PCT levels depend on the etiological agent, being significantly higher in Gram-negative BSI than in Gram-positive or Candida BSIs, although PCT is insufficient to make an etiologic diagnosis when used alone [10]. Persistently high PCT values may indicate a persistence of the infectious state and/or a reduced response to antibiotic treatment. In addition, it should be considered that patients with an infection and impaired responsiveness of the immune system could show persistently low PCT values [26]. In both cases, the absence of a Delta-PCT could indicate an early risk of mortality. On the contrary, Delta-PCT often correlates with clinical improvement of the infectious picture. It can be used as a marker of efficacy of antibiotic treatment, even for an early de-escalation in order to reduce antibiotics side effects, as demonstrated in ICU studies [27,28].

In the present sample of IM septic patients, the accuracy of Delta-PCT was better in terms of specificity/PPV, than sensitivity/NPV. In other words, it is a biomarker with better "rule-out" than "rule-in" performances.

The present study confirms our previous observation on severe vitamin D deficiency as independent predictor of death. This observation is in line with a recent meta-analysis, that showed that lower vitamin D at admission was independently associated with increased risk or mortality in patients with sepsis, even applying different diagnostic criteria for sepsis (SIRS, Sepsis-2, or Sepsis-3) [29]. However, this observation requires future epidemiological studies to understand whether low vitamin D levels represent a causal factor for sepsis due to reduced immune function or an epiphenomenon due to increased tissue utilization associated with inflammation [25]. Vitamin D is able to induce the expression of antibacterial proteins and to enhance the environment in which they function [30]. Thus, the increased susceptibility to infections among patients with vitamin D deficiency could be explained by reduced bacterial killing activity in several cell types. Severe vitamin D deficiency could also be directly involved in "freezing" the individual's immune response capacity, in the context of sepsis itself [26]. This observation could confirm the susceptibility of Internal Medicine patients (e.g., comorbid, elderly, and institutionalized) with severe vitamin D deficiency to infections, sepsis, and poor sepsis-related outcomes. However, the observed accuracy of vitamin D deficiency was "low".

Limitations of the present study are represented by the small sample size and the monocentric IM population. Moreover, results of our analysis have not been adjusted for potential confounders (e.g., age and sex), given their lack of influence observed in the main paper [4]. In any case, our observations need to be validated on a larger sample.

5. Conclusions

Sepsis is increasingly diagnosed in Internal Medicine wards. The management of septic patients with multiple comorbidities represents a real challenge due to the complexity of the syndrome and the high heterogeneity of septic populations. Even few and relatively easy assessments of biomarkers can be of help for patients' outcome in certain conditions. Within this context, Delta-PCT and vitamin D could play a promising role for predicting the prognosis of septic patients admitted to Internal Medicine wards.

Author Contributions: Conceptualization, A.T., M.P. and A.M.; methodology, A.G., G.A. and S.D.C.; formal analysis, A.C.; investigation, A.T., M.I., G.P., C.V.V. and V.Z.; data curation, A.T. and M.P.; writing—original draft preparation, A.T., M.P. and A.M.; writing—review and editing, A.T., A.C., M.P., M.I., G.P., C.V.V., V.Z., A.G., G.A., S.D.C. and A.M.; project administration, A.M. The I.M.S.S.G. worked on the feasibility of the project. All authors have read and agreed to the published version of the manuscript.

Funding: This research received no external funding.

Institutional Review Board Statement: Not applicable.

Informed Consent Statement: Informed consent was waived due to the observational, non-interventional design of the study.

Data Availability Statement: Data supporting reported results may be provided on reasonable request.

Conflicts of Interest: The authors declare no conflict of interest.

References

1. Reinhart, K.; Daniels, R.; Kissoon, N.; Machado, F.R.; Schachter, R.D.; Finfer, S. Recognizing Sepsis as a Global Health Priority-A WHO Resolution. *N. Engl. J. Med.* **2017**, *377*, 414–417. [CrossRef]
2. Rudd, K.E.; Johnson, S.C.; Agesa, K.M.; Shackelford, K.A.; Tsoi, D.; Kievlan, D.R.; Colombara, D.V.; Ikuta, K.S.; Kissoon, N.; Finfer, S.; et al. Global, Regional, and National Sepsis Incidence and Mortality, 1990–2017: Analysis for the Global Burden of Disease Study. *Lancet* **2020**, *395*, 200–211. [CrossRef]
3. Zaccone, V.; Tosoni, A.; Passaro, G.; Vallone, C.V.; Impagnatiello, M.; Li Puma, D.D.; De Cosmo, S.; Landolfi, R.; Mirijello, A.; Internal Medicine Sepsis Study Group. Sepsis in Internal Medicine Wards: Current Knowledge, Uncertainties and New Approaches for Management Optimization. *Ann. Med.* **2017**, *49*, 582–592. [CrossRef]
4. Mirijello, A.; Tosoni, A.; Zaccone, V.; Impagnatiello, M.; Passaro, G.; Vallone, C.V.; Cossari, A.; Ventura, G.; Gambassi, G.; De Cosmo, S.; et al. MEDS Score and Vitamin D Status Are Independent Predictors of Mortality in a Cohort of Internal Medicine Patients with Microbiological Identified Sepsis. *Eur. Rev Med Pharmacol. Sci.* **2019**, *23*, 4033–4043. [CrossRef]
5. Tosoni, A.; Addolorato, G.; Gasbarrini, A.; De Cosmo, S.; Mirijello, A.; Internal Medicine Sepsis Study Group. Predictors of Mortality of Bloodstream Infections among Internal Medicine Patients: Mind the Complexity of the Septic Population! *Eur. J. Intern. Med.* **2019**, *68*, e22–e23. [CrossRef] [PubMed]
6. Assicot, M.; Gendrel, D.; Carsin, H.; Raymond, J.; Guilbaud, J.; Bohuon, C. High Serum Procalcitonin Concentrations in Patients with Sepsis and Infection. *Lancet* **1993**, *341*, 515–518. [CrossRef]
7. Bartoletti, M.; Antonelli, M.; Bruno Blasi, F.A.; Casagranda, I.; Chieregato, A.; Fumagalli, R.; Girardis, M.; Pieralli, F.; Plebani, M.; Rossolini, G.M.; et al. Procalcitonin-Guided Antibiotic Therapy: An Expert Consensus. *Clin. Chem. Lab. Med.* **2018**, *56*, 1223–1229. [CrossRef] [PubMed]
8. Yunus, I.; Fasih, A.; Wang, Y. The Use of Procalcitonin in the Determination of Severity of Sepsis, Patient Outcomes and Infection Characteristics. *PLoS ONE* **2018**, *13*, e0206527. [CrossRef]
9. Bassetti, M.; Russo, A.; Righi, E.; Dolso, E.; Merelli, M.; D'Aurizio, F.; Sartor, A.; Curcio, F. Role of Procalcitonin in Predicting Etiology in Bacteremic Patients: Report from a Large Single-Center Experience. *J. Infect. Public Health* **2020**, *13*, 40–45. [CrossRef]

10. Cortegiani, A.; Misseri, G.; Ippolito, M.; Bassetti, M.; Giarratano, A.; Martin-Loeches, I.; Einav, S. Procalcitonin Levels in Candidemia versus Bacteremia: A Systematic Review. *Crit. Care* **2019**, *23*, 190. [CrossRef] [PubMed]
11. Tosoni, A.; Paratore, M.; Piscitelli, P.; Addolorato, G.; De Cosmo, S.; Mirijello, A.; Internal Medicine Sepsis Study Group. The Use of Procalcitonin for the Management of Sepsis in Internal Medicine Wards: Current Evidence. *Panminerva Med.* **2020**, *62*, 54–62. [CrossRef] [PubMed]
12. Adams, J.S.; Hewison, M. Unexpected Actions of Vitamin D: New Perspectives on the Regulation of Innate and Adaptive Immunity. *Nat. Clin. Pract. Endocrinol. Metab.* **2008**, *4*, 80–90. [CrossRef] [PubMed]
13. Koekkoek, W.A.C.K.; van Zanten, A.R.H. Vitamin D Deficiency in the Critically Ill. *Ann. Med.* **2016**, *48*, 301–304. [CrossRef]
14. Quraishi, S.A.; De Pascale, G.; Needleman, J.S.; Nakazawa, H.; Kaneki, M.; Bajwa, E.K.; Camargo, C.A.; Bhan, I. Effect of Cholecalciferol Supplementation on Vitamin D Status and Cathelicidin Levels in Sepsis: A Randomized, Placebo-Controlled Trial. *Crit. Care Med.* **2015**, *43*, 1928–1937. [CrossRef]
15. De Pascale, G.; Vallecoccia, M.S.; Schiattarella, A.; Di Gravio, V.; Cutuli, S.L.; Bello, G.; Montini, L.; Pennisi, M.A.; Spanu, T.; Zuppi, C.; et al. Clinical and Microbiological Outcome in Septic Patients with Extremely Low 25-Hydroxyvitamin D Levels at Initiation of Critical Care. *Clin. Microbiol. Infect.* **2016**, *22*, 456.e7–456.e13. [CrossRef]
16. Ala-Kokko, T.I.; Mutt, S.J.; Nisula, S.; Koskenkari, J.; Liisanantti, J.; Ohtonen, P.; Poukkanen, M.; Laurila, J.J.; Pettilä, V.; Herzig, K.-H.; et al. Vitamin D Deficiency at Admission Is Not Associated with 90-Day Mortality in Patients with Severe Sepsis or Septic Shock: Observational FINNAKI Cohort Study. *Ann. Med.* **2016**, *48*, 67–75. [CrossRef] [PubMed]
17. Levy, M.M.; Fink, M.P.; Marshall, J.C.; Abraham, E.; Angus, D.; Cook, D.; Cohen, J.; Opal, S.M.; Vincent, J.-L.; Ramsay, G.; et al. 2001 SCCM/ESICM/ACCP/ATS/SIS International Sepsis Definitions Conference. *Crit. Care Med.* **2003**, *31*, 1250–1256. [CrossRef]
18. Seymour, C.W.; Liu, V.X.; Iwashyna, T.J.; Brunkhorst, F.M.; Rea, T.D.; Scherag, A.; Rubenfeld, G.; Kahn, J.M.; Shankar-Hari, M.; Singer, M.; et al. Assessment of Clinical Criteria for Sepsis: For the Third International Consensus Definitions for Sepsis and Septic Shock (Sepsis-3). *JAMA* **2016**, *315*, 762–774. [CrossRef]
19. Holick, M.F.; Binkley, N.C.; Bischoff-Ferrari, H.A.; Gordon, C.M.; Hanley, D.A.; Heaney, R.P.; Murad, M.H.; Weaver, C.M.; Endocrine Society. Evaluation, Treatment, and Prevention of Vitamin D Deficiency: An Endocrine Society Clinical Practice Guideline. *J. Clin. Endocrinol. Metab.* **2011**, *96*, 1911–1930. [CrossRef]
20. Amrein, K.; Schnedl, C.; Holl, A.; Riedl, R.; Christopher, K.B.; Pachler, C.; Urbanic Purkart, T.; Waltensdorfer, A.; Münch, A.; Warnkross, H.; et al. Effect of High-Dose Vitamin D3 on Hospital Length of Stay in Critically Ill Patients with Vitamin D Deficiency: The VITdAL-ICU Randomized Clinical Trial. *JAMA* **2014**, *312*, 1520–1530. [CrossRef]
21. Trongtrakul, K.; Feemuchang, C. Prevalence and Association of Vitamin D Deficiency and Mortality in Patients with Severe Sepsis. *Int. J. Gen. Med.* **2017**, *10*, 415–421. [CrossRef]
22. The R Project for Statistical Computing. Available online: https://www.r-project.org/ (accessed on 2 February 2021).
23. Papadimitriou-Olivgeris, M.; Psychogiou, R.; Garessus, J.; Camaret, A.D.; Fourre, N.; Kanagaratnam, S.; Jecker, V.; Nusbaumer, C.; Monnerat, L.B.; Kocher, A.; et al. Predictors of Mortality of Bloodstream Infections among Internal Medicine Patients in a Swiss Hospital: Role of Quick Sequential Organ Failure Assessment. *Eur. J. Intern. Med.* **2019**, *65*, 86–92. [CrossRef] [PubMed]
24. Pieralli, F.; Vannucchi, V.; Mancini, A.; Antonielli, E.; Luise, F.; Sammicheli, L.; Turchi, V.; Para, O.; Bacci, F.; Nozzoli, C. Procalcitonin Kinetics in the First 72 Hours Predicts 30-Day Mortality in Severely Ill Septic Patients Admitted to an Intermediate Care Unit. *J. Clin. Med. Res.* **2015**, *7*, 706–713. [CrossRef] [PubMed]
25. Schuetz, P.; Beishuizen, A.; Broyles, M.; Ferrer, R.; Gavazzi, G.; Gluck, E.H.; González Del Castillo, J.; Jensen, J.-U.; Kanizsai, P.L.; Kwa, A.L.H.; et al. Procalcitonin (PCT)-Guided Antibiotic Stewardship: An International Experts Consensus on Optimized Clinical Use. *Clin. Chem. Lab. Med.* **2019**, *57*, 1308–1318. [CrossRef]
26. Feuerecker, M.; Sudhoff, L.; Crucian, B.; Pagel, J.-I.; Sams, C.; Strewe, C.; Guo, A.; Schelling, G.; Briegel, J.; Kaufmann, I.; et al. Early Immune Anergy towards Recall Antigens and Mitogens in Patients at Onset of Septic Shock. *Sci. Rep.* **2018**, *8*, 1754. [CrossRef] [PubMed]
27. Georgopoulou, A.-P.; Savva, A.; Giamarellos-Bourboulis, E.J.; Georgitsi, M.; Raftogiannis, M.; Antonakos, N.; Apostolidou, E.; Carrer, D.-P.; Dimopoulos, G.; Economou, A.; et al. Early Changes of Procalcitonin May Advise about Prognosis and Appropriateness of Antimicrobial Therapy in Sepsis. *J. Crit. Care* **2011**, *26*, 331.e1–331.e7. [CrossRef]
28. Schuetz, P.; Wirz, Y.; Sager, R.; Christ-Crain, M.; Stolz, D.; Tamm, M.; Bouadma, L.; Luyt, C.E.; Wolff, M.; Chastre, J.; et al. Effect of Procalcitonin-Guided Antibiotic Treatment on Mortality in Acute Respiratory Infections: A Patient Level Meta-Analysis. *Lancet Infect. Dis.* **2018**, *18*, 95–107. [CrossRef]
29. Li, Y.; Ding, S. Serum 25-Hydroxyvitamin D and the risk of mortality in adult patients with Sepsis: A meta-analysis. *BMC Infect. Dis.* **2020**, *20*, 189. [CrossRef]
30. Hewison, M. Antibacterial Effects of Vitamin D. *Nat. Rev. Endocrinol.* **2011**, *7*, 337–345. [CrossRef]

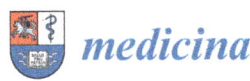

Review

Presepsin as Early Marker of Sepsis in Emergency Department: A Narrative Review

Andrea Piccioni [1], Michele Cosimo Santoro [1,*], Tommaso de Cunzo [2], Gianluca Tullo [2], Sara Cicchinelli [1], Angela Saviano [2], Federico Valletta [2], Marco Maria Pascale [1], Marcello Candelli [1], Marcello Covino [1,2] and Francesco Franceschi [1,2]

1. Emergency Medicine Fondazione Policlinico Universitario A. Gemelli IRCCS, 00168 Rome, Italy; andrea.piccioni@policlinicogemelli.it (A.P.); sara.cicchinelli@policlinicogemelli.it (S.C.); marcomaria.pascale@policlinicogemelli.it (M.M.P.); marcello.candelli@policlinicogemelli.it (M.C.); marcello.covino@policlinicogemelli.it (M.C.); francesco.franceschi@policlinicogemelli.it (F.F.)
2. Fondazione Policlinico Universitario A. Gemelli IRCCS, Università Cattolica del Sacro Cuore, 00168 Rome, Italy; tomdecunzo@gmail.com (T.d.C.); gianlucatullo@gmail.com (G.T.); saviange@libero.it (A.S.); fede.valletta@gemelli.com (F.V.)
* Correspondence: michelecosimo.santoro@policlinicogemelli.it

Abstract: The diagnosis and treatment of sepsis have always been a challenge for the physician, especially in critical care setting such as emergency department (ED), and currently sepsis remains one of the major causes of mortality. Although the traditional definition of sepsis based on systemic inflammatory response syndrome (SIRS) criteria changed in 2016, replaced by the new criteria of SEPSIS-3 based on organ failure evaluation, early identification and consequent early appropriated therapy remain the primary goal of sepsis treatment. Unfortunately, currently there is a lack of a foolproof system for making early sepsis diagnosis because conventional diagnostic tools like cultures take a long time and are often burdened with false negatives, while molecular techniques require specific equipment and have high costs. In this context, biomarkers, such as C-Reactive Protein (CRP) and Procalcitonin (PCT), are very useful tools to distinguish between normal and pathological conditions, graduate the disease severity, guide treatment, monitor therapeutic responses and predict prognosis. Among the new emerging biomarkers of sepsis, Presepsin (P-SEP) appears to be the most promising. Several studies have shown that P-SEP plasma levels increase during bacterial sepsis and decline in response to appropriate therapy, with sensitivity and specificity values comparable to those of PCT. In neonatal sepsis, P-SEP compared to PCT has been shown to be more effective in diagnosing and guiding therapy. Since in sepsis the P-SEP plasma levels increase before those of PCT and since the current methods available allow measurement of P-SEP plasma levels within 17 min, P-SEP appears a sepsis biomarker particularly suited to the emergency department and critical care.

Keywords: Presepsin; sepsis; emergency department; critical care; ICU

1. Introduction

The diagnosis and treatment of sepsis have always been a challenge for the physician, especially in critical care setting. Indeed, sepsis is one of the major causes of mortality in both emergency department (ED) and intensive care unit (ICU), due to main difficulty of early recognition and appropriate identification of the etiology [1–3]. In many cases, infections are characterized by signs and symptoms that can overlap with other acute disease, therefore differential diagnosis is crucial, but often demanding, and leads to a double issue. On the one hand, the untimely identification of a sepsis leads to a therapeutic delay with a consequent increase in mortality; on the other hand, often patients are treated with unnecessary antibiotic therapy, which is one of the main causes of antibiotic resistance [4–6]. The traditional definition of sepsis, since 1992 referred to as the presence or suspected infection associated with a systemic inflammatory response syndrome (SIRS) [7], changed in 2016, replaced by the new criteria of SEPSIS-3 [8], so that sepsis is currently defined as infection with organ dysfunction, assessed by the Sequential Organ Failure Assessment (SOFA score), while the previous expression "severe sepsis" is no longer adopted to increase predictive accuracy [9]; however, early identification and consequent early appropriated therapy remain a cornerstone of sepsis treatment. In clinical practice the diagnosis of sepsis is based on tools such as cultures, which take a long time and are often burdened with false negatives, while the use of molecular techniques requires specific equipment and skilled operators, thus entailing very high costs [5,10]. Therefore, currently there is a lack of a foolproof system for making early sepsis diagnosis. In this context, biomarkers, defined as objectively measurable characteristics of biological processes, are very useful tools to distinguish between normal and pathological conditions, graduate the disease severity, guide treatment, monitor therapeutic responses and predict prognosis [11,12]. Alongside the more widely spread and employed markers, such as C-Reactive Protein (CRP) and Procalcitonin (PCT), there are new ones emerging, among which P-SEP appears to be the most promising [13]. The purpose of this review is to search, by consulting electronic databases, the main studies performed in the last 10 years concerning the use of P-SEP in sepsis, with particular attention to those concerning the usefulness of P-SEP in the emergency department.

2. Methods and Results

We checked medical literature of the last 10 years to find P-SEP related studies and reports. The following electronic databases were systematically searched: MEDLINE-PubMed, Web of Science, Scopus, and the Cochrane Central Register of Controlled Trials (CENTRAL). The search strings were:

- Presepsin AND sepsis
- Presepsin AND emergency department
- Presepsin AND critical care
- Presepsin AND ICU

The search strategy was limited to English language articles. We mainly focused on randomized placebo-control studies, followed by case-control studies, observational (both retrospective or prospective), and finally systematic reviews and meta-analysis. The article selection process was carried out independently by two reviewers (MCS and TdC). Additional manual scrutiny carried out from the references of the selected articles was performed in order to identify other potentially relevant studies.

We identified a total of 224 studies deemed to be relevant for the issues in stake (Table 1). Among these, 166 articles are clinical trials, of which 4 are randomized controlled trials. The remaining articles consist in 38 reviews, and 13 systematic reviews and meta-analysis (Table 2). As summarized in Table 2, the meta-analysis performed in 2015 mainly focused on validating the diagnostic value of P-SEP in sepsis, while the meta-analysis conducted between 2016 and 2019 analyzed the prognostic value of P-SEP in comparison and in combination with other biomarkers of sepsis, especially the more common used C-RP and PCT [14–26].

Table 1. List of studies.

Type	n°
Total studies	224
Review	38
Systematic review and meta-analysis	13
Clinical trial	162
Randomized controlled trial	4

Table 2. Systematic review and meta-analysis.

Author	Year	Patients	Results
Zhang, J. et al. [14]	2015	3052	P-SEP is an effective diagnostic marker for sepsis (DOR 18)
Wu, J. et al. [15]	2015	2159	P-SEP is an effective diagnostic marker for sepsis (DOR 21.73)
Zheng, Z. et al. [16]	2015	1757	P-SEP is an effective diagnostic marker for sepsis (DOR 14.25)
Tong, X. et al. [17]	2015	3109	P-SEP is an effective diagnostic marker for sepsis (DOR 21.56)
Liu, Y. et al. [18]	2016	10438	PCT, CRP, IL6, sTREM-1, P-SEP, LBP and CD64 have similar diagnostic accuracy in detecting sepsis (AUC 0.85, 0.77, 0.79, 0.85, 0.88, 0.71 and 0.96 respectively)
Wu, C.C. et al. [19]	2017	3470	P-SEP is a good predictor for sepsis (DOR 16) but there is no significant variations compared to PCT (14) or CRP (13)
Yang, H.S. et al. [20]	2018	1617	P-SEP can predict mortality in patients with sepsis (SMD survivors/non-survivors 0.92)
Ruan, L. et al.[21]	2018	2661	Combination of PCT and CRP (DOR 79) or P-SEP alone (864) have better diagnostic power than CRP (19) and PCT (31) alone in neonatal sepsis
Yoon, S.H. et al. [22]	2019	308	P-SEP has higher diagnostic accuracy than PCT or CRP in detecting sepsis in children (OR 32.87, 11.8 and 4.63 respectively)
Kondo, Y. et al. [23]	2019	3012	Diagnostic accuracy in detecting infection is similar for PCT and P-SEP (sensibility 0.80 and 0.84, specificity 0.75 and 0.73 respectively)
Parri, N. et al. [24]	2019	636	Diagnostic accuracy of P-SEP resulted high in detecting neonatal sepsis (DOR 120.94)
van Maldeghem, I. et al. [25]	2019	1369	P-SEP is an effective diagnostic marker for sepsis in neonates (AUC 0.9639)
Zhu, Y. et al. [26]	2019	1561	PCT and P-SEP are both an effective diagnostic marker for sepsis (DOR 10 and 9 respectively)

3. Current Data on Presepsin as a Biomarker for Sepsis

3.1. Presepsin

P-SEP is the subtype of the soluble form of CD14 (sCD14-ST); more precisely, P-SEP is the 13 KDa N-terminal fragment of soluble form of CD14 (sCD14), cleaved by cathepsin D in plasma, and involved in activating the innate immune system. [27]. Especially in the last decade, several studies have shown increases in response to bacterial infections and decreases after healing or effective treatment [6,14], so that P-SEP is considered a new biomarker, effective in early recognition of different types of infections [28,29]. As known, infections activate the host's immune system, usually distinguished into innate and an adaptive: while adaptive needs several days to be effective, an innate system provides an immediate response mainly through the alternative complement system and phagocytosis [30–32]. Both systems need to recognize the pathogens, but the innate one carries out recognition through different receptors, that are already predetermined, placed on the immune effector cell surface [33,34], able to recognizing a wide range of antigens on the surface of most microbial pathogens [35]. CD14 is 55 KDa transmembrane glycoprotein acting as a coreceptor, placed on the monocytes and macrophages cell surface, belonging to the family of Toll-like receptors (TLRs), which play a role in the identification of several Gram-positive and Gram-negative bacterial ligands [31,36]. In particular, the recognition of Lipopolysaccharide (LPS), present on the Gram-negative bacteria surface, requires the association of the Lipoprotein Binding Protein (LBP), which presents the LPS at CD14; the CD14-LPS-LBP complex stimulates intra-cellular signals that promote the expression of genes involved in the immune response such as cytokines production by effector cells [37]. CD14 exists in two forms: one bound to the membrane (mCD14) of monocyte and macrophage cells, and a soluble one (sCD14) present in the plasma, where it is cleaved by cathepsin D into a fragment of 13 kDa (sCD14-ST), precisely named, released in the general circulation by proteolysis and exocytosis [13,37] (Figure 1).

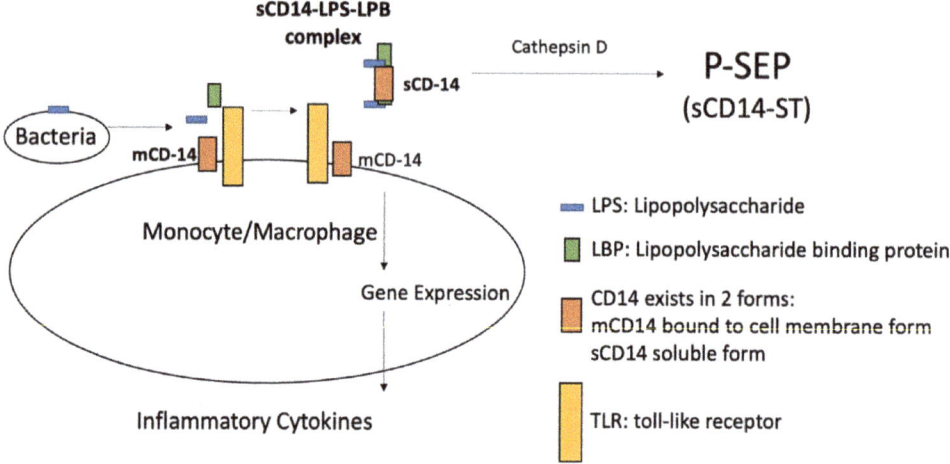

Figure 1. P-SEP is the 13 KDa N-terminal fragment of soluble form of CD14 (sCD14), cleaved by cathepsin D in plasma, and involved in activating the innate immune system.

3.2. Presepsin Measurement

Since P-SEP is released during the activation of the immune system, it is essential to have a rapid and accurate method to measure P-SEP plasma level and establish a cut-off, which allows distinguishing sick individuals from healthy ones [38]. The method initially developed was a conventional two-step ELISA assay, measuring P-SEP in a range of 3–150 ng/mL, but requiring a total assay time of 4 h and most importantly showing low accuracy. Subsequently, producing a one-step instead of a two-step method and using recombinant P-SEP instead of recombinant CD14, Thermo Fisher developed a faster ELISA, resulting in a reduction of the total assay time from 4 to 1.5 h and a change in range of 0.05–3.00 ng/mL (or 50–3000 ng/L) instead of 3-150 ng/mL (obtained with the previous two-step ELISA) [39]. Based on chemiluminescence enzyme immunoassay (CLEIA) in combination with MAGTRATION technology, PATHFAST (Mitsubishi Chemical) is an innovative, highly sensitive and fully automated method, which allows the measurement of P-SEP plasma levels, using whole blood samples, able to provide results within 17 min in six samples simultaneously [40,41]. This feature, together with the non-interference by other analytes such as hemoglobin, bilirubin, lipids, makes PATHFAST a very useful tool in critical areas, especially in an emergency department, where rapid quantitative results are required.

3.3. Diagnostic Significance of Presepsin in Sepsis

The results of several prospective multicenter trials, manly conducted in the last decade, have shown that, using a cut-off value of 600 ng/L, P-SEP plasma levels are significantly elevated in patients with bacterial infection compared to non-bacterial infections, with sensitivity and specificity of 87.8% and 81.4%, respectively [42–45]. Another study has shown that using a cut off of 670, sensitivity and specificity were reported to be 70.3% and 81.3%, respectively, while at a cut off value of 864 ng/L, sensitivity and specificities were 71.4% and 63.8%, respectively [46]. Several studies reported that a cut off of 600 ng/mL is not able to discriminate between Gram positive and Gram-negative and was not related to the positivity or negativity of blood cultures, while in 2015 in the multicentric randomized trial ALBIOS Masson et al. found that at a baseline concentration of 946 ng/L plasma P-SEP levels are higher in patients with Gram-negative than in Gram-positive bacterial infections [47]; it is hypothesized that this is due to the role played by P-SEP in the formation of the CD14-LPS-LBP complex. The ALBIOS trial also reported that the P-SEP value (mean ± standard deviation), in the healthy, SIRS and sepsis group, was 258.7 ± 92.53 ng/L, 430.0 ± 141.33 ng/L and 1508.3 ± 866.6 ng/L respectively [47]. However, in a 2015 meta-analysis, Wu et al. reported that P-SEP has only moderate diagnostic accuracy in differentiating sepsis from other non-septic inflammatory conditions, suggesting that the results should be interpreted with caution and further studies are needed before considering P-SEP as a definitive marker for the diagnosis of sepsis [15].

3.4. Prognostic Significance of Presepsin in Sepsis

The change in P-SEP plasma levels is a solid prognostic and therapeutic tool in hospitalized patients, however the P-SEP measured on arrival in the emergency department can be useful in risk stratification [48,49], especially for Gram-negative bacterial infection, probably due to the sCD14-ST role in the sepsis cascade as a receptor for LPS [50]. In a 2018 meta-analysis, including 10 studies with a total of 1617 patients, Yang et al. reported that P-SEP plasma levels in the first sampling (within 24 h) was significantly lower among survivors than non-survivors (I^2 = 79%, p < 0.01) [20], while in the subgroups, divided by severity of sepsis or infection site, P-SEP was consistently higher in non-survivors. In hospitalized patients, many studies show that in severe sepsis (according to the definition prior to SEPSIS-3) or septic shock, the reduction in P-SEP plasma levels is associated with an increased survival and indicates the effectiveness of the antibiotic therapy, with P-SEP tending to decline by day 7 in patients with positive blood cultures and appropriate antibiotic therapy. Speculatively, high P-SEP plasma levels in the seventh day is considered due to inappropriate or ineffective therapy even with positive blood cultures (mostly multidrug-resistant bacteria), and is associated with increased mortality, the onset of complications, such as prolonged need for ventilation and inotropic agents, therefore a prolonged length to stay in ICU, as well as the presence of acute or acute on chronic kidney injury. [46,51,52]. In a study conducted in ICU patients, P-SEP was effective in predicting sepsis with a sensitivity and specificity values of 84.6% and 62.5%, respectively, which were significantly related to APACHE II score (p-value = 0.016) [53].

3.5. Presepsin Compared to C-RP and PCT: Alone or in Company?

Recently, several studies have focused on the role of new and emerging biomarkers of sepsis, such as proadrenomedullin, interleukin-6 (IL-6), CD 64, the soluble form of triggering receptor expressed on myeloid cells-1 (sTREM-1) [54], however most of the studies were carried out comparing P-SEP with C-RP and PCT, which to date remain the most widely diffuse markers of sepsis in clinical practice [26]. The diagnostic and prognostic efficacy of P-SEP has been analyzed in different clinical settings not only as an alternative, but also in combination with C-RP and PCT; these comparative studies have reported controversial results [55–59]. In 2017, Kim et al. reported that, using a cutoff of 2455 ng/L, P-SEP is better than PCT in predicting mortality of sepsis at 30 days (AUC of 0.684 versus 0.513), being higher in non survivors than in survivors [55], while in another 2015 study, using a cut off of 413 ng/L for diagnosing bacterial infections in ICU patients, Godnic et al. reported that P-SEP has a higher AUC compared to PCT (0.705 vs. 0.630) but lower than C-RP (0.705 vs. 0.734) [53]. In 2016, Plesko et al. reported that in hematologic patients the association of P-ESP with IL-6 increases sensitivity compared to the use of P-SEP alone in detecting sepsis, while the association of P-SEP with PCT and C-RP did not show better accuracy than P-SEP alone in detecting sepsis in this type of patient [60]. Klouche et al. reported greater specificity of P-SEP and PCT in combination for the diagnosis of sepsis, septic shock and pneumonia, compared to using PCT alone or P-SEP alone [61].

3.6. Presepsin in Pediatric Bacterial Infection

Numerous studies have investigated the diagnostic and prognostic role of P-SEP in different type of infections in children, such as early (EOS) and late onset sepsis (LOS) in preterm infants, particularly meningitis and pneumonia, but also infections in febrile neutropenic patients affected by onco-hematological neoplasms [6,24,25,45,62–68]. In neonatal sepsis P-SEP compared to PCT has been shown to be more effective in diagnosing and guiding therapy [62]. In the EOS at the cutoff of 539 ng/L, P-SEP has showed a sensitivity of 80% and specificity of 75%, while in the LOS at the cutoff of 885 ng/L, P-SEP demonstrated a sensitivity of 94% and a specificity of 100% [21,22,69]. In the pediatric setting, mean P-SEP plasma levels in healthy infants are much higher (720 ng/L) than in healthy adults, probably due to the passage after birth from the intrauterine environment to the new external environment rich in foreign antigens, which activates the innate immune system [69].

3.7. Presepsin in Fungal Infection

Several recent studies have shown that fungi are responsible for about 20% of all cases of sepsis, with a fatal outcome reaching 80% [70]. For this reason, in recent years there has been a growing attention towards fungal sepsis, the differential diagnosis of which from bacterial sepsis is often very challenging since the clinical manifestations can be overlapped. The main issue of fungal infections concerns neutropenic patients suffering from onco-hematological neoplasms and immunosuppressed patients. In this category of patients, more recently in 2019, several studies have demonstrated the usefulness of P-SEP in combination with PCT and C-RP in the diagnosis of bacterial and fungal infections. Stoma et al. reported that in hematological patients undergoing stem cell transplantation a cutoff of 218 ng/L is indicative of bacteremia [71], while elevation of C-RP associated with plasma P-ESP in the normal range predicts a fungal infection in immunocompromised patients [50]. Other studies have confirmed that a fungal infection can be predicted by the combination of increased P-SEP plasma levels with little or no alteration in PCT [72] and that plasma PSP levels are related to the severity of sepsis [73].

3.8. Presepsin Significance in SARS-CoV-2 Infection

Some studies published in 2020 reported that P-SEP is effective in risk stratification in patients with SARS-CoV-2 pneumonia, but further studies are needed to solidify this assertion. In a case series of six patients with SARS-CoV-2 pneumonia, Fukada et al. found that elevated P-SEP plasma levels can predict evolution towards ARDS [74], and Zaninotto et al. confirmed the effectiveness the prognostic value of P-SEP in 75 patients with SARS-CoV-2 pneumonia admitted to infectious disease ward and ICU [75].

3.9. Presepsin in Emergency Department

The critical area setting, especially ED, is particularly suited to reveal the potential greater utility of P-SEP over PCT in the early diagnosis of sepsis. Several studies have shown that P-SEP has diagnostic and prognostic power substantially similar to PCT, but, unlike PCT, P-SEP increases earlier in bacterial infection and can be measured effectively and accurately within 17 min directly in the emergency department [53]. A 2013 prospective study, conducted on 859 consecutive ED patients with at least two SIRS criteria (as defined prior to SEPIS-3), showed that P-SEP plasma levels is useful both for the diagnosis and for prognosis of sepsis, since P-SEP has been shown to be effective in stratifying the severity of sepsis, septic shock and in predicting mortality at 28 days. This study showed that the sensitivity, specificity, positive predictive value (PPV), negative predictive value (NPV) and diagnostic accuracy vary according to the cutoff used for P-SEP plasma levels. Using a cutoff of 449 ng/L P-SEP grades the severity of sepsis with sensitivity of 82.4%, specificity of 72.4%, PPV of 71.3% and NPV of 83.2% with a predictive accuracy of 77.0%; using a cutoff of 550 ng/L P-SEP predicts septic shock with sensitivity, specificity, PVV and NPV of 85.7%, 63.6%, 28.5% and 96.3%, respectively, and a predictive accuracy of 66.8%;

using a cutoff of 556 ng/mL P-SEP predicts mortality at 28 days with sensitivity of 62.2%, specificity of 66.8%, PPV of 48.3%, NPV of 78.0% and predictive accuracy of 65.3% [44]. In 2015, Carpio et al. performed another single-center prospective observational study, including 120 patients with SIRS or sepsis criteria (prior to SEPSIS-3) and 123 healthy controls, confirmed that P-SEP at a cutoff of 581 ng/L is effective in diagnosing sepsis, graduating severity of disease and differentiating between SIRS and sepsis in ED, with sensitivity of 61% and specificity of 100% [49]. Also in this study, as in the previous one, the performance of P-SEP varies according to the cutoff considered: using a cutoff of 273 ng/L, a sensitivity of 95.5% and specificity of 21.7% were found, while using a cutoff of 686 ng/L these values were 46.5% and 91.3%, respectively. A study performed by de Guadiana Romualdo et al. in 2014, including 226 patients admitted to the ED with SIRS criteria, of which 37 had positive blood culture (bacteremic SIRS group) and 189 had negative blood culture (non-bacteremic SIRS group), reported sensitivity, specificity, PPV and NVP values of 81.1%, 63%, 30% and 94.4%, respectively, for the diagnosis of SIRS using a cutoff of 729 ng/L [57]. In 2017 the same author examined a cohort of 223 admitted in ED for suspected sepsis using two different P-SEP cutoffs, 312 and 849 ng/L, and found sensitivity values of 97.1% and of 67.1% and specificity values of 16.9% and 80.8%, respectively [58]. It has been reported that, using a 101.6 ng/L cutoff, P-SEP, measured at the time of diagnosis in the ED 24 h before admission to the ICU, has values of sensitivity, specificity, PPV and NPV of 81.9%, 96.5%, 82.4% and 96.3%, respectively, thus allowing for better management in both severe sepsis and septic shock [22,59]. The different cutoff values reported in the different studies are likely due to heterogeneity regarding the clinical setting (ED, ICU), the sepsis criteria adopted (before or after SEPSIS-3) and the type of sample (plasma, serum or whole blood) for the measurement of the P-SEP.

3.10. Presepsin Use Caveat

There are several clinical conditions in which special care must be taken in interpreting altered P-SEP plasma levels [50]. The more common diagnostic limitation of P-SEP is likely renal failure. Since the kidney is involved in the P-SEP excretion, the P-SEP plasma levels are increased in patients with renal failure. For this reason, the cutoffs must be adapted in patients with chronic kidney disease and/or on hemodialysis treatment [76]. P-SEP is also affected by the translocation of intestinal microbial flora [77]. Some pathophysiological conditions, such as age (newborns and elderly individuals, especially if suffering from renal failure) or burns [78] can influence P-SEP plasma levels, which may be higher even in the absence of disease [76], while further investigations are needed to define the influence of steroid use on P-SEP [27]. All these conditions must be considered to avoid an incorrect diagnosis of sepsis and consequently inappropriate treatments.

4. Discussion and Conclusions

The diagnosis and treatment of sepsis have always been a challenge for the physician, especially in critical care setting such as emergency department, and currently sepsis remains one of the major causes of mortality. Although the traditional definition of sepsis based on systemic inflammatory response syndrome (SIRS) criteria changed in 2016, replaced by the new criteria of SEPSIS-3 based on organ failure evaluation, early identification and consequent early appropriated therapy remain the primary goal of sepsis treatment. Among the new emerging biomarkers of sepsis, P-SEP appears to be the most promising. The studies examined demonstrate that P-SEP is a valid and reliable biomarker of bacterial sepsis, especially Gram-negative bacteria, and it is also a tool effective in evaluating the efficacy of therapy since the P-SEP plasma levels decrease when therapy is effective and increase when therapy is ineffective. It also emerges that P-SEP has a diagnostic and prognostic power substantially comparable to PCT, even if not all authors agree on the diagnostic accuracy; many currently recommend not to use P-SEP alone, but in combination with other sepsis markers, as well as traditional diagnostic tools like cultures. Furthermore, in some clinical conditions, such as renal failure, P-SEP plasma levels can be altered in the absence of sepsis, so that different P-SEP cutoffs are reported. Studies performed in pediatric setting have shown that P-SEP is a more effective than PCT in diagnosing neonatal sepsis. In critical areas, in particular the emergency department, P-SEP appears to be the most promising sepsis marker, due to earlier plasma levels increase than PCT, and the currently available assays, which allow for obtaining the P-SEP plasma levels within 17 min, thus allowing an early recognition and therapy of sepsis already in ED. Further studies are needed to better define diagnostic cutoffs and better evaluate the diagnostic and prognostic utility of P-SEP compared to PCT in the emergency department.

Author Contributions: Conceptualization, A.P. and M.C.S.; Methodology, T.d.C. and G.T.; Software, M.C. (Marcello Candelli) and M.C. (Marcello Covino); Validation, A.P. and M.C.S. and F.F.; Formal Analysis, M.C.S. and A.S.; Investigation, S.C. and M.M.P.; Resources, F.V.; Data Curation, M.C.S.; Writing—Original Draft Preparation, A.P. and M.C.S. and F.V. Writing—Review & Editing, A.P. and M.C.S.; Visualization, M.C. (Marcello Covino); Supervision, F.F. All authors have read and agreed to the published version of the manuscript.

Funding: This research received no external funding.

Institutional Review Board Statement: The study was conducted according to the guidelines of the Declaration of Helsinki. Ethical review and approval were waived for this study, because it is a review.

Informed Consent Statement: Not applicable.

Data Availability Statement: Not applicable.

Conflicts of Interest: The authors declare no conflict of interest.

References

1. Ulla, M.; Pizzolato, E.; Lucchiari, M.; Loiacono, M.; Soardo, F.; Forno, D.; Morello, F.; Lupia, E.; Moiraghi, C.; Mengozzi, G.; et al. Diagnostic and prognostic value of presepsin in the management of sepsis in the emergency department: A multicenter prospective study. *Crit. Care* **2013**, *17*, R168. [CrossRef] [PubMed]
2. Balci, C.; Sungurtekin, H.; Gürses, E.; Sungurtekin, U.; Kaptanoğlu, B. Usefulness of procalcitonin for diagnosis of sepsis in the intensive care unit. *Crit. Care* **2002**, *7*, 85–90. [CrossRef] [PubMed]
3. Harbarth, S.; Holeckova, K.; Froidevaux, C.; Pittet, D.; Ricou, B.; Grau, G.E.; Vadas, L.; Pugin, J.; Network, G.S. Diagnostic value of procalcitonin, interleukin-6, and in- terleukin-8 in critically ill patients admitted with suspected sepsis. *Am. J. Respir. Crit. Care Med.* **2001**, *164*, 396–402. [CrossRef]
4. Yusa, T.; Tateda, K.; Ohara, A.; Miyazaki, S. New possible biomarkers for diagnosis of infections and diagnostic distinction between bacterial and viral infections in children. *J. Infect. Chemother.* **2017**, *23*, 96–100. [CrossRef] [PubMed]
5. Alizadeh, N.; Memar, M.Y.; Moaddab, S.R.; Kafil, H.S. Aptamer-assisted novel technologies for detecting bacterial pathogens. *Biomed. Pharmacother.* **2017**, *93*, 737–745. [CrossRef]
6. Leli, C.; Ferranti, M.; Marrano, U.; Al Dhahab, Z.S.; Bozza, S.; Cenci, E.; Mencacci, A. Diagnostic accuracy of presepsin (sCD14-ST) and procalcitonin for prediction of bacteraemia and bacterial DNAaemia in patients with suspected sepsis. *J. Med. Microbiol.* **2016**, *65*, 713–719. [CrossRef] [PubMed]
7. Bone, R.C.; Balk, R.A.; Cerra, F.B.; Dellinger, R.P.; Fein, A.M.; Knaus, W.A.; Schein, R.M.; Sibbald, W.J. Definitions for sepsis and organ failure and guidelines for the use of innovative therapies in sepsis. *Chest* **1992**, *101*, 1644–1655. [CrossRef] [PubMed]
8. Singer, M.; Deutschman, C.S.; Seymour, C.W.; Shankar-Hari, M.; Annane, D.; Bauer, M.; Bellomo, R.; Bernard, G.R.; Chiche, J.-D.; Coopersmith, C.M.; et al. The Third International Consensus Definitions for Sepsis and Septic Shock (Sepsis-3). *JAMA* **2016**, *315*, 801–810. [CrossRef]
9. Cecconi, M.; Evans, L.; Levy, M.; Rhodes, A. Sepsis and septic shock. *Lancet* **2018**, *392*, 75–87. [CrossRef]
10. Labib, M.; Berezovski, M.V. Electrochemical aptasensors for microbial and viral pathogens. *Adv. Biochem. Eng. Biotechnol.* **2014**, *140*, 155–181. [CrossRef]
11. Biron, B.M.; Ayala, A.; Lomas-Neira, J.L. Biomarker insight biomarkers for sepsis: What is and what might be? *Biomark Insights* **2015**, *10* (Suppl. 4), 7–17.
12. Pierrakos, C.; Vincent, J.-L. Sepsis biomarkers: A review. *Crit. Care* **2010**, *14*, R15. [CrossRef]
13. Chenevier-Gobeaux, C.; Borderie, D.; Weiss, N.; Mallet-Coste, T.; Claessens, Y.-E. Presepsin (sCD14-ST), an innate immune response marker in sepsis. *Clin. Chim. Acta* **2015**, *450*, 97–103. [CrossRef]
14. Zhang, J.; Hu, Z.-D.; Song, J.; Shao, J. Diagnostic Value of Presepsin for Sepsis. A Systematic Review and Meta-Analysis. *Medicine* **2015**, *94*, e2158. [CrossRef] [PubMed]
15. Wu, J.; Hu, L.; Zhang, G.; Wu, F.; He, T. Accuracy of Presepsin in Sepsis Diagnosis: A Systematic Review and Meta-Analysis. *PLoS ONE* **2015**, *10*, e0133057. [CrossRef] [PubMed]

16. Zheng, Z.; Jiang, L.; Ye, L.; Gao, Y.; Tang, L.; Zhang, M. The accuracy of presepsin for the diagnosis of sepsis from SIRS: A systematic review and meta-analysis. *Ann. Intensive Care* **2015**, *5*, 48. [CrossRef] [PubMed]
17. Tong, X.; Cao, Y.; Yu, M.; Han, C. Presepsin as a diagnostic marker for sepsis: Evidence from a bivariate meta-analysis. *Ther. Clin. Risk Manag.* **2015**, *11*, 1027–1033. [CrossRef]
18. Liu, Y.; Hou, J.-h.; Li, Q.; Chen, K.-j.; Wang, S.-N.; Wang, J.-m. Biomarkers for diagnosis of sepsis in patients with systemic inflammatory response syndrome: A systematic review and meta-analysis. *SpringerPlus* **2016**, *5*, 2091. [CrossRef]
19. Wu, C.-C.; Lan, H.-M.; Han, S.-T.; Chaou, C.-H.; Yeh, C.-F.; Liu, S.-H.; Li, C.-H.; Blaney, G.N.; Liu, Z.-Y.; Chen, K.-F. Comparison of diagnostic accuracy in sepsis between presepsin, procalcitonin, and C-reactive protein: A systematic review and meta-analysis. *Ann. Intensiv. Care* **2017**, *7*, 1–16. [CrossRef]
20. Yang, H.S.; Hur, M.; Yi, A.; Kim, H.; Lee, S.; Kim, S.-N. Prognostic value of presepsin in adult patients with sepsis: Systematic review and meta-analysis. *PLoS ONE* **2018**, *13*, e0191486. [CrossRef]
21. Ruan, L.; Chen, G.-Y.; Liu, Z.; Zhao, Y.; Xu, G.-Y.; Li, S.-F.; Li, C.-N.; Chen, L.-S.; Tao, Z. The combination of procalcitonin and C-reactive protein or presepsin alone improves the accuracy of diagnosis of neonatal sepsis: A meta-analysis and systematic review. *Crit. Care* **2018**, *22*, 1–9. [CrossRef]
22. Yoon, S.H.; Kim, E.H.; Kim, H.Y.; Ahn, J.G. Presepsin as a diagnostic marker of sepsis in children and adolescents: A systemic review and meta-analysis. *BMC Infect Dis.* **2019**, *19*, 760. [CrossRef]
23. Kondo, Y.; Umemura, Y.; Hayashida, K.; Hara, Y.; Aihara, M.; Yamakawa, K. Diagnostic value of procalcitonin and presepsin for sepsis in critically ill adult patients: A systematic review and meta-analysis. *J. Intensiv. Care* **2019**, *7*, 1–13. [CrossRef] [PubMed]
24. Parri, N.; Trippella, G.; Lisi, C.; De Martino, M.; Galli, L.; Chiappini, E. Accuracy of presepsin in neonatal sepsis: Systematic review and meta-analysis. *Expert Rev. Anti. Infect Ther.* **2019**, *17*, 223–232. [CrossRef]
25. Van Maldeghem, I.; Nusman, C.M.; Visser, D.H. Soluble CD14 subtype (sCD14-ST) as biomarker in neonatal early-onset sepsis and late-onset sepsis: A systematic review and meta-analysis. *BMC Immunol.* **2019**, *20*, 17. [CrossRef]
26. Zhu, Y.; Li, X.; Guo, P.; Chen, Y.; Li, J.; Tao, T. The accuracy assessment of presepsin (sCD14-ST) for mortality prediction in adult patients with sepsis and a head-to-head comparison to PCT: A meta-analysis. *Ther. Clin. Risk Manag.* **2019**, *15*, 741–753. [CrossRef] [PubMed]
27. Memar, M.Y.; Baghi, H.B. Presepsin: A promising biomarker for the detection of bacterial infections. *Biomed. Pharmacother.* **2019**, *111*, 649–656. [CrossRef] [PubMed]
28. Memar, M.Y.; Alizadeh, N.; Varshochi, M.; Kafil, H.S. Immunologic biomarkers for diagnostic of early-onset neonatal sepsis. *J. Matern. Neonatal Med.* **2017**, *32*, 143–153. [CrossRef]
29. Sandquist, M.; Wong, H.R. Biomarkers of sepsis and their potential value in diagnosis, prognosis and treatment. *Expert Rev. Clin. Immunol.* **2014**, *10*, 1349–1356. [CrossRef] [PubMed]
30. Vanaja, S.K.; Rathinam, V.A.; Fitzgerald, K.A. Mechanisms of inflammasome activation: Recent advances and novel insights. *Trends Cell Biol.* **2015**, *25*, 308–315. [CrossRef]
31. Lonez, C.; Irvine, K.; Pizzuto, M.; Schmidt, B.I.; Gay, N.J.; Ruysschaert, J.-M.; Gangloff, M.; Bryant, C.E. Critical residues involved in Toll-like receptor 4 activation by cationic lipid nanocarriers are not located at the lipopolysaccharide-binding interface. *Cell. Mol. Life Sci.* **2015**, *72*, 3971–3982. [CrossRef]
32. Iwasaki, A.; Medzhitov, R. Control of adaptive immunity by the innate immune system. *Nat. Immunol.* **2015**, *16*, 343–353. [CrossRef]
33. Akira, S.; Uematsu, S.; Takeuchi, O. Pathogen recognition and innate immunity. *Cell* **2006**, *124*, 783–801. [CrossRef]
34. Nonaka, M.; Yoshizaki, F. Evolution of the complement system. *Mol. Immunol.* **2004**, *40*, 897–902. [CrossRef]
35. Barton, G.M.; Medzhitov, R. Control of adaptive immune responses by Toll-like receptors. *Curr. Opin. Immunol.* **2002**, *14*, 380–383. [CrossRef]
36. Van Der Mark, V.A.; Ghiboub, M.; Marsman, C.; Zhao, J.; Van Dijk, R.; Hiralall, J.K.; Ho-Mok, K.S.; Castricum, Z.; De Jonge, W.J.; Elferink, R.P.J.O.; et al. Phospholipid flippases attenuate LPS-induced TLR4 signaling by mediating endocytic retrieval of Toll-like receptor 4. *Cell. Mol. Life Sci.* **2017**, *74*, 715–730. [CrossRef] [PubMed]
37. Yuk, J.-M.; Jo, E.-K. Toll-like Receptors and Innate Immunity. *J. Bacteriol. Virol.* **2011**, *41*, 225–235. [CrossRef]
38. Zou, Q.; Wen, W.; Zhang, X.-C. Presepsin as a novel sepsis biomarker. *World J. Emerg. Med.* **2014**, *5*, 16–19. [CrossRef]
39. Shirakawa, K.; Naitou, K.; Hirose, J.; Takahashi, T.; Furusako, S. Prese-psin [sCD14-ST]: Development and evaluation of one-step ELISA with a new standard that is similar to the form of presepsin in septic patients. *Clin. Chem. Lab. Med.* **2011**, *49*, 937–939. [CrossRef]
40. Okamura, Y.; Yokoi, H. Development of a point-of-care assay system for measurement of presepsin (sCD14-ST). *Clin. Chim. Acta* **2011**, *412*, 2157–2161. [CrossRef]
41. Novelli, G.; Morabito, V.; Ferretti, G.; Pugliese, F.; Ruberto, F.; Venuta, F.; Poli, L.; Rossi, M.; Berloco, P. Pathfast Presepsin Assay for Early Diagnosis of Bacterial Infections in Surgical Patients: Preliminary Study. *Transplant. Proc.* **2013**, *45*, 2750–2753. [CrossRef] [PubMed]
42. Pugni, L.; Pietrasanta, C.; Milani, S.; Vener, C.; Ronchi, A.; Falbo, M.; Arghittu, M.; Mosca, F. Presepsin (Soluble CD14 Subtype): Reference Ranges of a New Sepsis Marker in Term and Preterm Neonates. *PLoS ONE* **2015**, *10*, e0146020. [CrossRef] [PubMed]

43. Endo, S.; Suzuki, Y.; Takahashi, G.; Shozushima, T.; Ishikura, H.; Murai, A.; Nishida, T.; Irie, Y.; Miura, M.; Iguchi, H.; et al. Usefulness of presepsin in the diagnosis of sepsis in a multicenter prospective study. *J. Infect. Chemother.* **2012**, *18*, 891–897. [CrossRef] [PubMed]
44. Liu, B.; Chen, Y.-X.; Yin, Q.; Zhao, Y.-Z.; Li, C.-S. Diagnostic value and prognostic evaluation of Presepsin for sepsis in an emergency department. *Crit. Care* **2013**, *17*, R244. [CrossRef] [PubMed]
45. Topcuoğlu, S.; Arslanbuga, C.; Gursoy, T.; Aktas, A.; Karatekin, G.; Uluhan, R.; Ovali, F. Role of presepsin in the diagnosis of late-onset neonatal sepsis in preterm infants. *J. Matern. Neonatal Med.* **2015**, *29*, 1–6. [CrossRef]
46. Vodnik, T.; Kaljevic, G.; Tadic, T.; Majkic-Singh, N. Presepsin (sCD14-ST) in pre-operative diagnosis of abdominal sepsis. *Clin. Chem. Lab. Med.* **2013**, *51*, 2053–2062. [CrossRef]
47. Masson, S.; Caironi, P.; Fanizza, C.; Thomae, R.; Bernasconi, R.; Noto, A.; Oggioni, R.; Pasetti, G.S.; Romero, M.; Tognoni, G.; et al. Circulating presepsin (soluble CD14 subtype) as a marker of host response in patients with severe sepsis or septic shock: Data from the multicenter, randomized ALBIOS trial. *Intensiv. Care Med.* **2015**, *41*, 12–20. [CrossRef]
48. Popa, T.O.; Cimpoeşu, D. Dorobăţ CM: Diagnostic and prognostic value of presepsin in the emergency department. *Rev Med. Chir. Soc. Med. Nat. Iasi.* **2015**, *119*, 69–76.
49. Carpio, R.; Zapata, J.; Spanuth, E.; Hess, G. Utility of presepsin (sCD14-ST) as a diagnostic and prognostic marker of sepsis in the emergency department. *Clin. Chim. Acta* **2015**, *450*, 169–175. [CrossRef]
50. Velissaris, D.; Zareifopoulos, N.; Karamouzos, V.; Karanikolas, E.; Pierrakos, C.; Koniari, I.; Karanikolas, M. Presepsin as a Diagnostic and Prognostic Biomarker in Sepsis. *Cureus* **2021**, *13*, 15019. [CrossRef]
51. Kweon, O.J.; Choi, J.-H.; Park, S.K.; Park, A.J. Usefulness of presepsin (sCD14 sub- type) measurements as a new marker for the diagnosis and prediction of disease severity of sepsis in the Korean population. *J. Crit. Care* **2014**, *29*, 965–970. [CrossRef]
52. Memar, M.Y.; Ghotaslou, R.; Samiei, M.; Adibkia, K. Antimicrobial use of reactive oxygen therapy: Current insights. *Infect. Drug Resist.* **2018**, *11*, 567–576. [CrossRef] [PubMed]
53. Godnic, M.; Stubljar, D.; Skvarc, M.; Jukic, T. Diagnostic and prognostic value of sCD14-ST—presepsin for patients admitted to hospital intensive care unit (ICU). *Wien. Klin. Wochenschr.* **2015**, *127*, 521–527. [CrossRef] [PubMed]
54. Hung, S.-K.; Lan, H.-M.; Han, S.-T.; Wu, C.-C.; Chen, K.-F. Current Evidence and Limitation of Biomarkers for Detecting Sepsis and Systemic Infection. *Biomedicines* **2020**, *8*, 494. [CrossRef] [PubMed]
55. Kim, H.; Hur, M.; Moon, H.-W.; Yun, Y.-M.; Di Somma, S.; Network, G. Multi-marker approach using procalcitonin, presepsin, galectin-3, and soluble suppression of tumorigenicity 2 for the prediction of mortality in sepsis. *Ann. Intensiv. Care* **2017**, *7*, 27. [CrossRef]
56. Madenci, Ö.Ç.; Yakupoğlu, S.; Benzonana, N.; Yücel, N.; Akbaba, D.; Kaptanağası, A.O. Evaluation of soluble CD14 subtype (presepsin) in burn sepsis. *Burns* **2014**, *40*, 664–669. [CrossRef]
57. De Guadiana Romualdo, L.G.; Torrella, P.E.; González, M.V.; Sánchez, R.J.; Holgado, A.H.; Freire, A.O.; Acebes, S.R.; Otón, M.D.A. Diagnostic accuracy of pre-sepsin (soluble CD14 subtype) for prediction of bacteremia in patients with systemic inflammatory response syndrome in the Emergency Department. *Clin. Biochem.* **2014**, *47*, 505–508. [CrossRef]
58. Romualdo, L.G.D.G.; Torrella, P.E.; Acebes, S.R.; Otón, M.D.A.; Sánchez, R.J.; Holgado, A.H.; Santos, E.J.; Freire, A.O. Diagnostic accuracy of presepsin (sCD14-ST) as a biomarker of infection and sepsis in the emergency department. *Clin. Chim. Acta* **2017**, *464*, 6–11. [CrossRef]
59. Enguix-Armada, A.; Escobar-Conesa, R.; García-De La Torre, A.; De La Torre- Prados, M.V. Usefulness of several biomarkers in the management of septic patients: C- reactive protein, procalcitonin, presepsin and mid-regional pro-adrenomedullin. *Clin. Chem. Lab. Med. (CCLM)* **2016**, *54*, 163–168. [CrossRef]
60. Plesko, M.; Suvada, J.; Makohusova, M.; Waczulikova, I.; Behulova, D.; Vasilenkova, A.; Vargova, M.; Stecova, A.; Kaiserova, E.; Kolenova, A. The role of CRP, PCT, IL-6 and presepsin in early diagnosis of bacterial infectious complications in paediatric haemato-oncological patients. *Neoplasma* **2016**, *63*, 752–760. [CrossRef]
61. Klouche, K.; Cristol, J.P.; Devin, J.; Gilles, V.; Kuster, N.; Larcher, R.; Amigues, L.; Corne, P.; Jonquet, O.; Dupuy, A.M. Diagnostic and prognostic value of soluble CD14 subtype (Presepsin) for sepsis and community-acquired pneumonia in ICU patients. *Ann. Intensiv. Care* **2016**, *6*, 1–11. [CrossRef] [PubMed]
62. Iskandar, A.; Arthamin, M.Z.; Indriana, K.; Anshory, M.; Hur, M.; Di Somma, S.; Network, O.B.O.T.G. Comparison between presepsin and procalcitonin in early diagnosis of neonatal sepsis. *J. Matern. Neonatal Med.* **2018**, *32*, 3903–3908. [CrossRef] [PubMed]
63. Kumar, N.; Dayal, R.; Singh, P.; Pathak, S.; Pooniya, V.; Goyal, A.; Kamal, R.; Mohanty, K.K. A Comparative Evaluation of Presepsin with Procalcitonin and CRP in Diagnosing Neonatal Sepsis. *Indian J. Pediatr.* **2019**, *86*, 177–179. [CrossRef] [PubMed]
64. Baraka, A.; Zakaria, M. Presepsin as a diagnostic marker of bacterial infections in febrile neutropenic pediatric patients with hematological malignancies. *Int. J. Hematol.* **2018**, *108*, 184–191. [CrossRef] [PubMed]
65. El Gendy, F.M.; El-Mekkawy, M.S.; Saleh, N.Y.; Habib, M.S.E.-D.; Younis, F.E. Clinical study of Presepsin and Pentraxin3 in critically ill children. *J. Crit. Care* **2018**, *47*, 36–40. [CrossRef] [PubMed]
66. Mussap, M.; Puxeddu, E.; Puddu, M.; Ottonello, G.; Coghe, F.; Comite, P.; Cibecchini, F.; Fanos, V. Soluble CD14 subtype (sCD14-ST) presepsin in premature and full term critically ill newborns with sepsis and SIRS. *Clin. Chim. Acta* **2015**, *451*, 65–70. [CrossRef]

67. Koh, H.; Aimoto, M.; Katayama, T.; Hashiba, M.; Sato, A.; Kuno, M.; Makuuchi, Y.; Takakuwa, T.; Okamura, H.; Hirose, A. Diagnostic value of levels of presepsin (so-luble CD14-subtype) in febrile neutropenia in patients with hematological dis- orders. *J. Infect. Chemother.* **2016**, *22*, 466–471. [CrossRef]
68. Poggi, C.; Bianconi, T.; Gozzini, E.; Generoso, M.; Dani, C. Presepsin for the Detection of Late-Onset Sepsis in Preterm Newborns. *Pediatrics* **2015**, *135*, 68–75. [CrossRef]
69. Kollmann, T.R.; Levy, O.; Montgomery, R.; Goriely, S. Innate Immune Function by Toll-like Receptors: Distinct Responses in Newborns and the Elderly. *Immunity* **2012**, *37*, 771–783. [CrossRef]
70. Badiee, P.; Hashemizadeh, Z. Opportunistic invasive fungal infections: Diagnosis & clinical management. *Indian J. Med. Res.* **2014**, *139*, 195–204.
71. Stoma, I.; Karpov, I.; Uss, A.; Krivenko, S.; Iskrov, I.; Milanovich, N.; Vlasenkova, S.; Lendina, I.; Belyavskaya, K.; Cherniak, V. Combination of sepsis biomarkers may indicate an invasive fungal infection in haematological patients. *Biomarkers* **2019**, *24*, 401–406. [CrossRef]
72. Lippi, G.; Cervellin, G. Can presepsin be used for screening invasive fungal infections? *Ann. Transl. Med.* **2019**, *7*, 87. [CrossRef]
73. Bamba, Y.; Moro, H.; Aoki, N.; Koizumi, T.; Ohshima, Y.; Watanabe, S. Increased presepsin levels are associated with the severity of fungal bloodstream infections. *PLoS ONE* **2019**, *13*, e0206089. [CrossRef] [PubMed]
74. Fukada, A.; Kitagawa, Y.; Matsuoka, M.; Sakai, J.; Imai, K.; Tarumoto, N.; Orihara, Y.; Kawamura, R.; Takeuchi, S.; Maesaki, S.; et al. Presepsin as a predictive biomarker of severity in COVID-19: A case series. *J. Med. Virol.* **2021**, *93*, 99–101. [CrossRef] [PubMed]
75. Zaninotto, M.; Mion, M.M.; Cosma, C.; Rinaldi, D.; Plebani, M. Presepsin in risk stratification of SARS-CoV-2 patients. *Clin. Chim. Acta* **2020**, *507*, 161–163. [CrossRef] [PubMed]
76. Nagata, T.; Yasuda, Y.; Ando, M.; Abe, T.; Katsuno, T.; Kato, S.; Tsuboi, N.; Matsuo, S.; Maruyama, S. Clinical Impact of Kidney Function on Presepsin Levels. *PLoS ONE* **2015**, *10*, e0129159. [CrossRef]
77. Sargentini, V.; Ceccarelli, G.; D'Alessandro, M.; Collepardo, D.; Morelli, A.; D'Egidio, A.; Mariotti, S.; Nicoletti, A.M.; Evangelista, B.; D'Ettorre, G.; et al. Presepsin as a potential marker for bacterial infection relapse in critical care patients. A preliminary study. *Clin. Chem. Lab. Med.* **2014**, *53*, 567–573. [CrossRef] [PubMed]
78. Hayashi, M.; Yaguchi, Y.; Okamura, K.; Goto, E.; Onodera, Y.; Sugiura, A.; Suzuki, H.; Nakane, M.; Kawamae, K.; Suzuki, T. A case of extensive burn without sepsis showing high level of plasma presepsin (sCD14-ST). *Burn. Open* **2017**, *1*, 33–36. [CrossRef]

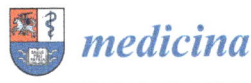

Review

Proadrenomedullin in Sepsis and Septic Shock: A Role in the Emergency Department

Andrea Piccioni [1], Angela Saviano [1,*], Sara Cicchinelli [1], Federico Valletta [1], Michele Cosimo Santoro [1], Tommaso de Cunzo [1], Christian Zanza [1], Yaroslava Longhitano [2], Gianluca Tullo [1], Pietro Tilli [1], Marcello Candelli [1], Marcello Covino [1] and Francesco Franceschi [1]

1. Emergency Department, Fondazione Policlinico Universitario A. Gemelli, IRCCS, 00168 Roma, Italy; andrea.piccioni@policlinicogemelli.it (A.P.); sara.cicchinelli@policlinicogemelli.it (S.C.); fede.valletta@gmail.com (F.V.); michelecosimo.santoro@policlinicogemelli.it (M.C.S.); tomdecunzo@gmail.com (T.d.C.); christian.zanza@live.it (C.Z.); gianlucatullo@gmail.com (G.T.); pietro.tilli@policlinicogemelli.it (P.T.); marcello.candelli@policlinicogemelli.it (M.C.); marcello.covino@policlinicogemelli.it (M.C.); francesco.franceschi@policlinicogemelli.it (F.F.)
2. Dietetics and Clinical Nutrition Unit, Department of Internal Medicine, University of Genoa, IRCCS Polyclinic Hospital San Martino, 16132 Genoa, Italy; lon.yaro@gmail.com
* Correspondence: saviange@libero.it

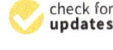

Abstract: Sepsis and septic shock represent a leading cause of mortality in the Emergency Department (ED) and in the Intensive Care Unit (ICU). For these life-threating conditions, different diagnostic and prognostic biomarkers have been studied. Proadrenomedullin (MR-proADM) is a biomarker that can predict organ damage and the risk of imminent death in patients with septic shock, as shown by a large amount of data in the literature. The aim of our narrative review is to evaluate the role of MR-proADM in the context of Emergency Medicine and to summarize the current knowledge of MR-proADM as a serum indicator that is useful in the Emergency Department (ED) to determine an early diagnosis and to predict the long-term mortality of patients with sepsis and septic shock. We performed an electronic literature review to investigate the role of MR-proADM in sepsis and septic shock in the context of ED. We searched papers on PubMed®, Cochrane®, UptoDate®, and Web of Science® that had been published in the last 10 years. Data extracted from this literature review are not conclusive, but they show that MR-proADM may be helpful as a prognostic biomarker to stratify the mortality risk in cases of sepsis and septic shock with different degrees of organ damage, guiding emergency physicians in the diagnosis and the succeeding therapeutic workup. Sepsis and septic shock are conditions of high complexity and have a high risk of mortality. In the ED, early diagnosis is crucial in order to provide an early treatment and to improve patient survival. Diagnosis and prognosis are often the result of a combination of several tests. In our opinion, testing for MR-proADM directly in the ED could contribute to improving the prognostic assessment of patients, facilitating the subsequent clinical management and intensive treatment by the emergency physicians, but more studies are needed to confirm these results.

Keywords: sepsis; septic shock; proadrenomedullin; MR-proADM; procalcitonin; emergency department

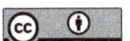
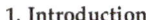

1. Introduction

Sepsis and septic shock are life-threatening medical emergencies characterized by severe systemic inflammation and organ dysfunction due to an excessive response to infections that may lead to death [1–6]. The definition of sepsis includes a dysregulated systemic inflammation, acute multi-organ dysfunction (i.e., cardiovascular, respiratory, and renal systems), and a deregulated immune response to a microbial invasion of the blood that is responsible of organ failure [7–10]. The mortality rate ranges from 15–25% [7]. Septic shock is sepsis characterized by a state of hypotension and hyperlactatemia, refractory to adequate fluid volume resuscitation that leads to hypoperfusion abnormalities, oliguria, and the alteration of mental status [7]. Septic shock has a mortality rate that ranges from 30–50% [7]. The early identification of sepsis and septic shock is essential for immediate treatment [1,2] and for the reduction of the patient mortality rate [10,11]. Sepsis can affect people of all ages [2–4]. Therapy for sepsis should be personalized and tailored according to the patient's needs. Many biomarkers such as procalcitonin (PCT) or interleukin (IL)-6 or IL-18 are used in clinical practice to facilitate the diagnosis of sepsis [5,6]. Novel biomarkers such as proadrenomedullin (MR-proADM), kallistatin, testican-1, and presepsin have been introduced to assess the severity of sepsis and to predict the organ damage and the risk of imminent death [5]. As of now, a golden standard biomarker in terms of the diagnosis and prognosis for sepsis and septic shock has not been found. The aim of our narrative review is to evaluate the role of MR-proADM as a biomarker of sepsis in the context of emergency medicine and to summarize the current knowledge about MR-proADM in sepsis and septic shock as a potential biomarker to achieve an early diagnosis and to predict the long-term mortality of patients directly in the ED.

2. Literature Research

We performed an electronic literature review to investigate the role of MR-proADM in sepsis and septic shock. We searched papers on PubMed®, Cochrane®, UptoDate®, and Web of Science®. No ethical approval was necessary to perform this review. The principal words we included in the search were "severe sepsis" OR "sepsis", OR "septic shock", AND "procalcitonin", AND/OR "pro-adrenomedullin", OR "MR-proADM", AND/OR "IL-6", AND/OR "systemic inflammation", AND/OR "organ failure", AND/OR "infections", AND "diagnostic biomarkers" AND "prognostic biomarkers", OR "bacteria-induced sepsis", AND/OR Emergency Department (ED) OR Emergency Medicine. Our search was based on clinical trials, meta-analysis, randomized controlled trials, reviews, and systematic reviews if available. We extracted data from comprehensive studies based on the new definition of sepsis and septic shock and reviewed the role of serum MR-proADM as a diagnostic and/or prognostic biomarker according to the available literature. We summarized the main studies, exploring the role of MR-proADM with the investigated cut-off value (nmol/L) (when available). No exclusion criteria (patient age, gender, comorbidities, admission to ICU, etc.) were applied. We also searched studies performed in the context of emergency medicine/ED. Papers were initially selected by title and abstract and then by the availability of the full text. We reviewed the results of the studies on the basis of the total number of patients, levels of MD-proADM, outcomes, management in the ED or Intensive Care Unit (ICU), and use of MD-proADM or other biomarkers or stratification scores of the severity of the patient's condition. We investigated a total of 16 manuscripts from 2013 to 2021. The limitation of our review is the heterogeneity of the studies (type of patients included, design of study, endpoints).

3. Role of MR-proADM in ICU and in ED

Several authors have investigated the role of MR-proADM in patients with sepsis and septic shock. MR-proADM is a stable and detectable fragment of 48-amino acids derived from ADM (a 52-amino acid peptide and member of the calcitonin family) that is mainly produced by vascular endothelial cells and smooth muscle cells. ADM and MR-proADM have effects on vasodilatation (on artery and vein), natriuresis, bronchodilatation, and they have influences on cardiac contractility and glomerular filtration [11], which are involved in some clinical manifestations of sepsis and septic shock as refractory hypotension. MR-proADM has a half-life that is longer than ADM and can be more easily detected in blood compared to ADM, which is rapidly cleared from the circulation.

Most of the reported studies found that MR-proADM was a reliable biomarker that could serve as an early predictor of high mortality risk. In fact, levels of MR-proADM can potentially reflect the severity of organ dysfunction, even in the first stages of the disease, in the progression of systemic inflammatory response, in the movement from sepsis to septic shock, and in the mortality risk of septic patients [11,12]. A prospective observational study conducted with 213 septic patients showed that MR-proADM was able to predict system dysfunction (respiratory, coagulation, renal, neurological, and cardiovascular) and was well-correlated with Sequential Organ Failure Assessment (SOFA) score components [13]. The same results were obtained by Onal et al. [11], who concluded that MR-proADM could be a good alternative to SOFA score. L. Buendgens and his team [14] designed a prospective study to assess the role of MR-proADM in a cohort of 203 ICU patients and 66 healthy controls that they followed for a period of 26 months. They demonstrated that MR-proADM values were higher in critically ill patients—especially in those with sepsis progression—with a close correlation with other markers of systemic inflammation and endothelial dysfunction. Moreover, MR-proADM levels correlated with scores for disease severity (Acute Physiology and Chronic Health Disease Classification System (APACHE II), SOFA, and Simplified Acute Physiology Score (SAPS2)). The best cut-off value that was found by these authors to identify patients at high mortality risk was of 1.4 nmol/L [14]. Similar results were also reported by Gonzales Del Castillo et al. [15] in a larger study of 684 patients admitted to the ED for a suspected infection.

The abovementioned authors found that MR-proADM was able to identify those hiding an underlying severe condition and who were at high risk for delayed or insufficient initial treatment. In addition, authors compared several biomarkers (MR-proADM, C-reactive protein (CRP), PCT, and lactate) and clinical scores (SOFA, quick SOFA, and National early warning score (NEWS)), concluding that MR-proADM could help identify patients with low NEWS or quick SOFA values but who were at high risk for sepsis progression, helping in the initial treatment choices [15]. A prospective observational study of 657 patients with an acute infection conducted by Haang et al. [16] reported that the combination of MR-proADM and SOFA-score would better improve the stratification risk of patients for 30-day mortality (area under the curve (AUC) 0.87) than the SOFA-score alone (AUC 0.81). The authors defined a MR-proADM threshold value of 1.75 nmol/L as a prognostic value for 30-day mortality (sensitivity 81%, specificity 75%, and negative predictive value 98%) [16].

Spoto et al. [2] conducted a study on 571 septic patients and reported that MR-proADM has a strong correlation with a high risk of 90-day mortality, with a cut-off of 3.39 nmol/L for septic patients and a cut-off value of 4.33 nmol/L for shock patients. In another prospective study of 209 patients with a clinical sepsis diagnosis, S. Spoto [17] et al. showed that MR-proADM had an important function in predicting the development of organ failure over 24 h [17]. Significant evidence of MR-proADM prognostic reliability was also provided by a prospective observational study conducted in a sample of 326 patients with sepsis or septic shock by Andaluz-Ojeda [18] and his coworkers. Their results showed that MR-proADM was an optimal biomarker for the early identification of patients who had a high-risk of mortality, even if these patients who initially had a moderate clinical severity [18]. Such evidence further strengthens the role of MR-proADM as a prognostic factor for mortality in critical illness, but this evidence also shows how its inclusion in the first evaluation of septic patients with a moderate clinical condition is able to predict later organ dysfunction. Schuetz et al. [19] conducted a prospective, multicenter study including 7132 patients and revealed that MR-proADM improved the models that predict ICU admission for patients with sepsis and septic shock. In a cohort of 128 septic patients in the ED, Travaglino et al. [20] proved that MR-proADM was correlated with the APACHE score. Chris-Crain et al. [21] proved that MR-proADM was a good prognostic biomarker in critically ill patients with sepsis. However, a neat cut-off value for the identification of septic patients with a high mortality risk has not yet been found, and more studies are needed to finally set a threshold that can be standardized.

4. Discussion

Sepsis and septic shock are medical emergencies that require a proper diagnosis and appropriate management from the moment of admission to the ED. In fact, sepsis and septic shock carry a high mortality risk for patients [7,10,16]. Many factors contribute to the complexity of these conditions. Among them, the over-activation and dysregulation of the innate immune system in response to a blood microbial invasion is a topic of great interest in order to better define the most targeted therapeutic strategy. The innate immune system expresses some receptors that are able to recognize the signaling of damage or infection as damage-associated molecular patterns (DAMPs) or pathogen-associated molecular patterns (PAMPs). DAMPs and PAMPs, which are binding receptors of the innate immune cells, lead to the release of many pro-inflammatory cytokines and molecules such as tumor necrosis factor-α (TNF-α), interleukin-6 (IL-6), and interleukin-1β (IL-1β) followed by the release of acute phase proteins such as CRP, PCT, and MR-proADM [22]. In the context of the ED, it is important to have easily measurable biomarkers that can produce an indication level of the patient's severity level in order to modulate the priority and the intensity of the patient's care. Literature studies [5,6] have investigated the role, both diagnostic and prognostic, of some biomarkers such as PCT, IL-6, IL-18, presepsin, etc., in patients with sepsis and septic shock without finding conclusive results. MR-proADM seems to be a good biomarker in assessing a patient's initial state, evolution, and prognosis. Moreover, MR-proADM may be a good alternative to the sequential organ failure assessment (SOFA) score. In the context of the ED, especially in the case of overcrowding, the administration of a simple blood test may be more practical compared to the collection of a multitude of data to calculate a score. MD-proADM has shown a strong ability to predict localized bacterial infections and to make a differentiatial diagnosis of sepsis from SIRS in patients with hematologic malignancies [23]. More studies are underway to explore the pathophysiological profile of MD-proADM regarding the release kinetics and the blood clearance time in order to reduce the risk of false-positive or -negative results and to avoid confounding and misleading mistakes in interpretation.

Moreover, the best cut-off value of MR-proADM for the early diagnosis of sepsis and for predicting patient prognosis has not yet been clarified. More studies are required to better define it for use in clinical practice and directly in the ED.

Some other molecules proposed as ideal predictor biomarkers of sepsis include CD64, the soluble receptors of myeloid cells (sTREM)-1, the soluble urokinase-type plasminogen activator receptor (suPAR), and pentraxin-3, but they are still far from application in the ED. Recent advances in technology are now focusing on microbiome and non-coding RNAs [22], some of which, for example miR-21, contribute to inflammatory responses and multi-organ dysfunction (i.e., kidney, lung, and liver) during sepsis [24,25]. Moreover, several models and scoring systems involving the combination of biomarkers are in progress [26–29]. They seem to have interesting diagnostic and prognostic performance, but they need confirmation through more trials. Our review has some limitations. The analyzed studies often extrapolated conclusions about MR-proADM based on a combination of different biomarkers and/or scores and not from the analysis of MR-proADM alone. Moreover, most of research studies included in the present work were not conducted in the ED and were conducted in the ICU. The population sample and design of the studies were often not homogeneous. Due to these considerations, it is essential to perform more studies in the context of ED and to identify good biomarkers or a combination of biomarkers and their cut off values that are able to promptly recognize the different phenotypes of septic patients in order to stratify the most urgent patients in order to improve the quality of care and survival, starting directly from the ED. The summary of studies exploring the role of MR-proADM can be seen in Table 1.

Table 1. Summary of studies exploring the role of proadrenomedullin (MR-proADM).

Authors	Type of Study	Number of Patients and Time of Enrollment	Evidence	Cut-Off (nmol/L)
Spoto S [2] et al. Microb Pathog 2019	Retrospective observational study in adults	571 (2012–2018)	MR-proADM has a strong correlation with 90-day mortality	3.39 (for sepsis) and 4.33 (for septic shock)
Li [3] et al. Med Intensiva 2018	Systematic review and meta-analysis of thirteen studies in adults	2556 (1999—2017)	MR-proADM might predict the prognosis of septic patients	unknown
Fahmey [4] et al. Korean J Pediatr 2018	Prospective observational pediatric study	60 septic newborns vs. 30 healthy neonates (May 2016–January 2017)	MR-proADM: valid biomarker for neonatal sepsis. High levels were associated with mortality and the disease's outcome.	4.3
Enguix-Armada [12] et al. Clin Chem Lab Med 2016	Prospective observational study in adults	388 (2015)	MR-proADM is useful in the management of septic patients (measured in the first 24 h after ICU admission)	unknown
Andrés C [13] et al. Eur J Clin Invest 2020	Prospective observational study in adults	213 (2019–2020)	MR-proADM correlates with the largest number of Sequential Organ Failure Assessment (SOFA) score components and with organ dysfunction	1.4
Buendgens L [14] et al. Mediators Inflamm 2020	Prospective observational study in adults	269 (2018–2020)	MR-proAMD values are higher in critical septic patients and correlates with other markers of systemic inflammation and severity scores	0.05
Gonzalez Del Castillo J [15] et al. Crit Care 2019	Prospective observational study in adults	684 (May–July 2018)	MR-proADM identifies patients hiding an underlying severe condition and who are at high risk for delayed or insufficient initial treatment	1.77
Haag E [16] et al. Clin Chem Lab Med 2021	Prospective observational study in adults	657 (2019)	MR-proADM plus SOFA-score provide a better risk stratification than SOFA alone	1.75
Spoto S [17] et al. Sci Rep 2020	Prospective observational study in adults	209 (May 2014–June 2018)	MR-proADM anticipates organ failure in septic patients	1
Andaluz-Ojeda D [18] et al. Ann Intensive Care 2017	Prospective observational study in adults	326 (April 2013–January 2016)	MR-proADM predicts mortality in patients with sepsis at an early clinical stage	0.8
Schuetz [19] et al. Crit Care 2015	Review in adult patients	4 studies (March 2013–October 2014)	MR-proADM: prognostic marker that may improve site of care decisions	unknown
Kim [22] et al. Infect Chemother 2020	Review in adult patients	9 studies (1985–2020)	MR-proADM predicts 28-day mortality in septic patients	unknown
Al Shuaibi [23] et al. Clin Infect Dis 2013	Control observational study in adults	340 (June 2009–December 2010)	MR-proADM is useful in the management of febrile patients with hematologic malignancies. It localized bacterial infection and differentiated sepsis from SIRS	0.91 median level in septic patients (range: 0.05–8.78) 0.79 median level in non-septic patients (range: 0.05–6.48)
Valenzuela-Sánchez [25] et al. Minerva Anestesiol 2019	Prospective observational single-center study in adults	20 ICU-patients (June 2011–January 2013)	MR-proADM helped to identify sepsis in patients admitted to ICU. After 48 h of admission, it was associated with death risk	1.425 (before ICU admission) 5.626 (48 hours after)
Viaggi [26] et al. PLoS One 2018	Prospective observational study in adults	64 (12 March–25 June 2016)	MR-proADM anticipates the modification of several scores (SOFA, Pitt, and CPIS) related to organ dysfunction	1.1
De La Torre-Prados [27] et al. Minerva Anestesiol 2016	Prospective observational study in adults	100 (January–December 2011)	MR-proADM correlates with 28-day mortality in septic shock patients	unknown

5. Conclusions

Data extracted from this narrative literature review showed that MR-proADM may be helpful as a prognostic biomarker to stratify the mortality risk in cases of sepsis and septic shock with different degrees of organ damages directly in the ED. Sepsis and septic shock are conditions of high complexity and high mortality-risk. In the ED, early diagnosis is crucial to provide early treatment and to improve patient survival. Diagnosis and prognosis are often the result of a combination of several tests. In our opinion, testing MR-proADM directly in the ED could help emergency physicians to facilitate the subsequent clinical management and intensive treatment of septic patients with better patient survival results.

Author Contributions: Conceptualization, A.P. and A.S.; methodology, S.C. and F.V.; software, M.C. (Marcello Candelli) and M.C. (Marcello Covino); validation, A.P., F.F. and Y.L.; formal analysis, M.C. and G.T.; investigation, T.d.C. and P.T.; resources, C.Z.; data curation, M.C.S.; writing—original draft preparation, A.S., S.C. and F.V.; writing—review and editing, A.P. and A.S.; visualization, Y.L.; supervision, F.F. All authors have read and agreed to the published version of the manuscript.

Funding: This research received no external funding.

Institutional Review Board Statement: Not applicable.

Informed Consent Statement: Not applicable.

Data Availability Statement: Not applicable.

Conflicts of Interest: The authors declare no conflict of interest.

References

1. Dugar, S.; Choudhary, C.; Duggal, A. Sepsis and septic shock: Guideline-based management. *Clevel. Clin. J. Med.* **2020**, *87*, 53–64. [CrossRef] [PubMed]
2. Spoto, S.; Fogolari, M.; De Florio, L.; Minieri, M.; Vicino, G.; Legramante, J.; Lia, M.S.; Terrinoni, A.; Caputo, D.; Constantino, S.; et al. Procalcitonin and MR-proAdrenomedullin combination in the etiological diagnosis and prognosis of sepsis and septic shock. *Microb. Pathog.* **2019**, *137*, 103763. [CrossRef]
3. Li, Q.; Wang, B.S.; Yang, L.; Peng, C.; Ma, L.B.; Chai, C. Assessment of adrenomedullin and proadrenomedullin as predictors of mortality in septic patients: A systematic review and meta-analysis. *Med. Intensiv.* **2018**, *42*, 416–424. [CrossRef]
4. Fahmey, S.S.; Mostafa, H.; Elhafeez, N.A.; Hussain, H. Diagnostic and prognostic value of proadrenomedullin in neonatal sepsis. *Korean J. Pediatr.* **2018**, *61*, 156–159. [CrossRef]
5. Mierzchala-Pasierb, M.; Lipinska-Gediga, M.; Fleszar, M.G.; Lesnik, P.; Placzkowska, S.; Serek, P.; Wisniewski, J.; Gamian, A.; Krzystek-Korpacka, M. Altered profiles of serum amino acids in patients with sepsis and septic shock—Preliminary findings. *Arch. Biochem. Biophys.* **2020**, *691*, 108508. [CrossRef]
6. Mierzchala-Pasierb, M.; Krzystek-Korpacka, M.; Lesnik, P.; Adamik, B.; Placzkowska, S.; Serek, P.; Gamian, A.; Lipinska-Gediga, M. Interleukin-18 serum levels in sepsis: Correlation with disease severity and inflammatory markers. *Cytokine* **2019**, *120*, 22–27. [CrossRef]
7. Hotchkiss, R.S.; Moldawer, L.L.; Opal, S.M.; Reinhart, K.; Turnbull, I.R.; Vincent, J.L. Sepsis and septic shock. *Nat. Rev. Dis. Prim.* **2016**, *2*, 16045. [CrossRef]
8. Evans, T. Diagnosis and management of sepsis. *Clin. Med.* **2018**, *18*, 146–149. [CrossRef]
9. Angus, D.C.; Van der Poll, T. Severe sepsis and septic shock. *N. Engl. J. Med.* **2013**, *369*, 2063. [CrossRef] [PubMed]
10. Zhang, Z.; Smischney, N.J.; Zhang, H.; Poucke, S.V.; Argaud, L.; Kim, W.Y.; Spapen, H.D.; Rocco, J.R. AME evidence series 001-The Society for Translational Medicine: Clinical practice guidelines for diagnosis and early identification of sepsis in the hospital. *J. Thorac. Dis.* **2016**, *8*, 2654–2665. [CrossRef] [PubMed]
11. Önal, U.; Valenzuela-Sánchez, F.; Vandana, K.E.; Rello, J. Mid-Regional Pro-Adrenomedullin (MR-proADM) as a Biomarker for Sepsis and Septic Shock: Narrative Review. *Healthcare* **2018**, *6*, 110. [CrossRef]
12. Enguix-Armada, A.; Escobar-Conesa, R.; García-De La Torre, A.; De La Torre-Prados, M.V. Usefulness of several biomarkers in the management of septic patients: C-reactive protein, procalcitonin, presepsin and mid-regional pro-adrenomedullin. *Clin. Chem. Lab. Med.* **2016**, *54*, 163–168. [CrossRef] [PubMed]
13. Andrés, C.; Andaluz-Ojeda, D.; Cicuendez, R.; Munoz-Bellvis, L.; Aldecoa, C.; Bermejo-Martin, J.F. MR-proADM to detect specific types of organ failure in infection. *Eur. J. Clin. Investig.* **2020**, *50*, e13246. [CrossRef] [PubMed]
14. Buendgens, L.; Yagmur, E.; Ginsberg, A.; Weiskirchen, R.; Wirtz, T.; Jhaisha, S.A.; Eisert, A.; Luedde, T.; Trautwein, C.; Tacke, F.; et al. Midregional Proadrenomedullin (MRproADM) Serum Levels in Critically Ill Patients Are Associated with Short-Term and Overall Mortality during a Two-Year Follow-Up. *Mediat. Inflamm.* **2020**, *2020*, 7184803. [CrossRef]

15. Gonzalez Del Castillo, J.; Wilson, D.C.; Clemente-Callejo, C.; Gonzales, V.; Llopis-Roca, F. On behalf of the INFURG-SEMES investigators. Biomarkers and clinical scores to identify patient populations at risk of delayed antibiotic administration or intensive care admission. *Crit. Care* **2019**, *23*, 335. [CrossRef]
16. Haag, E.; Gregoriano, C.; Molitor, A.; Kloter, M.; Kutz, A.; Mueller, B.; Schuetz, P. Does mid-regional pro-adrenomedullin (MR-proADM) improve the sequential organ failure assessment-score (SOFA score) for mortality-prediction in patients with acute infections? Results of a prospective observational study. *Clin. Chem. Lab. Med.* **2021**, *59*, 1165–1176. [CrossRef]
17. Spoto, S.; Nobile, E.; Carnà, E.P.R.; Fogolari, M.; Caputo, D.; De Florio, L.; Valeriani, E.; Benvenuto, D.; Constantino, S.; Ciccozzi, M.; et al. Best diagnostic accuracy of sepsis combining SIRS criteria or qSOFA score with Procalcitonin and Mid-Regional pro-Adrenomedullin outside ICU. *Sci. Rep.* **2020**, *10*, 16605. [CrossRef]
18. Andaluz-Ojeda, D.; Nguyen, H.B.; Meunier-Beillard, N.; Gandia, F.; Bermejo-Martin, J.F.; Charles, P.E. Superior accuracy of mid-regional proadrenomedullin for mortality prediction in sepsis with varying levels of illness severity. *Ann. Intensiv. Care* **2017**, *7*, 15. [CrossRef]
19. Schuetz, P.; Hausfater, P.; Amin, D.; Amin, A.; Haubitz, S.; Faessler, L.; Kutz, A.; Conca, A.; Reutlinger, B.; Canavaggio, P.; et al. TRIAGE Study group. Biomarkers from distinct biological pathways improve early risk stratification in medical emergency patients: The multinational, prospective, observational TRIAGE study. *Crit. Care* **2015**, *19*, 377. [CrossRef] [PubMed]
20. Travaglino, F.; De Berardinis, B.; Magrini, L.; Bongiovanni, C.; Candelli, M.; Silveri, N.G.; Legramante, J.; Galante, A.; Salerno, G.; Cardelli, P.; et al. Utility of Procalcitonin (PCT) and Mid Regional pro-Adrenomedullin (MR-proADM) in Risk Stratification of Critically Ill Febrile Patients in Emergency Department (ED). A Comparison with APACHE II Score. *BMC Infect. Dis.* **2012**, *12*, 184. [CrossRef]
21. Christ-Crain, M.; Morgenthaler, N.G.; Struck, J.; Harbarth, S.; Bergmann, A.; Müller, B. Mid-Regional pro-Adrenomedullin as a Prognostic Marker in Sepsis: An Observational Study. *Crit. Care* **2005**, *9*, R816–R824. [CrossRef]
22. Kim, M.H.; Choi, J.H. An Update on Sepsis Biomarkers. *Infect. Chemother.* **2020**, *52*, 1–18. [CrossRef]
23. Al Shuaibi, M.; Bahu, R.R.; Chaftari, A.M.; Chaftari, A.M.; Wohoush, I.A.; Shomali, W.; Jiang, Y.; Debiane, L.; Raad, S.; Jabbour, J.; et al. Pro-adrenomedullin as a novel biomarker for predicting infections and response to antimicrobials in febrile patients with hematologic malignancies. *Clin. Infect. Dis.* **2013**, *56*, 943–950. [CrossRef] [PubMed]
24. Zhu, M.; Wang, X.; Gu, Y.; Wang, F.; Li, L.; Qiu, X. MEG3 overexpression inhibits the tumorigenesis of breast cancer by downregulating miR-21 through the PI3K/Akt pathway. *Arch. Biochem. Biophys.* **2019**, *661*, 22–30. [CrossRef] [PubMed]
25. Valenzuela-Sánchez, F.; Valenzuela-Méndez, B.; Bohollo de Austria, R.; Rodriguez-Gutierrez, J.F.; Estella-Garcia, A.; Fernandez-Ruiz, L.; Gonzalez-Garcia, M.; Rello, J. Plasma levels of mid-regional pro-adrenomedullin in sepsis are associated with risk of death. *Minerva Anestesiol.* **2019**, *85*, 366–375. [CrossRef] [PubMed]
26. Viaggi, B.; Poole, D.; Tujjar, O.; Marchiani, S.; Ognibene, A.; Finazzi, S. Mid regional pro-adrenomedullin for the prediction of organ failure in infection. Results from a single centre study. *PLoS ONE* **2018**, *13*, e0201491. [CrossRef] [PubMed]
27. DE LA Torre-Prados, M.V.; Garcia-DE LA Torre, A.; Enguix, A.; Mayor-Reyes, M.; Nieto-González, M.; Garcia-Alcantara, A. Mid-regional pro-adrenomedullin as prognostic biomarker in septic shock. *Minerva Anestesiol.* **2016**, *82*, 760–766. [PubMed]
28. Lundberg, O.H.; Bergenzaun, L.; Rydén, J.; Rosenqvist, M.; Melander, O.; Chew, M.S. Adrenomedullin and endothelin-1 are associated with myocardial injury and death in septic shock patients. *Crit. Care* **2016**, *20*, 178. [CrossRef]
29. Singer, M.; Deutschman, C.S.; Seymour, C.W.; Shankar-Hari, M.; Martin, G.S.; Opal, S.M.; Van der Poll, T.; Vincent, J.L.; Angus, D.C. The Third International Consensus Definitions for Sepsis and Septic Shock (Sepsis-3). *JAMA* **2016**, *315*, 801–810. [CrossRef]

Article

Diagnostic Accuracy and Prognostic Value of Neutrophil-to-Lymphocyte and Platelet-to-Lymphocyte Ratios in Septic Patients outside the Intensive Care Unit

Silvia Spoto [1], Domenica Marika Lupoi [1], Emanuele Valeriani [1], Marta Fogolari [2,*], Luciana Locorriere [1], Giuseppina Beretta Anguissola [1], Giulia Battifoglia [1], Damiano Caputo [3], Alessandro Coppola [3], Sebastiano Costantino [1], Massimo Ciccozzi [4] and Silvia Angeletti [2]

1. Diagnostic and Therapeutic Medicine Department, University Campus Bio-Medico of Rome, 00128 Roma, Italy; s.spoto@unicampus.it (S.S.); domenicamarika.lupoi@unicampus.it (D.M.L.); e.valeriani@unicampus.it (E.V.); l.locorriere@unicampus.it (L.L.); g.beretta@unicampus.it (G.B.A.); g.battifogliaa@gmail.com (G.B.); s.costantino@unicampus.it (S.C.)
2. Unit of Clinical Laboratory Science, University Campus Bio-Medico of Rome, 00128 Roma, Italy; s.angeletti@unicampus.it
3. Department of Surgery, University Campus Bio-Medico of Rome, 00128 Roma, Italy; d.caputo@unicampus.it (D.C.); a.coppola@unicampus.it (A.C.)
4. Unit of Medical Statistics and Molecular Epidemiology, University Campus Bio-Medico of Rome, 00128 Roma, Italy; m.ciccozzi@unicampus.it
* Correspondence: m.fogolari@unicampus.it; Tel.: +39-0622-541-1461

Abstract: *Background and Objectives*: The aim of this study was to evaluate the diagnostic accuracy and prognostic value of neutrophil-to-lymphocyte (NLR) and platelet-to-lymphocyte (PLR) ratios and to compare them with other biomarkers and clinical scores of sepsis outside the intensive care unit. *Materials and methods*: In this retrospective study, 251 patients with sepsis and 126 patients with infection other than sepsis were enrolled. NLR and PLR were calculated as the ratio between absolute values of neutrophils, lymphocytes, and platelets by complete blood counts performed on whole blood by *Sysmex* XE-9000 (Dasit, Italy) following the manufacturer's instruction. *Results*: The best NLR value in diagnosis of sepsis was 7.97 with sensibility, specificity, AUC, PPV, and NPV of 64.26%, 80.16%, 0.74 ($p < 0.001$), 86.49%, and 53.18%, respectively. The diagnostic role of NLR significantly increases when PLR, C-reactive protein (PCR), procalcitonin (PCT), and mid-regional pro-adrenomedullin (MR-proADM) values, as well as systemic inflammatory re-sponse syndrome (SIRS), sequential organ failure assessment (SOFA), and quick-sequential organ failure assessment (qSOFA) scores, were added to the model. The best value of NLR in predicting 90-day mortality was 9.05 with sensibility, specificity, AUC, PPV, and NPV of 69.57%, 61.44%, 0.66 ($p < 0.0001$), 28.9%, and 89.9%, respectively. Sensibility, specificity, AUC, PPV, and NPV of NLR increase if PLR, PCR, PCT, MR-proADM, SIRS, qSOFA, and SOFA scores are added to NLR. *Conclusions*: NLR and PLR represent a widely useful and cheap tool in diagnosis and in predict-ing 90-day mortality in patients with sepsis.

Keywords: neutrophil-to-lymphocyte; platelet-to-lymphocyte; C-reactive protein; procalcitonin; MR-proAdrenomedullin; systemic inflammatory response syndrome; sequential organ failure assessment; quick-sequential organ failure assessment; sepsis; septic shock

1. Introduction

Sepsis is a systemic syndrome induced by infection and leading to a widespread inflammation up to septic shock, multi organ failure, and death [1,2]. Patients with bacteriemia, sepsis, and septic shock presented a high mortality rate ranging from 25% to 30% and 40% to 50%, respectively [3,4]. Patients' prognosis and mortality rate, however, are strictly affected by a timely performed clinical and laboratory diagnosis as well as by proper therapeutic management [5–7].

Blood cultures represent the gold standard for microbiological diagnosis of sepsis [6]. Unfortunately, they yielded positive results in just a third of cases and may require several days for positivization even if newer and more expensive molecular techniques are used (e.g., polymerase chain reaction and mass spectroscopy) [8–18].

To overcome these issues, several scores such as SIRS and qSOFA were introduced in clinical practice to help diagnosis, disease severity stratification, and prognostic evaluation [5,19,20]. Adding laboratory biomarkers increases the usefulness of these scores in guiding clinical and therapeutic choices [12–26]. Among these, C-reactive protein (PCR, ≥ 5 mg/dL), procalcitonin (PCT, ≥ 0.5 ng/mL), and mid-regional pro-adrenomedullin (MR-proADM, ≥ 1.50 nmol/L) showed the highest diagnostic and prognostic power, but they were expensive and not widely available [15,26–29]. Conversely, the neutrophil-to-lymphocyte ratio (NLR) represents a widely available, inexpensive, and easily performed marker that has been recently evaluated for its diagnostic and prognostic role in sepsis. NLR early expresses the relationship between innate (neutrophils) and adaptive cellular immune response (lymphocytes) during pathological states. [30]. Mean NLR values below 2 (1,6) are representative of healthy people (without differences in sex category or race) [30,31], while it may increase up to values of >10 in sepsis and >20 in septic shock, with good sensibility and specificity [30–44]. NLR seems to also vary in relation to different bacterial pathogens, with the lowest and highest values in Gram-positive and Gram-negative or polymicrobial sepsis, respectively [37–39].

NLR, however, may be affected by some clinical condition or therapies resulting in false positive (e.g., corticosteroids) or false negative (e.g., chemotherapy, radiotherapy, antibiotic therapy, Cachexia) results [31].

Along with NLR, the monocyte-to-lymphocyte ratio (MLR), the platelet-to-lymphocyte ratio (PLR), and the mean platelet volume-to-platelet count (MPV/PC) ratio have been studied recently, but the results are contrasting [30–39].

The aim of this study was to evaluate the diagnostic accuracy and prognostic value of NLR, PLR, and MLR in patients with sepsis and septic shock outside the intensive care unit (ICU) and to compare them with C-reactive protein (CRP), PCT, MR-proADM, *SIRS*, qSOFA, and SOFA scores.

Furthermore, we evaluated the role of NLR in aetiological diagnosis of sepsis and on length of stay stratification.

2. Materials and Methods

The study was approved on 23 July 2016 by the Ethical Committee of the University Hospital Campus Bio-Medico of Rome (28.16 TS Com Et CBM). All methods were performed in accordance with the relevant guidelines and regulations. Informed consent was not required for the retrospective design of the study.

2.1. Patients Selection and Study Design

Consecutive patients with clinically suspected sepsis or septic shock admitted to the Diagnostic and Therapeutic Medicine Department and General Surgery of the University Hospital Campus Bio-Medico of Rome were retrospectively enrolled between May 2014 and February 2021.

Exclusion criteria were age < 18 years and pregnancy.

The control group included patients with infection, but without sepsis admitted to the Diagnostic and Therapeutic Medicine Department between May 2014 and February 2021.

Diagnosis of sepsis was performed according to the Third Consensus Conference Criteria of 2016 when qSOFA or SOFA scores were ≥ 2 from the baseline in the presence of an infection.

Bloodstream infection was defined as any positive blood culture for pathogens. Pneumonia was defined based on a positive pathogen respiratory culture and other Infectious

Diseases Society of America (IDSA) diagnostic criteria [45]. Patients with positive urine cultures were identified as cases based on the CDC National Healthcare Safety Network (NHSN) UTI case definitions [46].

Baseline patients' characteristics were retrospectively collected form medical records including demographic information (age, sex category), presence of comorbidities (cardiovascular, pulmonary, kidney, liver disease), immune status (active malignancy or other causes of an immunosuppression), immunosuppressive treatments (corticosteroids, antibiotics), laboratory values (complete blood count, NLR, PLR, MLR, PCR, PCT, MR-proADM), and clinical scores (e.g., SIRS, qSOFA, SOFA).

2.2. Laboratory and Microbiological Parameters

Complete blood counts (CBCs) were performed on whole blood by *Sysmex* XE-9000 (Dasit, Italy) following the manufacturer's instruction. NLR, PLR, and MLR were calculated by the ratio between absolute values of neutrophils, lymphocytes, monocytes, respectively, and that of platelets.

CRP protein was measured by Alinity c (Abbott, diagnostics) following the manufacturer's instruction.

PCT and MR-proADM plasma concentrations were measured by an automated Kryptor analyzer, using a time-resolved amplified cryptate emission (TRACE) technology assay (Kryptor PCT; Brahms AG; Hennigsdorf, Germany) with commercially available immunoluminometric assays (Brahms) [5,21,25,26].

Blood specimens from patients were collected in BACTEC bottles containing anaerobic or aerobic broth and resins. Blood culture bottles were incubated in BACTEC FX instrument (Becton Dickinson, Meylan, France) until they were positive for bacterial growth or for a maximum of 5 days. Positive samples were cultivated in selective agar media. Growing colonies were identified by MALDI-TOF (Brahms) [5,21,25,26]. Selective and non-selective media were used for microbiological cultures.

2.3. Statistical Analysis

Data were analysed using Med-Calc 11.6.1.0 statistical package (MedCalc Software, Mariakerke, Belgium). Receiver operating characteristic (ROC) analysis was performed among independent variables associated with sepsis to define the cutoff point for NLR, PLR, plasma PCR, PCT, MR-proADM, SIRS, SOFA, and qSOFA score values. ROC curves and areas under the curve (AUCs) were calculated for all markers and compared in patients with sepsis or septic shock versus control patients.

$\chi 2$ for proportions test was used to compare the relative percentage of patients with positivity and/or negativity to SIRS criteria, SOFA score, qSOFA score, and other demographic characteristics of septic patients and control patients.

Positive predictive value (PPV) and negative predictive value (NPV) were calculated for each variable, based on sensitivity, specificity, and disease prevalence. Younden Index was used for cut-off selection.

The multivariate logistic regression model is performed to evaluate the association between all evaluable laboratory markers and 90-day mortality.

Mann–Whitney test was used for median values' comparison. p-value < 0.05 was considered significant.

3. Results

3.1. Baseline Patients' Characteristics

Demographic and clinical characteristics of patients with sepsis (251 patients) and the control group (126 patients) are reported in Table 1.

Patients with sepsis were younger than the control group (73 vs. 80, $p = 0.001$), while roughly half of the patients in both groups were male (52.6 vs. 50.4%, $p = 0.771$).

Table 1. Baseline patients' characteristics.

Variables	Patients with Sepsis N = 251	Patients without Sepsis N = 126	p-Value
Age, y	73.0 (65.0, 80.0)	80.0 (68.5, 86.0)	0.001
Male sex, n (%)	132 (52.6)	63 (50.4)	0.771
Steroid use, n (%)	62 (24.8)	27 (21.6)	0.577
Ongoing chemotherapy, n (%)	7 (2.8)	1 (0.8)	0.376
Septic shock, n (%)	100 (39.8)	0 (0.0)	<0.001
Smoke history (%)			<0.001
Never	180 (71.7)	55 (44.0)	
Former	61 (24.3)	52 (41.6)	
Current	10 (4.0)	18 (14.4)	
Diabetes mellitus type 2, n (%)	56 (22.3)	29 (23.0)	0.981
Cancer, n (%)	92 (36.7)	30 (23.8)	0.016
Lung disease, n (%)	58 (23.1)	43 (34.1)	0.031
Heart disease, n (%)	137 (54.6)	74 (59.2)	0.459
Liver disease, n (%)	24 (9.6)	8 (6.3)	0.390
Chronic kidney disease, n (%)	73 (29.1)	34 (27.0)	0.760
Chronic cerebrovascular disease, n (%)	68 (27.1)	19 (15.1)	0.013
SIRS, median values [IQR]	2 (1, 3)	0 (0, 1)	<0.001
q-SOFA, median values [IQR]	2 (1, 2)	0 (0, 0)	<0.001
SOFA, median values [IQR]	4 (2, 6)	2 (1, 3)	<0.001
NLR, median [IQR]	10.7 (6.3, 18.7)	5.4 (3.7, 7.4)	<0.001
PLR, median [IQR]	228.7 (147.8, 407.9)	219.7 (147.1, 308.2)	0.049
CRP, median [IQR]	107.5 (41.8, 173.7)	8.5 (2.3, 16.5)	<0.001
PCT, median [IQR]	1.2 (0.4, 5.2)	0.1 (0.1, 0.3)	<0.001
MR-proADM, median [IQR]	1.2 (0.8, 1.9)	2.8 (1.8, 4.5)	<0.001
Lenght of stay, median [IQR]	15.0 (11.0, 25.5)	10.0 (7.0, 13.0)	<0.001
ICU admission, n (%)	47 (18.7)	0 (0.0)	<0.001
90-day mortality	69 (27.5)	1 (0.8)	<0.001

The vast majority of baseline patients' characteristics were similar between septic patients and control group (Table 1), except for the presence of presence of cancer and chronic lung disease that was more (36.7% vs. 23.8%, $p = 0.016$) and less frequent (23.1 vs. 34.1, $p = 0.031$), respectively, in the former.

In septic patients, median SIRS, qSOFA, and SOFA scores' values were 2 (IQR, 1 to 3), 2 (IQR, 1 to 2), and 4 (IQR, 2 to 6), respectively. One hundred out of 251 patients (39.8%) had septic shock and 47 out of 251 patients (18.7%) required ICU transfer during hospitalization.

The median length of stay was higher in septic patients than the control group (15 days (IQR, 11 to 26) vs. 10 days (IQR 7 to 13), $p \leq 0.001$) and a significantly higher proportion of patients with sepsis died during 90-day follow-up (27.5% vs. 0.8%, $p < 0.001$).

3.2. Diagnostic Role of NLR

For the diagnosis of sepsis, the best value of NLR was 7.97 with sensibility of 64.26%, specificity of 80.16%, AUC of 0.74 ($p < 0.001$), PPV of 86.49%, and NPV of 53.18%. The ROC curve is reported in Figure 1A. In Table 2, the diagnostic role of NLR is compared with that of PLR, PCR, PCT, and MR-proADM, as well as with that of SIRS, q-SOFA, and SOFA scores. MLR did not reach a significant role in the diagnosis of sepsis.

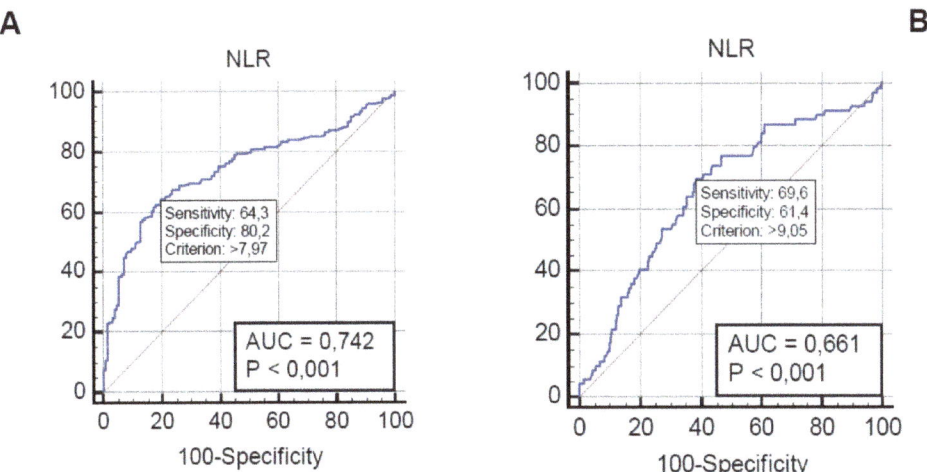

Figure 1. (**A**) Receiver operating characteristic (ROC) curve analysis, showing neutrophil-to-lymphocyte (NLR) ability to differentiate Scheme 7.97. (**B**) ROC curve analysis, showing NLR ability in to predict 90-day mortality in septic patients; the best value of NRL was 9.05.

Table 2. Diagnostic role of NLR by ROC curve analysis.

Model	Cut-Off	Sensibility	Specificity	AUC	p	PPV	NPV
NLR	7.97	64.26	80.16	0.74	<0.001	86.49	53.18
PLR	370.59	29.3	92.1	0.56	0.037	87.99	39.72
PCR	37.88	78.75	93.51	0.92	<0.0001	95.93	60.46
PCT	0.41	79.6	81.00	0.88	<0.001	89.26	60.67
MR-proADM	1.83	80.1	74.6	0.86	<0.0001	85.51	66.68
SIRS	≥2	67.3	89.7	0.57	<0.001	96.77	43.30
q-SOFA	≥2	51.4	99.2	0.87	<0.001	99.23	50.21
SOFA	≥2	69.7	71.4	0.77	<0.001	82.94	54.21

Area under the curve (AUC); positive predictive value (PPV); negative predictive value (NPV). NLR, neutrophil-to-lymphocyte; PLR, platelet-to-lymphocyte; PCR, C-reactive protein; PCT, procalcitonin; MR-proADM, mid-regional pro-adrenomedullin; SIRS, systemic inflammatory response syndrome; SOFA, sequential organ failure assessment.

The diagnostic role of NLR significantly increases when PCR, PCT, and MR-proADM values, as well as SIRS, qSOFA, and SOFA scores, were added to the model (Table 3).

When just PCT and MR-proADM are considered in the diagnosis of sepsis, the model reached a PPV of 96% and a NPV of 69%. PPV and NPV for SIRS ≥2, qSOFA ≥2, and SOFA ≥2 were 96.77% and 43.3%, 99.23 and 50.21%, and 82.94% and 54.21%, respectively.

The best values of PPV and NPV are reached when NLR, PLR, and SIRS scores (99.7% and 94%, respectively), or NLR, PLR, and qSOFA scores (99.9% and 95.6%, respectively), are included in the model.

NLR, MLR, and PLR did not show a significant role in aetiological diagnosis of sepsis. Conversely, our results confirm the role of PCT in aetiological diagnosis of sepsis with higher values in Gram-negative versus Gram-positive bacteria ($p = 0.0022$). Furthermore, MR-proADM values are significantly higher in Gram-negative ($p = 0.037$) and polymicrobial ($p = 0.037$) than Gram-positive sepsis.

Table 3. Comparison of the diagnostic role of NLR with other inflammatory markers or clinical scores: positive predictive value (PPV) and negative predictive value (NPV).

Model *	PPV	NPV
NLR	86.49	53.18
PLR	87.99	39.73
PCR	95.93	69.46
PCT	89.26	66.68
MR-proADM	85.52	66.68
SIRS	96.77	43.31
qSOFA	99.23	50.21
SOFA	82.94	54.21
NLR + PLR	96.00	83.00
NLR + PCR	98.70	59.00
NLR + PCT	96.49	61.50
NLR + ADM	95.30	63.30
NLR + SIRS	98.90	81.00
NLR + q-SOFA	99.70	76.00
NLR + SOFA	94.00	73.00
NLR + PLR + SIRS	99.70	94.00
NLR + PLR + q-SOFA	99.90	95.60
NLR + PLR + SOFA	98.30	91.60

* Cut-off values: NLR, 7.97; PLR, 370.59; PCR, 37.88 mg/dL; PCT, 0.41 ng/mL; MRproADM, 1.83 ng/mL; SIRS, q-SOFA, SOFA ≥ 2. NLR, neutrophil-to-lymphocyte; PLR, platelet-to-lymphocyte; PCR, C-reactive protein; PCT, procalcitonin; MR-proADM, mid-regional pro-adrenomedullin; SIRS, systemic inflammatory response syndrome; SOFA, sequential organ failure assessment.

3.3. Role of NLR in Predicting 90-Day Mortality

The best value of NLR in predicting 90-day mortality was 9.05, with sensibility, specificity, AUC, PPV, and NPV of 69.57%, 61.44%, 0.66 ($p < 0.0001$), 28.9%, and 89.9%, respectively. The ROC curve is reported in Figure 1B.

The prognostic role of NLR in comparison with that of PLR, PCR, PCT, and MR-proADM values, as well as with that of SIRS, qSOFA, and SOFA scores, is listed in Table 4.

Table 4. Role of NLR in predicting 90-day mortality.

Model	Cut-Off	Sensibility	Specificity	AUC	p	PPV	NPV
NLR	9.05	69.57	61.44	0.66	<0.001	71.40	89.90
PCR	37.88	83.33	52.35	0.67	<0.001	27.90	93.40
PCT	0.39	90.00	47.00	0.70	<0.001	27.98	95.36
MR-proADM	3.21	76.50	71.40	0.79	<0.001	38.20	92.92
SIRS	≥2	44.29	79.80	0.72	<0.001	33.33	86.26
q-SOFA	≥2	25.70	91.48	0.80	<0.001	40.90	84.20
SOFA	≥2	92.86	52.44	0.82	<0.001	30.80	96.98

Area under the curve (AUC); positive predictive value (PPV); negative predictive value (NPV). NLR, neutrophil-to-lymphocyte; PCR, C-reactive protein; PCT, procalcitonin; MR-proADM, mid-regional pro-adrenomedullin; SIRS, systemic inflammatory response syndrome; SOFA, sequential organ failure assessment.

Sensibility, specificity, AUC, PPV, and NPV of NLR increase if PLR, PCR, PCT, MR-proADM, SIRS, qSOFA, and SOFA scores are added to NLR (Table 5).

MLR was not statistically significant in the 90-day mortality prediction.

Multivariate logistic regression model including all evaluable laboratory markers showed as just MR-proADM is significantly associated with 90-day mortality (Table 6).

Table 5. Improvement of the prognostic role of NLR with further biomarkers or clinical scores: positive predictive value (PPV) and negative predictive value (NPV) reached by the association of different biomarkers and clinical scores.

Model *	PVV	NPV
NLR	28.9	89.9
NLR + MR-proADM	52.0	50.0
NLR + SIRS	95.0	86.0
NLR + q-SOFA	96.0	88.0
NLR + SOFA	94.6	89.9

* Cut-off values: NLR, 9.05; MRproADM, 3.21 ng/mL; SIRS, q-SOFA, SOFA ≥2. NLR, neutrophil-to-lymphocyte; MR-proADM, mid-regional pro-adrenomedullin; SIRS, systemic inflammatory response syndrome; SOFA, sequential organ failure assessment.

Table 6. Multivariate logistic regression model for 90-day mortality.

Model	OR (95% CI)	p-Values
NLR	1.002 (0.968 to 1.037)	0.912
PLR	0.999 (0.997 to 1.000)	0.142
MLR	0.952 (0.489 to 1.753)	0.878
CRP	0.998 (0.994 to 1.002)	0.270
PCT	0.989 (0.966 to 1.006)	0.226
MRproADM	1.406 (1.219 to 1.657)	<0.001

4. Discussion

The results of this study showed that NLR values of 7.97 had a good diagnostic accuracy, whereas a value of 9.05 allowed a prognostic stratification of patients with sepsis that is increased by the association with PLR values of 370.59. Conversely to PCT and MR-proADM, NLR did not help identify the type of bacterial pathogen responsible for sepsis. MLR evaluation did not yield significant results.

Patients with sepsis presented a higher 90-day mortality (27.5%) and need for ICU transfer (18.7%) than the control group. However, these proportions of patients resulted lower than data available from previous studies, where mortality and ICU transfer reached values as high as 37.5% and 80.8%, respectively [47].

Performing a complete blood count and calculating NLR and PLR in a clinical suspicion of sepsis may, therefore, help the clinician in diagnostic evaluation and prognostic stratification of patients with significant values of sensibility, specificity, PPV, NPV, and AUC ($p < 0.0001$). These latter values were similar to the values of PCT >0.41 and MR-proADM >1.83 and are increased by the association with PLR values (PPV of 96% and NPV of 83%) and clinical score of sepsis such as SIRS (PPV of 99.7% and NPV of 94.0%), qSOFA (PPV of 99.9% and NPV of 95.6%), and SOFA (PPV 98.3% and NPV on 91.6%). In our study, the association between NLR and SIRS or qSOFA reached higher diagnostic power than the association between NLR and SOFA. This may be related to the clinical setting; our patients, indeed, were hospitalized in a medical ward and outside the ICU.

Furthermore, the best values of NLR, CRP, PCT, and MR-proADM for a diagnosis of sepsis were lower than the values reported from previous studies (10, 5 mg/dL, 0.5 ng/mL, and 1.5 nmol/L respectively) [5,25,26,28,30–44]. This may be related to a prompt laboratory evaluation performed immediately after the suspicion of sepsis. These biomarkers, indeed, have a turnaround time of less than an hour for complete blood count and one hour for CRP, PCT, and MR-proADM. A prompt availability of these biomarkers may reduce the delay between the diagnosis of sepsis and the administration of an effective treatment.

As for sepsis diagnosis, NLR values of 9.05 showed a good role in prognostic stratification in terms of 90-day mortality. This is increased by its combination with both MR-proADM (PPV of 52% and NPV of 50%) and clinical scores of sepsis such as SIRS (PPV of 95% and NPV of 86%), q-SOFA (PPV of 96% and NPV of 88%), and SOFA (PPV of 94.6% and NPV of 55.7%).

Knowing that, the shorter the time between clinical presentation and diagnosis, the better the patients' prognosis, NLR may ameliorate septic patients' management. This, latter, further increases when the clinical score such as SIRS and qSOFA is used in association with NLR.

The results of our study certainly showed that a prompt and accurate diagnosis of sepsis may be achieved by the use of rapid, cheap, and widely performed biomarkers, as well as in those clinical setting where the use of other biomarkers may be not available or too expensive. Outside the ICU, adding information derived by these biomarkers to clinical score such as SIRS or qSOFA reached a diagnostic accuracy of about 100%.

A limitation of the study is the monocentric enrollment of patients, which should be expanded in the future to be multicentric, thus increasing the number of patients, which is limited to 251 in this first study.

5. Conclusions

NLR is a good, rapid, cheap, and widely performed biomarker useful in diagnosis and prognostic stratification of patients with sepsis. The association of NLR with other biomarkers and clinical scores further increases these characteristics. Only the association between clinical signs and several biomarkers may help increase the diagnostic sensibility of sepsis and predict disease severity and mortality. Biomarkers must be performed in supporting a clinical diagnosis. We hope that the use of NLR may improve the management and ameliorate the prognosis of patients with sepsis.

Author Contributions: Conceptualization, S.S. and S.A.; Methodology, S.S. and S.A.; Software, D.M.L. and E.V.; Validation, L.L., G.B.A., M.F., and E.V.; Formal analysis, S.S. and E.V.; Investigation, D.M.L. and E.V.; Data curation, S.S.; writing—original draft preparation, S.S., S.A., and E.V.; writing—review and editing, S.S., S.A., and E.V.; visualization, M.F., M.C., D.C., A.C., G.B., and S.C.; supervision, S.S., M.C., and S.C.; project administration, S.S. All authors have read and agreed to the published version of the manuscript.

Funding: This research received no external funding.

Institutional Review Board Statement: The study was conducted according to the guidelines of the Declaration of Helsinki and approved by the Ethical Committee of the University Hospital Campus Bio-Medico of Rome (28.16 TS Com Et CBM).

Informed Consent Statement: Informed consent was not required for the retrospective design of the study.

Data Availability Statement: The data presented in this study are available on request from the corresponding author. The data are not publicly available due to their containing information that could compromise the privacy of research participants.

Conflicts of Interest: The authors declare no conflict of interest.

Abbreviations

AUCs	Areas under the curve
CBC	Complete blood counts
CRP	C-reactive protein
ICU	Intensive care unit
MR-proADM	Mid-regional pro-adrenomedullin
PCR	Polymerase chain reaction
PCT	Procalcitonin
PPV	Positive predictive value
NPV	Negative predictive value
ROC	Receiver operating characteristic
SIRS	Systemic inflammatory response syndrome
SOFA	Sequential sepsis-related organ failure assessment
WBC	White blood cell

References

1. Fleischmann, C.; Scherag, A.; Adhikari, N.K.J.; Hartog, C.S.; Tsaganos, T.; Schlattmann, P.; Angus, D.C.; Reinhart, K.; International Forum of Acute Care Trialists. Assessment of global incidence and mortality of hospital-treated sepsis. Current estimates and limitations. *Am. J. Respir. Crit. Care Med.* **2016**, *193*, 259–272. [CrossRef]
2. Churpek, M.M.; Snyder, A.; Han, X.; Sokol, S.; Pettit, N.; Howell, M.D.; Edelson, D.P. Quick sepsis-related organ failure assessment, systemic inflammatory response syndrome, and early warning scores for detecting clinical deterioration in infected patients outside the intensive care unit. *Am. J. Respir. Crit. Care Med.* **2017**, *195*, 906–911. [CrossRef]
3. Leibovici, L.; Greenshtain, S.; Cohen, O.; Mor, F.; Wysenbeek, A.J. Bacteremia in febrile patients. A clinical model for diagnosis. *Arch Intern Med* **1991**, *151*, 1801–1806. [CrossRef] [PubMed]
4. Bone, R.C.; Balk, R.A.; Cerra, F.B.; Dellinger, R.P.; Fein, A.M.; Knaus, W.A.; Schein, R.M.; Sibbald, W.J. Definitions for sepsis and organ failure and guidelines for the use of innovative therapies in sepsis. The ACCP/SCCM Consensus Conference Committee. American College of Chest Physicians/Society of Critical Care Medicine. *Chest* **1992**, *101*, 1644–1655. [CrossRef] [PubMed]
5. Spoto, S.; Nobile, E.; Rafano Carnà, E.P.; Fogolari, M.; Caputo, D.; De Florio, L.; Valeriani, E.; Benvenuto, D.; Costantino, S.; Ciccozzi, M.; et al. Best diagnostic accuracy of sepsis combining SIRS criteria or qSOFA score with Procalcitonin and Mid-Regional pro-Adrenomedullin outside ICU. *Sci. Rep.* **2020**, *10*, 16605. [CrossRef] [PubMed]
6. Levy, M.M.; Fink, M.P.; Marshall, J.C.; Abraham, E.; Angus, D.; Cook, D.; Cohen, J.; Opal, S.M.; Vincent, J.-L.; Ramsay, G. SCCM/ESICM/ACCP/ATS/SIS. 2001 SCCM/ESICM/ACCP/ATS/SIS International Sepsis Definitions Conference. *Crit. Care Med.* **2003**, *31*, 1250–1256.
7. Kopczynska, M.; Sharif, B.; Cleaver, S.; Spencer, N.; Kurani, A.; Lee, C.; Davis, J.; Durie, C.; Gubral, J.J.; Sharma, A.; et al. Red-flag sepsis and SOFA identifies different patient population at risk of sepsis-related deaths on the general ward. *Medicine* **2018**, *97*, e13238. [CrossRef] [PubMed]
8. Singer, M.; Deutschman, C.S.; Seymour, C.W.; Shankar-Hari, M.; Annane, D.; Bauer, M.; Bellomo, R.; Bernard, G.R.; Chiche, J.D.; Coopersmith, C.M.; et al. The third international consensus definitions for sepsis and septic shock (sepsis-3). *JAMA* **2016**, *315*, 801–810. [CrossRef]
9. Diekema, D.J.; Hsueh, P.-R.; Mendes, R.E.; Pfaller, M.A.; Rolston, K.V.; Sader, H.S.; Jones, R.N. The microbiology of bloodstream infection: 20-year trends from the SENTRY antimicrobial surveillance program. *Antimicrob. Agents Chemother.* **2019**, *63*, e00355-19. [CrossRef]
10. Sprung, C.L.; Schein, R.M.H.; Balk, R.A. The new sepsis consensus definitions: The good, the bad and the ugly. *Intensive Care Med.* **2016**, *42*, 2024–2026. [CrossRef] [PubMed]
11. Horeczko, T.; Green, J.P.; Panacek, E.A. Epidemiology of the systemic inflammatory response syndrome (SIRS) in the emergency department. *West J. Emerg. Med.* **2014**, *15*, 329–336. [CrossRef] [PubMed]
12. De Florio, L.; Riva, E.; Giona, A.; Dedej, E.; Fogolari, M.; Cella, E.; Spoto, S.; Lai, A.; Zehender, G.; Ciccozzi, M.; et al. MALDI-TOF MS Identification and Clustering Applied to Enterobacter Species in Nosocomial Setting. *Front. Microbiol.* **2018**, *14*, 9:1885. [CrossRef] [PubMed]
13. Angeletti, S.; Cella, E.; Prosperi, M.; Spoto, S.; Fogolari, M.; De Florio, L.; Antonelli, F.; Dedej, E.; De Flora, C.; Ferraro, E.; et al. Multi-drug resistant Pseudomonas aeruginosa nosocomial strains: Molecular epidemiology and evolution. *Microb. Pathog.* **2018**, *123*, 233–241. [CrossRef]
14. Cella, E.; Ciccozzi, M.; Lo Presti, A.; Fogolari, M.; Azarian, T.; Prosperi, M.; Salemi, M.; Equestre, M.; Antonelli, F.; Conti, A.; et al. Multi-drug resistant Klebsiella pneumoniae strains circulating in hospital setting: Whole-genome sequencing and Bayesian phylogenetic analysis for outbreak investigations. *Sci. Rep.* **2017**, *7*, 3534. [CrossRef] [PubMed]
15. Cancilleri, F.; Ciccozzi, M.; Fogolari, M.; Cella, E.; De Florio, L.; Berton, A.; Salvatore, G.; Dicuonzo, G.; Spoto, S.; Denaro, V.; et al. A case of methicillin-resistant Staphylococcus aureus wound infection: Phylogenetic analysis to establish if nosocomial or community acquired. *Clin. Case Rep.* **2018**, *6*, 871–874. [CrossRef]
16. Santini, D.; Ratta, R.; Pantano, F.; De Lisi, D.; Maruzzo, M.; Galli, L.; Biasco, E.; Farnesi, A.; Buti, S.; Sternberg, C.N.; et al. Outcome of oligoprogressing metastatic renal cell carcinoma patients treated with locoregional therapy: A multicenter retrospective analysis. *Oncotarget* **2017**, *7*, 100708–100716. [CrossRef]
17. Rizzo, S.; Galvano, A.; Pantano, F.; Iuliani, M.; Vincenzi, B.; Passiglia, F.; Spoto, S.; Tonini, G.; Bazan, V.; Russo, A.; et al. The effects of enzalutamide and abiraterone on skeletal related events and bone radiological progression free survival in castration resistant prostate cancer patients: An indirect comparison of randomized controlled trials. *Crit. Rev. Oncol. Hematol.* **2017**, *120*, 227–233. [CrossRef] [PubMed]
18. Vincent, J.L.; Sakr, Y.; Sprung, C.L.; Ranieri, V.M.; Reinhart, K.; Gerlach, H.; Moreno, R.; Carlet, J.; Le Gall, J.R.; Payen, D. Sepsis Occurrence in Acutely Ill Patients Investigators. Sepsis in European intensive care units: Results of the SOAP study. *Crit. Care Med.* **2006**, *34*, 344–353. [CrossRef]
19. Bates, D.W.; Sands, K.; Miller, E.; Lanken, P.N.; Hibberd, P.L.; Graman, P.S.; Schwartz, J.S.; Kahn, K.; Snydman, D.R.; Parsonnet, J.; et al. Predicting bacteremia in patients with sepsis syndrome. *J. Infect. Dis.* **1997**, *176*, 1538–1551. [CrossRef]
20. Sridharan, P.; Chamberlain, R.S. The efficacy of procalcitonin as a biomarker in the management of sepsis: Slaying dragons or tilting at windmills? *Surg. Infect.* **2013**, *14*, 489–511. [CrossRef]

21. Spoto, S.; Fogolari, M.; De Florio, L.; Minieri, M.; Vicino, G.; Legramante, J.; Lia, M.S.; Terrinoni, A.; Caputo, D.; Costantino, S.; et al. Procalcitonin and MR-proAdrenomedullin combination in the etiological diagnosis and prognosis of sepsis and septic shock. *Microb. Pathog.* **2019**, *137*, 103763. [CrossRef] [PubMed]
22. Briel, M.; Schuetz, P.; Mueller, B.; Young, J.; Schild, U.; Nusbaumer, C.; Périat, P.; Bucher, H.C.; Christ-Crain, M. Procalcitonin-guided antibiotic use vs a standard approach for acute respiratory tract infections in primary care. *Arch. Intern. Med.* **2008**, *168*, 2000–2007. [CrossRef]
23. Stolz, D.; Christ-Crain, M.; Bingisser, R.; Leuppi, J.; Miedinger, D.; Müller, C.; Huber, P.; Müller, B.; Tamm, M. Antibiotic treatment of exacerbations of COPD: A randomized, controlled trial comparing procalcitonin-guidance with standard therapy. *Chest* **2007**, *131*, 9–19. [CrossRef]
24. Larsen, F.F.; Petersen, J.A. Novel biomarkers for sepsis: A narrative review. *Eur. J. Intern. Med.* **2017**, *45*, 46–50. [CrossRef]
25. Spoto, S.; Valeriani, E.; Caputo, D.; Cella, E.; Fogolari, M.; Pesce, E.; Mulè, M.T.; Cartillone, M.; Costantino, S.; Dicuonzo, G.; et al. The role of procalcitonin in the diagnosis of bacterial infection after major abdominal surgery: Advantage from daily measurement. *Medicine* **2018**, *97*, e9496. [CrossRef]
26. Spoto, S.; Cella, E.; De Cesaris, M.; Locorriere, L.; Mazzaroppi, S.; Nobile, E.; Lanotte, A.M.; Pedicino, L.; Fogolari, M.; Costantino, S.; et al. Procalcitonin and MR-Proadrenomedullin Combination with SOFA and qSOFA Scores for Sepsis Diagnosis and Prognosis: A Diagnostic Algorithm. *Shock* **2018**, *50*, 44–52. [CrossRef]
27. Angeletti, S.; Ciccozzi, M.; Fogolari, M.; Spoto, S.; Lo Presti, A.; Costantino, S.; Dicuonzo, G. Procalcitonin and MR-proAdrenomedullin combined score in the diagnosis and prognosis of systemic and localized bacterial infections. *J. Infect.* **2016**, *72*, 395–398. [CrossRef] [PubMed]
28. Povoa, P.; Almeida, E.; Moreira, P.; Fernandes, A.; Mealha, R.; Aragao, A.; Sabino, H. C-reactive protein as an indicator of sepsis. *Intensive Care Med.* **1998**, *24*, 1052–1056. [CrossRef]
29. Reny, J.L.; Vuagnat, A.; Ract, C.; Benoit, M.O.; Safar, M.; Fagon, J.Y. Diagnosis and follow-up of infections in intensive care patients: Value of C-reactive protein compared with other clinical and biological variables. *Crit. Care Med.* **2002**, *30*, 529–535. [CrossRef]
30. de Jager, C.P.; van Wijk, P.T.; Mathoera, R.B.; de Jongh-Leuvenink, J.; van der Poll, T.; Wever, P.C. Lymphocytopenia and neutrophil-lymphocyte count ratio predict bacteremia better than conventional infection markers in an emergency care unit. *Crit. Care* **2010**, *14*, R192. [CrossRef] [PubMed]
31. de Jager, C.P.; Wever, P.C.; Gemen, E.F.; Kusters, R.; van Gageldonk-Lafeber, A.B.; van der Poll, T.; Laheij, R.J.F. The neutrophil-lymphocyte count ratio in patients with community-acquired pneumonia. *PLoS ONE* **2012**, *7*, e46561. [CrossRef]
32. Zhiwei, H.; Zhaoyin, F.; Wujun, H.; Kegang, H. Prognostic value of neutrophil-to-lymphocyte ratio in sepsis: A meta-analysis. *Am. J. Emerg. Med.* **2020**, *38*, 641–647.
33. Forget, P.; Khalifa, C.; Defour, J.P.; Latinne, D.; Van Pel, M.C.; De Kock, M. What is the normal value of the neutrophil-to-lymphocyte ratio? *BMC Res. Notes* **2017**, *10*, 12. [CrossRef] [PubMed]
34. Lee, J.S.; Kim, N.Y.; Na, S.H.; Youn, Y.H.; Shin, C.S. Reference values of neutrophil lymphocyte ratio, lymphocyte-monocyte ratio, platelet-lymphocyte ratio, and mean platelet volume in healthy adults in South Korea. *Medicine* **2018**, *97*, e11138. [CrossRef] [PubMed]
35. Jiang, J.; Liu, R.; Yu, X.; Yang, R.; Xu, H.; Mao, Z.; Wang, Y. The neutrophil-lymphocyte count ratio as a diagnostic marker for bacteraemia: A systematic review and meta-analysis. *Am. J. Emerg. Med.* **2019**, *37*, 1482–1489. [CrossRef]
36. Zhang, H.B.; Chen, J.; Lan, Q.F.; Ma, X.J.; Zhang, S.Y. Diagnostic values of red cell distribution width, platelet distribution width and neutrophil-lymphocyte count ratio for sepsis. *Exp. Ther. Med.* **2016**, *12*, 2215–2219. [CrossRef]
37. Laukemann, S.; Kasper, N.; Kulkarni, P.; Steiner, D.; Rast, A.C.; Kutz, A.; Felder, S.; Haubitz, S.; Faessler, L.; Huber, A.; et al. Can we reduce negative blood cultures with clinical scores and blood markers? Results from an observational cohort study. *Medicine* **2015**, *94*, e2264. [CrossRef]
38. Lowsby, R.; Gomes, C.; Jarman, I.; Lisboa, P.; Nee, P.A.; Vardhan, M.; Eckersley, T.; Saleh, R.; Mills, H. Neutrophil to lymphocyte count ratio as an early indicator of blood stream infection in the emergency department. *Emerg. Med. J.* **2015**, *32*, 531–534. [CrossRef] [PubMed]
39. Loonen, A.J.M.; de Jager, C.P.; Tosserams, J.; Kusters, R.; Hilbink, M.; Wever, P.C.; van den Brule, A.J. Biomarkers and molecular analysis to improve bloodstream infection diagnostics in an emergency care unit. *PLoS ONE* **2014**, *9*, e87315. [CrossRef]
40. Ljungstrom, L.; Pernestig, A.K.; Jacobsson, G.; Andersson, R.; Usener, B.; Tilevik, D. Diagnostic accuracy of procalcitonin, neutrophil-lymphocyte count ratio, C-reactive protein, and lactate in patients with suspected bacterial sepsis. *PLoS ONE* **2017**, *12*, e0181704. [CrossRef]
41. Russell, C.D.; Parajuli, A.; Gale, H.J.; Bulteel, N.S.; Schuetz, P.; de Jager, C.P.; Loonen, A.J.M.; Merekoulias, G.I.; Baillie, J.K. The utility of peripheral blood leucocyte ratios as biomarkers in infectious diseases: A systematic review and meta-analysis. *J. Infect.* **2019**, *78*, 339–348. [CrossRef] [PubMed]
42. Djordjevic, D.; Rondovic, G.; Surbatovic, M.; Stanojevic, I.; Udovicic, I.; Andjelic, T.; Zeba, S.; Milosavljevic, S.; Stankovic, N.; Abazovic, D.; et al. Neutrophil-to-Lymphocyte Ratio, Monocyte-to-Lymphocyte Ratio, Platelet-to-Lymphocyte Ratio, and Mean Platelet Volumeto- Platelet Count Ratio as Biomarkers in Critically Ill and Injured Patients: Which Ratio to Choose to Predict Outcome and Nature of Bacteremia? *Mediat. Inflamm.* **2018**, *2018*, 3758068.

43. Cheung, K.C.P.; Fanti, S.; Mauro, C.; Wang, G.; Nair, A.S.; Fu, H.; Angeletti, S.; Spoto, S.; Fogolari, M.; Romano, F.; et al. Preservation of microvascular barrier function requires CD31 receptor-induced metabolic reprogramming. *Nat. Commun.* **2020**, *11*, 3595. [CrossRef] [PubMed]
44. Angeletti, S.; Fogolari, M.; Morolla, D.; Capone, F.; Costantino, S.; Spoto, S.; De Cesaris, M.; Lo Presti, A.; Ciccozzi, M.; Dicuonzo, G. Role of neutrophil gelatinase-associated lipocalin in the diagnosis and early treatment of acute kidney injury in a case series of patients with acute decompensated heart failure: A case series. *Cardiol. Res. Pract.* **2016**, *2016*, 3708210. [CrossRef] [PubMed]
45. ATS. Guidelines for the management of adults with hospital acquired, ventilator-associated, and healthcare-associated pneumonia. *Am. J. Respir. Crit. Care. Med.* **2005**, *171*, 388–416. [CrossRef] [PubMed]
46. CDC. *Urinary Tract Infection (Catheter-Associated Urinary Tract Infection [CAUTI] and Non-Catheter-Associated Urinary Tract Infection [UTI]) and Other Urinary System Infection [USI]) Events*; Centers for Disease Control and Prevention: Atlanta, GA, USA, 2016.
47. Spoto, S.; Costantino, S.; Fogolari, M.; Valeriani, E.; Ciccozzi, M.; Angeletti, S. An algorithm of good clinical practice to reduce intra-hospital 90-day mortality and need for Intensive Care Unit transfer: A new approach for septic patient management. *Ital. J. Med.* **2020**, *14*, 14–21. [CrossRef]

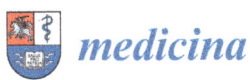

Editorial

Sepsis: New Challenges and Future Perspectives for an Evolving Disease—Precision Medicine Is the Way!

Antonio Mirijello [1,*] and Alberto Tosoni [2,*]

1. Internal Medicine Unit, Department of Medical Sciences, IRCCS Casa Sollievo della Sofferenza, 71013 San Giovanni Rotondo, Italy
2. Department of Internal Medicine and Gastroenterology, Fondazione Policlinico Universitario "A. Gemelli" IRCCS, 00168 Rome, Italy
* Correspondence: a.mirijello@operapadrepio.it (A.M.); alberto.tosoni@policlinicogemelli.it (A.T.); Tel.: +39-0882-410-600 (A.M.); +39-06-3015-1 (A.T.)

Sepsis still remains the leading cause of in-hospital death in the world [1,2]. In the very recent years, this condition became even more evident with the appearance of COVID-19, which has reached an unexpected burden in terms of morbidity and mortality worldwide [3]; the severe form of COVID-19 is characterized by multi-organ failure, mainly secondary to an inappropriate host response, which can be considered a full-fledged sepsis [4]. In addition, SARS-CoV-2 infection has been shown to be an independent risk factor for the development of bloodstream infection (BSI) and sepsis in hospitalized patients [5].

The knowledge in the field of sepsis has accumulated over time. Nevertheless, significant gaps in understanding the pathophysiological aspects and the management possibilities of this deadly condition are still present.

The Special Issue "New Strategies for Treatment of Sepsis" was thought as an opportunity to bring together high-quality manuscripts that showcase the current knowledge on the management of sepsis. We were particularly aware that several unmet needs still needed to be addressed: the comprehension of mechanisms underlying the development and progression of sepsis, the use of new diagnostic tools (including artificial intelligence) for a better and less invasive approach, and the development of antimicrobial strategies in order to effectively fight antimicrobial resistance [1].

The findings reported in the studies published as part of this Special Issue further confirm the potential beneficial role of a deep understanding of mechanisms underlying sepsis, both in reference to the characteristics of microbes and of hosts involved, which in their singularity go to outline different types of sepsis each time. In this way this Special Issue pave the way for future investigations aimed at further dissecting the impact of Precision Medicine as the leading strategy for treatment of sepsis.

Specifically, the article by Rossetti et al. comprehensively analyzed the substantial changes in the homeostasis of micronutrients connected with sepsis and its regulatory processes [6]. In particular, the roles of Vitamin D, Vitamin C, Thiamine and Zinc, all involved in inflammatory or immune response processes, were analyzed. Authors reviewed several studies, many of which have failed to achieve statistical significance or contradict each other. However, the main limitation of these studies, having mortality as outcome, is that the action of micronutrients on seriously ill patients may be less relevant, probably because the severity of organ failure is the result of several metabolic pathways that cannot be easily reverted. Research on this topic should consider reliable and clinically sensitive surrogate outcomes besides mortality, since in seriously ill patients the outcome is too often confused by concomitant factors.

On this connection, the article by Aisa-Alvarez et al. highlighted the antioxidant effect of Vitamin C, Vitamin E, N-acetylcysteine, and Melatonin in patients with septic shock determining the SOFA score and measuring antioxidant markers in plasma [7].

Other secondary outcomes were measured on day 28th including mortality due to any cause, ventilator-free days, ICU-free days, and hospital-free days. The results showed that antioxidant therapy associated with standard therapy reduces multi-organ failure, oxidative stress, and inflammation in patients with septic shock. The strengths of this study are certainly the monitoring of the plasma levels of the micronutrients administered, the evident paucity of treatment-associated side effects, a rapid assessment of patients that allowed to start the administration of micronutrients in a much faster way compared to other comparable studies. Moreover, this is the first study in which the use of Melatonin has been tested in humans with septic shock.

Back to pathophysiological aspects of sepsis, the study by Cutuli et al. analyzed the possibility of both pharmacological and extracorporeal immune modulation in critically ill septic patients [8]. In the last few years, an increasing body of evidence has demonstrated that the administration of immune modulating drugs can mitigate both pro- and anti-inflammatory bursts due to an infection and should be considered as a complementary therapy to be associated with appropriate etiologic therapies (e.g., source infection control and antibiotics). However, the real application of this complementary treatment is still a matter of debate due to controversial results between laboratory and clinical trials. Trials may be inconclusive or discordant with each other due to the great heterogeneity of septic patients enrolled [9]. It is mandatory to push towards a personalized approach trying to distinguish the peculiar characteristics of each septic patient, in order to better choose and monitor the therapy to be tested and the effects to be evaluated.

Pursuing a personalized medicine of septic patients, which also includes the differentiation of types of sepsis and the context in which they develop, the article by Bertozzi et al. gives a detailed description of Neutropenic Enterocolitis (NE) and its frequent association with sepsis [10]. NE is an acute alteration of the intestinal mucosa, mainly of the colon, which develops in immunocompromised patients with a history of cancer and chemotherapy in the previous month, particularly treated with those agents that cause mucositis such as taxanes. This condition has an extremely high lethality rate (79% of patients with histologically confirmed NE died after a median survival of 1 day) and septicemia occurs frequently. The demonstration of an altered intestinal mucosal barrier would seem to support the hypothesis of translocation as a prerequisite for subsequent bacteremia, sepsis, and multi-organ failure.

The study by Perrotta et al. describes the case of a patient affected by thrombotic thrombocytopenic purpura (TTP) admitted to an ICU after developing a hospital-acquired SARS-CoV-2 interstitial pneumonia, further complicated by a K. Pneumoniae NDM sepsis [11]. The antibiotic treatment was effective not only for the treatment of sepsis, but also for intestinal decolonization. This is the first report in literature on intestinal decontamination using the ceftazidime/avibactam + aztreonam combination as treatment for Klebsiella pneumoniae NDM sepsis. This article allows a reflection on the risk of bacteremia related to intestinal colonization with KPC-Kp and on the possibility that a specific acquired condition such as SARS-CoV-2 infection may increase this risk, either through a direct mechanism of infection at intestinal level, either following the use of immuno-modulatory therapies, both capable of increasing bacterial translocation in the intestinal tract.

On this connection, again with a view to a personalized medicine that allows managing the infection in the context of the patient's singularity, the study by Murri et al. acquires relevance [12]. It took into consideration the management of candidemia and the frequent overtreatment of this condition. Indeed, overtreatment may be associated with several disadvantages: possible increase in antifungal resistance, drugs-related adverse events and high costs. The intervention of a stewardship program associated with a biomarker such as beta-D-glucan has been shown to be effective in reducing the excessive duration of treatment without impacting length of hospitalization or mortality.

Another thriving line of research concerns diagnostic tools for an early and accurate diagnosis of sepsis, taking into account not only the type of infection and the characteristics of host, but also the context in which the patient is being managed.

Covino et al. retrospectively analyzed a monocentric cohort of patients presenting to ED with fever, over a 10-year period, and subsequently hospitalized [13]. The aim of this study was to ascertain whether PCT determination at ED could improve patient's prognosis with respect to those with no PCT assessment. As main result, in the whole sample of 12.062 evaluated patients, the PCT-guided management was not associated with a better outcome. However, two subgroups of patients showed a clinical benefit from this approach: those who received a final diagnosis of bloodstream infection and those with a qSOFA ≥ 2. At a closer look, this work underlines the importance of PCT in the management of the septic patient, rather than in its early diagnosis.

Even though literature data recommend the use prediction scores to early recognize those patients at risk for sepsis and poor in-hospital outcome, there is still a significant burden of uncertainty on the optimal prognostic score to be used (e.g. qSOFA, SOFA, SIRS, EWS). Sozio and Colleagues focused their research on the most accurate predictor of in-hospital mortality outcome in septic patients presenting to the ED [14]. Their retrospective monocentric study included 1014 patients admitted to two ED in Tuscany, Italy, for suspected sepsis. Among them the diagnosis of sepsis was confirmed in 651 patients, while 363 received an alternative diagnosis. A Bayesian mean multivariate logistic regression model identified septic shock and positive qSOFA as independent risk factors for in-hospital mortality while hyperthermia was a protective factor. In other words, the absence of fever could identify sicker patients who are not able to properly respond to infection (anergy), thus at higher risk of mortality.

Shifting the gaze from the ED setting to that of Internal Medicine departments, the management of patients with a septic state and a bloodstream infection still represents a challenge for the heterogeneity of the population and the scarcity of literature data on the optimal management.

Our research group focused on the prognostic accuracy of delta-PCT (a reduction of PCT > 50% after 48 h, >75% after 72 h, and >85% after 96 h) in predicting mortality of Internal Medicine patients with microbiological identified sepsis [15]. In a sample of 80 patients with at least two available PCT determinations, those patients with Delta-PCT showed a significantly higher proportion of survival both at 28-days and 90-days. Delta-PCT can therefore be used to predict the prognosis of septic patients admitted to internal medicine wards.

The possible application of new diagnostic markers was evaluated by Piccioni et al. who reviewed the current literature on the use of presepsin and proadrenomedullin in the setting of ED [16,17]. Presepsin is a fragment of the soluble form of CD14 (sCD14), after being cleaved by plasma cathepsin D; it contributes to the activation of the innate immune response. Proadrenomedullin derives from the degradation of adrenomedullin into a fragment of 48-amino acids; it is mainly produced by endothelium and smooth muscle cells and exerts its effects on vasodilatation, bronchodilatation, promoting diuresis and myocardial contractility. Levels of these two peptides rise during bloodstream infections, thus they have been proposed in the setting of early identification of septic and critical patients. However, their ability to add significant information compared to those given by PCT is still matter of debate. In any case, given that a single biomarker cannot give an unfailing and absolute answer in the setting of prognostication [9], expanding diagnostic possibilities is warranted.

Similarly, Spoto and Colleagues tested the diagnostic accuracy and prognostic validity of neutrophil-to-lymphocyte (NLR) and platelet-to-lymphocyte (PLR) ratios in comparison with other biomarkers of sepsis in non-ICU wards [18]. They found them good, rapid and cheap biomarkers to help clinician in the identification and prognostic stratification of patients with sepsis.

In summary, the field of sepsis is exceptionally diverse and it is a rapidly growing area of research and development.

We, the Co-Guest-Editors of this Special Issue, are thankful to all the authors and reviewers who have contributed to this issue by sharing their knowledge, findings and time.

Author Contributions: A.M. and A.T. equally worked on the conceptualization, writing, review and editing of the paper. Members of Internal Medicine Sepsis Study Group participated in the writing and revision process. All authors have read and agreed to the published version of the manuscript.

Funding: This research received no external funding.

Conflicts of Interest: The authors declare no conflict of interest.

References

1. Mirijello, A.; Tosoni, A.; On Behalf of The Internal Medicine Sepsis Study Group. New Strategies for Treatment of Sepsis. *Medicina* **2020**, *56*, 527. [CrossRef] [PubMed]
2. Belsky, J.B.; Wira, C.R.; Jacob, V.; Sather, J.E.; Lee, P.J. A review of micronutrients in sepsis: The role of thiamine, l-carnitine, vita-min C, selenium and vitamin D. *Nutr. Res. Rev.* **2018**, *31*, 281–290. [CrossRef] [PubMed]
3. Wiersinga, W.J.; Rhodes, A.; Cheng, A.C.; Peacock, S.J.; Prescott, H.C. Pathophysiology, Transmission, Diagnosis, and Treatment of Coronavirus Disease 2019 (COVID-19): A Review. *JAMA* **2020**, *324*, 782–793. [CrossRef]
4. Koçak Tufan, Z.; Kayaaslan, B.; Mer, M. COVID-19 and SEPSIS. *Turk. J. Med. Sci.* **2021**. [CrossRef]
5. Pasquini, Z.; Barocci, I.; Brescini, L.; Candelaresi, B.; Castelletti, S.; Iencinella, V.; Mazzanti, S.; Procaccini, G.; Orsetti, E.; Pallotta, F.; et al. Bloodstream infections in the COVID-19 era: Results from an Italian multi-centre study. *Int. J. Infect. Dis.* **2021**, *111*, 31–36. [CrossRef] [PubMed]
6. Rossetti, M.; Martucci, G.; Starchl, C.; Amrein, K. Micronutrients in Sepsis and COVID-19: A Narrative Review on What We Have Learned and What We Want to Know in Future Trials. *Medicina* **2021**, *57*, 419. [CrossRef] [PubMed]
7. Aisa-Alvarez, A.; Soto, M.E.; Guarner-Lans, V.; Camarena-Alejo, G.; Franco-Granillo, J.; Martínez-Rodríguez, E.A.; Gamboa Ávi-la, R.; Manzano Pech, L.; Pérez-Torres, I. Usefulness of Antioxidants as Adjuvant Therapy for Septic Shock: A Randomized Clinical Trial. *Medicina* **2020**, *56*, 619. [CrossRef] [PubMed]
8. Cutuli, S.L.; Carelli, S.; Grieco, D.L.; De Pascale, G. Immune Modulation in Critically Ill Septic Patients. *Medicina* **2021**, *57*, 552. [CrossRef] [PubMed]
9. Tosoni, A.; Addolorato, G.; Gasbarrini, A.; De Cosmo, S.; Mirijello, A.; Internal Medicine Sepsis Study Group. Predictors of mortality of bloodstream infections among internal medicine patients: Mind the complexity of the septic population! *Eur. J. Intern. Med.* **2019**, *68*, e22–e23. [CrossRef] [PubMed]
10. Bertozzi, G.; Maiese, A.; Passaro, G.; Tosoni, A.; Mirijello, A.; Simone, S.D.; Baldari, B.; Cipolloni, L.; La Russa, R. Neutropenic Enterocolitis and Sepsis: Towards the Definition of a Pathologic Profile. *Medicina* **2021**, *57*, 638. [CrossRef] [PubMed]
11. Perrotta, F.; Perrini, M.P. Successful Treatment of *Klebsiella pneumoniae* NDM Sepsis and Intestinal Decolonization with Ceftazidime/Avibactam Plus Aztreonam Combination in a Patient with TTP Complicated by SARS-CoV-2 Nosocomial Infection. *Medicina* **2021**, *57*, 424. [CrossRef] [PubMed]
12. Murri, R.; Lardo, S.; De Luca, A.; Posteraro, B.; Torelli, R.; De Angelis, G.; Giovannenze, F.; Taccari, F.; Pavan, L.; Parroni, L.; et al. Post-Prescription Audit Plus Beta-D-Glucan Assessment Decrease Echinocandin Use in People with Suspected Invasive Candidiasis. *Medicina* **2021**, *57*, 656. [CrossRef] [PubMed]
13. Covino, M.; Gallo, A.; Montalto, M.; De Matteis, G.; Burzo, M.L.; Simeoni, B.; Murri, R.; Candelli, M.; Ojetti, V.; Franceschi, F. The Role of Early Procalcitonin Determination in the Emergency Department in Adults Hospitalized with Fever. *Medicina* **2021**, *57*, 179. [CrossRef] [PubMed]
14. Sozio, E.; Bertini, A.; Bertolino, G.; Sbrana, F.; Ripoli, A.; Carfagna, F.; Giacinta, A.; Viaggi, B.; Meini, S.; Ghiadoni, L.; et al. Recognition in Emergency Department of Septic Patients at Higher Risk of Death: Beware of Patients without Fever. *Medicina* **2021**, *57*, 612. [CrossRef] [PubMed]
15. Tosoni, A.; Cossari, A.; Paratore, M.; Impagnatiello, M.; Passaro, G.; Vallone, C.V.; Zaccone, V.; Gasbarrini, A.; Addolorato, G.; De Cosmo, S.; et al. On behalf of the Internal Medicine Sepsis Study Group. Delta-Procalcitonin and Vitamin D Can Pre-dict Mortality of Internal Medicine Patients with Microbiological Identified Sepsis. *Medicina* **2021**, *57*, 331. [CrossRef] [PubMed]
16. Piccioni, A.; Santoro, M.C.; de Cunzo, T.; Tullo, G.; Cicchinelli, S.; Saviano, A.; Valletta, F.; Pascale, M.M.; Candelli, M.; Covino, M.; et al. Presepsin as Early Marker of Sepsis in Emergency Department: A Narrative Review. *Medicina* **2021**, *57*, 770. [CrossRef] [PubMed]
17. Piccioni, A.; Saviano, A.; Cicchinelli, S.; Valletta, F.; Santoro, M.C.; de Cunzo, T.; Zanza, C.; Longhitano, Y.; Tullo, G.; Tilli, P.; et al. Proadrenomedullin in Sepsis and Septic Shock: A Role in the Emergency Depart-ment. *Medicina* **2021**, *57*, 920. [CrossRef] [PubMed]
18. Spoto, S.; Lupoi, D.M.; Valeriani, E.; Fogolari, M.; Locorriere, L.; Beretta Anguissola, G.; Battifoglia, G.; Caputo, D.; Coppola, A.; Costantino, S.; et al. Diagnostic Accuracy and Prognostic Value of Neutrophil-to-Lymphocyte and Platelet-to-Lymphocyte Ratios in Septic Patients outside the Intensive Care Unit. *Medicina* **2021**, *57*, 811. [CrossRef] [PubMed]

MDPI
St. Alban-Anlage 66
4052 Basel
Switzerland
Tel. +41 61 683 77 34
Fax +41 61 302 89 18
www.mdpi.com

Medicina Editorial Office
E-mail: medicina@mdpi.com
www.mdpi.com/journal/medicina

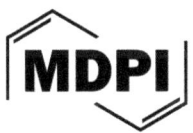

www.ingramcontent.com/pod-product-compliance
Lightning Source LLC
LaVergne TN
LVHW070607100526
838202LV00012B/587